Speech and Language Disorders Associated with Subcortical Pathology

Speech and Language Disorders Associated with Subcortical Pathology

Bruce E. Murdoch BSc(Hons), PhD, DSc
Head, School of Health and Rehabilitation Sciences,
The University of Queensland,
Director, Centre for Neurogenic Communication Disorders Research,
School of Health and Rehabilitation Sciences,
Brisbane,
Australia

Brooke-Mai Whelan BSp Path(Hons), PhD
Senior Research Fellow,
The University of Queensland,
Centre for Neurogenic Communication Disorders Research,
School of Health and Rehabilitation Sciences,
Brisbane,
Australia

WILEY-BLACKWELL
A John Wiley & Sons, Ltd., Publication

Wiley-Blackwell is an imprint of John Wiley & Sons, formed by the merger of Wiley's global Scientific, Technical and Medical business with Blackwell Publishing.

Registered office
John Wiley & Sons Ltd, The Atrium, Southern Gate, Chichester, West Sussex, PO19 8SQ, United Kingdom

Editorial office
John Wiley & Sons Ltd, The Atrium, Southern Gate, Chichester, West Sussex, PO19 8SQ, United Kingdom

For details of our global editorial offices, for customer services and for information about how to apply for permission to reuse the copyright material in this book please see our website at www. wiley.com/wiley-blackwell.

Wiley also publishes its books in a variety of electronic formats. Some content that appears in print may not be available in electronic books.

Designations used by companies to distinguish their products are often claimed as trademarks. All brand names and product names used in this book are trade names, service marks, trademarks or registered trademarks of their respective owners. The publisher is not associated with any product or vendor mentioned in this book. This publication is designed to provide accurate and authoritative information in regard to the subject matter covered. It is sold on the understanding that the publisher is not engaged in rendering professional services. If professional advice or other expert assistance is required, the services of a competent professional should be sought.

Library of Congress Cataloging-in-Publication Data

Murdoch, B. E., 1950–
  Speech and language disorders associated with subcortical pathology / Bruce E. Murdoch, Brooke-Mai Whelan.
    p. ; cm.
  Includes bibliographical references and index.
  ISBN 978-0-470-02573-4 (pbk. : alk. paper)   1. Language disorders–Pathophysiology.
2. Brain–Pathophysiology.   I. Whelan, Brooke-Mai.   II. Title.
  [DNLM: 1. Language Disorders–etiology.   2. Speech Disorders–etiology.   3. Brain Diseases–complications.   4. Cerebellum–physiopathology.   5. Cerebrum–physiopathology. WL 340.2 M974s 2009]
  RC423.M7385 2009
  616.85'5–dc22

                                                                                    2008049830

A catalogue record for this book is available from the British Library.

Set in 9.5/11.5pt Palatino by SNP Best-set Typesetter Ltd., Hong Kong
Printed in Singapore by Markono Print Media Pte Ltd

1   2009

Contents

Section A Introduction 1

1 Subcortical involvement in speech and language:
   an introduction and historical perspective 3

2 Neuroanatomy and functional neurology of the subcortical region 18

Section B Subcortical language disorders 61

3 Models of subcortical participation in language 63

4 Language disorders associated with striatocapsular and
   thalamic lesions 97

5 Pallidal and thalamic involvement in language: evidence from
   stereotactic surgical studies 112

6 A role for the subthalamic nucleus in language 137

7 Influence of the cerebellum on language function 162

8 Degenerative subcortical syndromes: aetiology, clinical features,
   medical treatment and associated language disorders 180

9 Assessment and treatment of subcortical language disorders 200

Section C Subcortical speech disorders 213

10 Role of the subcortical structures in speech motor control 215

11 Dysarthria associated with subcortical pathologies 244

12 Subcortical dysarthrias: assessment and treatment 275

Index 290

Section A   Introduction

1 Subcortical involvement in speech and language: an introduction and historical perspective

Introduction

Recent advances in our understanding of the connectivity of subcortical structures such as the basal ganglia and cerebellum with the cerebral cortex, combined with the development and introduction of advanced neuroimaging techniques, has, over the past two decades, forced a re-think of our concepts of the contribution of subcortical structures to speech and language function. In particular, there has been a growing realization that subcortical structures such as the thalamus, caudate nucleus, globus pallidus, subthalamic nucleus, substantia nigra and cerebellum, among others, not only contribute to the regulation and coordination of the motor aspects of speech production but also are important components of the neural circuits that regulate cognitive and linguistic function. Consequently, there is now much greater acceptance that subcortical structures participate in the regulation of language to a greater extent than proposed by various localizationist models of language function (e.g. Wernicke–Lichtheim model) that had their origins in phrenological theory in the early 1800s and the post-mortem studies of Broca (1861), Wernicke (1874) and Lichtheim (1885), each of which dominated our thinking in relation to language function throughout the twentieth century.

Gall (1809), through his introduction of the concept of phrenology, was the first person to propose a systematic relationship between specific psychological components of human behaviour and specific cerebral regions. According to phrenological theory, complex behaviours such as language, mathematical ability, musical ability and various aspects of human character (e.g. ambition, charity, etc.) were regulated in specific locations in the cerebral cortex. These specific cortical locations were thought to correspond to surface regions of the skull and accordingly the exterior of the skull was partitioned into regions that were believed to be the 'seat' of a 'faculty', with the size of these seats and the areas of the protuberances and lumps of the skull being innately determined in a given individual. Further, the area of each region was considered to be a measure of the complex behaviour or particular aspect of character regulated by that region. Although phrenology fell into disfavour, the underlying premise of phrenological theory, that all aspects of a complex behaviour (e.g. language) are regulated in an anatomically discrete, separable, area of the cerebral cortex, remained as an important component of influential models and theories of speech and language function (e.g. Wernicke–Lichtheim model) that dominated this field throughout the majority of the twentieth century. For example, Broca (1861) adhered to phrenological theory when he concluded that speech production was regulated in the anterior cortical region of the left cerebral hemisphere on the basis of his observation of a patient with a lesion in this region who was unable to speak except for production of a single monosyllable.

Unfortunately Broca overlooked the fact that his patient also had extensive subcortical damage and extensive non-linguistic motor impairment. Likewise, on the basis of his observation that patients who had suffered lesions in the second temporal gyrus of the cortex in the posterior left hemisphere had difficulty comprehending speech, Wernicke (1874) concluded that receptive linguistic ability was located in the posterior region of the left temporal gyrus. Lichtheim (1885) proposed a hypothetical pathway connecting Broca's and Wernicke's areas of the cerebral cortex, his revision of the Broca–Wernicke model, later recognized as the Wernicke–Lichtheim model persisting in textbooks and research literature to the present day. Importantly, the Wernicke–Lichtheim model plays down the importance of subcortical structures in language function, and implies that subcortical lesions only disrupt language if they cause disconnection between the major language centres of the cerebral cortex, as occurs for instance with disruption to the arcuate fasciculus in conduction aphasia.

More recently, localizationist models such as the Wernicke–Lichtheim model that neglect the contribution of subcortical structures to speech and language have been challenged, primarily because of their failure to account for emerging knowledge of the computational architecture of the human brain. Clinical evidence is now available to show that permanent loss of language does not occur without subcortical damage, even when Broca's and Wernicke's areas have been destroyed by lesions. For example, patients with extensive damage to Brocas's area generally recover linguistic ability, unless subcortical damage also occurs (Stuss and Benson, 1986; Dronkers et al., 1992; D'Esposito and Alexander, 1995). Patients suffering brain damage that involves subcortical structures but that leaves Broca's area alone can also manifest the signs and symptoms of Broca's aphasia (Alexander et al., 1987; Mega and Alexander, 1994). The case for Wernicke's aphasia appears to be similar, with reports of premorbid linguistic skills being recovered after complete destruction of Wernicke's area (Lieberman, 2000). Also, although the locus for brain damage associated with Wernicke's aphasia includes the posterior region of the left temporal gyrus (Wernicke's area) it often extends to the supramarginal and angular gyrus including involvement of the white matter below. As stated by D'Esposito and Alexander (1995) a purely cortical lesion that can produce Broca's or Wernicke's aphasia has never been documented. In contrast, numerous cliniconeuroradiological correlation studies reported in recent years have documented the occurrence of aphasic syndromes in association with subcortical lesions that apparently spare the cerebral cortex. Further details of the latter studies are outlined below.

Rather than being regulated by specific cortical sites, it is now recognized that complex behaviours such as talking and walking are mediated by neural circuits that link anatomically segregated populations of neurones in both subcortical and cortical regions of the human brain. In other words, complex behaviours such as talking and walking are regulated by neural circuits that constitute networks linking activity in many parts of the brain at both the cortical and subcortical levels, these networks therefore constituting the neural basis of complex behaviours. As Mesulam (1990) states 'complex behaviour is mapped at the level of multifocal neural systems rather than specific anatomical sites, giving rise to brain–behaviour relationships that are both localized and distributed' (p. 588). Although 'local operations' occur in particular areas of the brain (e.g. specific areas of the cerebral cortex or specific components of the basal ganglia system) these areas in themselves do not constitute an observable behaviour such as talking or walking. Rather these local processes form part of the neural 'computations' that when linked together in complex neural circuits (e.g. cortico-striato-thalamo-cortical loops; cerebrocortico-ponto-cerebellocortico-dentato-thalamo-cerebrocortical loops) manifest in behaviours such as talking, auditory comprehension, walking, etc. For example, the corpus striatum (caudate nucleus plus the lenticular nucleus), although best recognized for its role in the regulation of motor activities, is known to receive input from most areas of the cerebral cortex. In turn, output from the striatum is targeted not only at the primary motor cortex, but also specific areas of the premotor and prefrontal cortex, suggesting that the corpus striatum has the ability to influence not only motor control but also several types of cognitive, language and limbic function. Similarly it has been hypothesized that output from the lateral deep cerebellar nucleus (the dentate) influences not only motor areas of the cerebral cortex but also areas of the prefrontal cortex involved in language and cognition (Fabbro, 2000; Marien et al., 2001).

One consequence of specific areas of the brain being connected to multiple other areas to form complex neural circuits for the purpose of regulating complex behaviours is that lesions in specific areas of the brain can be associated with an ensemble of seemingly unrelated behavioural deficits. For example, a lesion in the substantia nigra is known to cause the syndrome of Parkinson's disease, involving symptoms that are primarily motoric (e.g. bradykinesia, tremor, rigidity) but also involving speech (see Chapter 11), and cognitive and linguistic deficits (see Chapter 8).

The premise that complex neural circuits that link anatomically segregated populations of neurones in both subcortical and cortical structures form the neural substrate of complex behaviours will constitute a unifying and repetitive theme throughout the various chapters of this volume. Specifically, later chapters will elaborate on and provide evidence of the importance of subcortical structures to human behaviours, particularly in the context of speech and language function.

This chapter will outline contemporary theories proposed to explain involvement of various subcortical structures in speech and language function and provide a historical context to their development.

Subcortical mechanisms in speech motor control: historical perspective

Speech production requires smooth coordination of orofacial, laryngeal and respiratory muscles. Clinical data indicate that initiation and precise execution of articulatory movements depend upon the integrity of various neural subsystems involving both cortical and subcortical brain structures, such as the primary motor cortex, supplementary motor area, basal ganglia and cerebellum. Consequently, damage to the basal ganglia and cerebellum produces well-described alterations in motor function, such as tremor, rigidity, akinesia or dysmetria, which may affect the speech-production mechanism.

Basal ganglia

Disorders of the basal ganglia are associated with a number of movement disorders which include Parkinson's disease, Huntington's disease, chorea, athetosis, dystonia and ballismus, among others. In general, movement disorders associated with basal ganglia lesions are classified into either hypokinetic disorders (e.g. Parkinson's disease) and hyperkinetic disorders (e.g. chorea, athetosis, dystonia). Hypokinetic disorders are characterized by significant impairments in movement initiation (akinesia) and reduction in velocity of voluntary movements (bradykinesia), and are usually accompanied by muscular rigidity and tremor at rest. By contrast, hyperkinetic disorders are characterized by excessive motor activity in the form of involuntary movements (dyskinesias) and varying degrees of hypotonia. In line with this division, motor speech disorders associated with basal ganglia lesions have been labelled hypokinetic or hyperkinetic dysarthria (Darley et al., 1975). Full description of the clinical features of hypo- and hyperkinetic dysarthria are presented in Chapter 11.

The major components of the basal ganglia include: the putamen and caudate nucleus, collectively known as the neostriatum; the globus pallidus; the substantia nigra pars compacta and pars reticulata; and the subthalamic nucleus (for a full description of the neuroanatomy of the basal ganglia and their connections see Chapter 2). Participation of the basal ganglia in the control of movement is a well-established idea dating back to the early part of the twentieth century when Wilson (1912) described a disease characterized by muscular rigidity, tremor and weakness with pathological changes in the liver and basal ganglia (hepatolenticular degeneration). Wilson (1912) noted that several features usually associated with damage to the pyramidal tracts were not present in this disease and postulated that the motor abnormalities were due to dysfunction of what he called an 'extrapyramidal motor system'. Further, Wilson (1912) proposed that the basal ganglia were the major constituents of this extrapyramidal motor system that he viewed to be parallel to and independent of the pyramidal (corticospinal) motor system. In a subsequent publication Wilson (1928) developed the view of two motor systems, the phylogenetically 'old' extrapyramidal system and the 'new' pyramidal system, the function of the former being automatic, postural, static and minimally modifiable and that of the pyramidal system being voluntary, phasic and readily modifiable.

Links between basal ganglia pathology and the occurrence of movement disorders had previously been suggested by Jackson (1868), who proposed that instability of activities of the striatum led to chorea. Hunt (1917, 1933) postulated further that large cells in the striatum and globus pallidus constituted the pallidal system which was the output of basal ganglia motor functions, and that lesions in the pallidal system caused Parkinsonism. He also postulated that small cells in the striatum inhibited large cells and lesions in the striatum released the pallidal system and resulted in chorea, while lesions involving both the pallidal system and small cells in the striatum produced athetosis.

In the 1960s and 1970s more modern anatomical techniques showed that the bulk of the basal ganglia output passed via the thalamus to motor cortical areas (Nauta and Mehler, 1966). Thus it appeared that the basal ganglia output was prepyramidal rather than extrapyramidal. This finding contributed to the development of hypotheses that the basal ganglia initiate movement via their output to the motor cortex. Currently, the basal ganglia are generally considered to be comprised of a group of 'input' structures (the caudate nucleus, putamen and ventral striatum) that receive direct input essentially from areas of the cerebral cortex and 'output' structures (the internal segment of the globus pallidus, the substantia nigra pars reticulata and the ventral pallidum) that project back to the cerebral cortex via the thalamus. Originally the striatum was considered to serve primarily to integrate diverse inputs from the entire cerebral cortex and to 'funnel' these influences via the ventrolateral thalamus to the primary motor cortex alone. This thinking was consistent with the view held at the time that the basal ganglia functioned primarily in the domain of motor control.

Based on recent research, it is now clear that output from the basal ganglia terminates in thalamic regions that gain access to a wider region of the frontal lobe than just the primary motor cortex, including areas thought to have cognitive functions (Alexander *et al.*, 1986; Middleton and Strick, 1994). Consequently, the original notion has been superseded by the view of the striatum as a 'multi-laned throughway' which forms part of a series of multi-segregated circuits connecting the cerebral cortex, the basal ganglia and the thalamus (Alexander *et al.*, 1986; Graybiel and Kimura, 1995; Middleton and Strick, 2000). Thus basal ganglia anatomy is characterized by their participation in multiple 'loops' with the cerebral cortex, each of which follows the basic route of cortex → striatum → globus pallidus/substantia nigra → thalamus → cortex in a unidirectional fashion.

Alexander *et al.* (1986) identified at least five separate, parallel corticobasal ganglion circuits according to the specific region of the frontal lobe that serves as a target for their thalamocortical projections. One of these circuits projected to the skeletomotor areas of the frontal cortex while another projected to the oculomotor areas. The three remaining circuits projected to non-motor areas of the frontal cortex, including the dorsolateral prefrontal area (Brodmann area 46), the lateral orbitofrontal cortex (Brodmann area 12) and the anterior cingulate/medial orbitofrontal cortices (Brodmann areas 24 and 13). Importantly, these circuits appear to be functionally segregated to a large extent, suggesting that structural convergence and functional integration occur within rather than between each of the identified circuits. Given the segregated nature of the corticobasal ganglia circuits, collectively they may be viewed as having a unified role in modulating the operations of the entire frontal lobe, thereby influencing such diverse frontal lobe processes as motor activities, behavioural, cognitive, language and even limbic processes. This anatomical arrangement, whereby the output from the basal ganglia gains access to multiple areas of the frontal lobe including non-motor areas, has profound consequences for the possible functional roles of the basal ganglia system and provides a basic neuroanatomical mechanism whereby these subcortical structures can influence aspects of behaviour, cognition and language as well as motor function.

Each corticobasal ganglia circuit has been proposed to contain a direct and indirect pathway from the striatum to the internal globus pallidus and substantia nigra pars reticulata, the output nuclei of the basal ganglia (Delong and Georgopoulos, 1981). This direct and indirect pathway theory makes it easy to explain various clinical signs of basal ganglia diseases, including hypo- and hyperkinetic movement disorders. Imbalance between the activity in the direct and indirect pathways and the resulting alterations in the activity of the internal segment of the globus pallidus and substantia nigra pars reticulata are thought to account for hypo- and hyperkinetic features of basal ganglia disorders, including hypo- and hyperkinetic dysarthria. The possible roles of the direct and indirect pathways in the development of the various hypo- and hyperkinetic movement disorders, including hypo- and hyperkinetic dysarthria, are discussed in detail in Chapter 10 of the present volume. Neuroanatomical details of each of these pathways are provided in Chapter 2.

Cerebellum

The most obvious signs of damage to the cerebellum are disturbances in motor function, characterized by incoordination of the limbs (dysmetria), wide-based gait, dysarthria and disturbed ocular movements (nystagmus). Consequently, the cerebellum has traditionally been viewed as a structure that contributes primarily to motor coordination and control. Although there are suggestions in the writings of Aristotle that the anatomical functions of the 'little brain' were known in ancient Greece, one of the first researchers to document the functions of the cerebellum was Gall (1809) who, in his cartographic scheme of psychological characteristics of the skull, designated the cerebellum as the organ of 'amativeness'. At the same time Luigi Rolando was the first researcher to report the outcome of removal of the cerebellum in animals. He noted that cerebellar lesions impaired posture and movement, leaving sensory and cognitive functions intact. Flourens (1824) continued experiments of cerebellar ablation in animals and demonstrated that 'all movements persist after ablation of the cerebellum; all that is missing is that they are not regular and coordinated' (p. 181). The physiological experiments conducted by Ludwig Edinger further confirmed that the cerebellum was involved in coordination of movements and maintenance of muscle-tonus and equilibrium.

The first systematic descriptions of the neurological symptoms specific to what was named 'the cerebellar syndrome' were provided by Babinski (1913) and Holmes (1917, 1922). Currently, cerebellar syndrome is considered to basically involve ataxia, hypotonia, dysmetria and essential tremor (Trouillas *et al.*, 1997). They described in detail the role of the cerebellum in the coordination of extremity movement, gait, posture, equilibrium and speech. In relation to speech, Holmes (1917, 1922) noted that acute and chronic cerebellar lesions may provoke alterations in both phonation and articulation. Darley *et al.* (1975) later classified this speech disorder as ataxic dysarthria, the predominant features of which include a breakdown in the articulatory and prosodic aspects of speech. Unlike some forms of dysarthria (e.g. flaccid dysarthria), where the speech disorder can be linked to deficits in individual muscles, ataxic dysarthria is associated with decomposition of complex movements arising from a breakdown in the coordinated action of the muscles of the speech-production apparatus to produce speech (for a complete description of the clinical features and neuropathophysiological basis of ataxic dysarthria see Chapter 11).

To be able to perform its primary function of synergistic coordination of muscular activity, the cerebellum requires extensive connections with other parts of the nervous system. Briefly, the cerebellum functions in part by comparing input from the motor cortex with information concerning the momentary status of muscle contraction, degree of tension of the muscle tendons, positions of parts of the body, and forces acting on the surfaces of the body originating from muscle spindles, Golgi tendon organs, etc., and then sending appropriate messages back to the motor cortex to ensure smooth, coordinated muscle function. Consequently, the cerebellum requires input from the motor cortex, muscle and joint receptors, receptors in the internal ear detecting changes in the position and rotation in the head, and skin receptors, among others. Conversely, pathways carrying signals from the cerebellum back to the cortex are also required to complete the cerebrocerebellar loop. Traditionally the output of cerebellar processing was thought to be directed at only a single cortical area, namely the primary motor cortex, consistent with the belief the corticocerebellar circuits function primarily in the domain of motor control. It is now known that the cerebellum is a relay for many segregated neural circuits involved in the control process of several physiological functions; for example, vestibulo-cerebellar-vestibular loops are involved in the regulation of equilibrium and ocular motility, while reticulo-cerebello-reticular loops are involved in muscle tone, the control process of posture and the regulation of many vegetative functions. Spino-cerebello-rubro-spinal loops subserve regulation of the motor apparatus at the spinal level.

The main loops involved in the regulation of voluntary movement and possibly cognitive and language functions are the cerebrocortico-ponto-cerebellocortico-dentato-thalamo-cerebrocortical loops (Middleton and Strick, 1997; Schmahmann, 1997) and the cerebrocortico-rubro-olivo-neodentato-cerebrocortical loops (Leiner *et al.*, 1993). Importantly, it is now recognized that the thalamo-cerebrocortical projections of these latter two loops project not only to the motor cortex but also to non-motor regions of the cerebral cortex, including the major speech/language centres, thereby providing a neuroanatomical basis for the cerebellum to influence functions such as cognition and language in addition to motor activities. The role of the cerebellum in language is further discussed briefly below and in detail in Chapter 7.

Motor speech disorders associated with subcortical pathology

It is well established that neurological disorders considered to be attributable primarily to lesions involving subcortical structures such as the basal ganglia and cerebellum are frequently associated with the occurrence of motor speech disorders, implying that these structures have a role in the normal regulation of the motor functioning of the speech musculature (Darley *et al.*, 1975; Murdoch, 1998). For instance, hypokinetic dysarthria, a motor speech disorder characterized by features such as monotony of pitch and loudness, decreased use of all vocal parameters for effecting stress and emphasis, breathy and harsh vocal quality, reduced vocal intensity, variable speech rate, including short rushes of speech or accelerated speech, consonant imprecision, impaired breath support for speech, reduction in phonation time, difficulty in the initiation of speech activities and inappropriate silences has been reported to occur in association with Parkinson's disease, a condition caused by nerve cell loss in the pigmented brain stem nuclei, most markedly the pars compacta of the substantia nigra (Darley *et al.*, 1975; Theodoros and Murdoch, 1998). Likewise, a variety of motor speech disorders collectively referred to as 'hyperkinetic dysarthria' may occur in association with the abnormal involuntary movements encountered in a range of other neurological conditions caused by neuropathological changes in the basal ganglia system, including chorea, dystonia, etc. (Darley *et al.*, 1975). Further, lesions to, or diseases of, the cerebellum or its afferent or efferent connections may disrupt the motor components of speech production at the segmental or suprasegmental level, giving rise to ataxic dysarthria, a motor speech disorder characterized by articulatory inaccuracy (imprecision of consonant production, irregular articulatory breakdowns and distorted vowels), prosodic excess (excess and equal stress, prolonged phonemes, prolonged intervals and slow rate), and phonatory-prosodic insufficiency (harshness, monopitch and monoloudness) (Murdoch and Theodoros, 1998).

In recent years, several models have been proposed in an attempt to further elucidate the contribution of subcortical structures to motor control, and to explain the occurrence of movement disorders subsequent to basal ganglia and cerebellar lesions. These models are discussed in Chapter 10.

Subcortical mechanisms in language: historical perspective

The basal ganglia and cerebellum are two groups of subcortical nuclei that have classically been regarded as motor structures. In addition to their role in motor functions, anatomical studies and clinical research conducted over the past two decades have increasingly implicated the basal ganglia and cerebellum in a range of behavioural functions, including several different types of cognitive, linguistic and limbic function. Consequently, the traditional view that the basal ganglia and cerebellum are only involved in motor functions has been challenged. A major reason for this reappraisal has been new information regarding basal ganglia and cerebellar connections with the cerebral cortex.

Recently reported anatomical studies have noted that these connections are organized into discrete, segregated neural circuits, or loops. Rather than simply enabling widespread cortical areas to gain access to the motor system, these loops reciprocally interconnect a large and diverse set of cerebral cortical areas with the basal ganglia and cerebellum, enabling the latter structures to influence a range of cognitive functions in addition to their more traditional motor roles. For example, Alexander *et al.* (1986) proposed that the output of the basal ganglia targeted not only the primary motor cortex, but also specific areas of the premotor and prefrontal cortex, thereby suggesting that the basal ganglia have the ability to influence not only motor control but also several different types of cognitive and limbic (e.g. memory) function. Similarly, it has been hypothesized that output from the lateral deep cerebellar nucleus (the dentate) influences not only motor areas of the cerebral cortex but also areas of the prefrontal cortex involved in language and cognition. Evidence to support this functional diversity of the basal ganglia and cerebellum comes from several sources, including neuroanatomical studies documenting the presence of extensive connections between the basal ganglia and cerebral cortex, animal studies reporting a range of behavioural correlates documented by single-cell recordings from basal ganglia neurones, observations of the behavioural effects of disease-induced lesions in the basal ganglia, clinico-neuroradiological studies documenting the presence of speech disorders and other behavourial deficits in association with subcortical lesions, the findings of studies based on functional neuroimaging, including positron emission tomography (PET) and functional magnetic resonance imaging (fMRI) and, more recently, observations of the behavioural effects of deep-brain stimulation and surgically induced lesions in the globus pallidus (pallidotomy), thalamus (thalamotomy) and subthalamic nucleus, carried out as part of the treatment for Parkinson's disease and other basal ganglia syndromes.

Role of the basal ganglia and thalamus in language: historical perspective

As outlined above, ever since the era of phrenological science the cerebral cortex has been considered the neural substrate of higher psychological function, including language. In keeping with this view, the standard 'associationist' anatomo-functional model of language organization was deeply rooted in cortical areas and their fibre connections (Lichtheim, 1885; Wernicke, 1874). According to this still influential model, linguistic representations are stored in discrete cortical areas and consequently subcortical brain lesions were thought to only produce language deficits if they disrupted the white matter fibres that connect the various cortical language centres.

Despite the emphasis on the cerebral cortex, evidence to suggest the occurrence of language disorders associated with subcortical brain lesions has been available since the late nineteenth century. More than a century ago, Broadbent (1872) proposed that words were 'generated' as motor acts in the basal ganglia. Marie (1906) challenged the traditional view of aphasia and described a clinical syndrome that he called 'anartria' secondary to dysfunction of a specific subcortical region involving the caudate nucleus, putamen, internal capsule and thalamus (Marie's quadrilateral space). Monakow (1914) also championed the participation of the lentiform nucleus in the pathogenesis of aphasia. Perusal of the monumental anatomo-clinical summaries published in the early twentieth century, such those by Moutier (1908), Henschen (1922) and Nielsen (1946), also reveals a number of cases of language disturbance associated with lesions apparently limited to subcortical structures. Unfortunately, these empirical data were subjected to radically different interpretations by the various authors. Moutier supported the '*quadrilatère*' proposed by his teacher Pierre Marie. In contrast Nielsen explicitly denied any role of subcortical structures in mental activities, interpreting his observations in strict adherence to the traditional Wernicke–Lichtheim model. Later Fisher (1959) described aphasia as a clinical feature in a patient with left-thalamic haemorrhage. Penfield and Roberts (1959) suggested that the thalamus had an integrative function in language processing.

Since the late 1970s the traditional view of language processing in the brain has been challenged by the findings of an increasing number of cliniconeuroradiological correlation studies that have documented the occurrence of adult language disorders in association with apparently subcortical vascular lesions. The introduction in recent decades of new neuroradiological methods for lesion localization *in vivo*, including computed tomography in the 1970s and more recently MRI, has led to an increasing number of reports in the literature of aphasia following subcortical lesions (for reviews of correlation studies *in vivo* see Alexander, 1989; Cappa and Vallar, 1992; Murdoch, 1996). In particular, these new neuroimaging techniques have allowed more precise identification and localization of subcortical lesion parameters (Alexander, *et al.*, 1987; Cappa and Wallesch, 1994) and hence the ability to evaluate the influence of specific lesions in producing motor and cognitive anomalies. Therefore, although the concept of subcortical aphasia remains somewhat controversial, recent years have seen a growing acceptance of a role for subcortical structures in language and the development of a range of theories that attempt to explain the nature of that role. These theories, largely developed on the basis of speech and language data collected from subjects who have had cerebrovascular accidents involving the thalamus or striato-capsular region, have been expressed as neuroanatomically based models. The most influential models of subcortical participation in language proposed to date include the Subcortical White Matter Pathways (Alexander *et al.*,1987), Response-Release Semantic Feedback (Crosson, 1985), Lexical Decision Making (Wallesch and Papagno, 1988) and Selective Engagement (Nadeau and Crosson, 1997) models. The Subcortical White Matter Pathways model dismisses a role for the subcortical nuclei in language and advocates cortico-cortical, corticostriatal, thalamocortical and corticobulbar white matter pathways as critical to the facilitation of auditory comprehension and verbal expression. In contrast, the Response-Release Semantic Feedback model proposes a role for subcortical structures in regulating the release of preformulated language segments from the cerebral cortex via a complex neural circuit called the cortico-striato-pallido-thalamo-cortical loop. Likewise, the Lexical Decision Making model also proposes a cortico-striato-pallido-thalamo-cortical loop as the neural platform for linguistic operations. Specifically, Wallesch and Papagno (1988) postulated that the subcortical components of the loop constitute a frontal lobe system comprised of parallel modules with integrative and decision-making capabilities rather than the simple neuroregulatory role proposed in Crosson's (1985) model. The Selective Engagement model represents the most contemporary schema of subcortical participation in language and principally proposes a frontal-inferior thalamic peduncle-nucleus reticularis-centrum medianum system to subserve the 'engagement' of cortical components which mediate attentional and behavioural processes, including language. In particular, the Selective Engagement model disputes a role for the basal ganglia in language and redefines non-specific thalamic nuclei (i.e. nucleus reticularis, centrum medianum and parafascicular nucleus) as critical to the mediation of language (a full discussion of the above models of subcortical participation in language is presented in Chapter 3). Although the basal ganglia, thalamus and subcortical white matter pathways represent the subcortical structures which have been afforded the most consideration within contemporary models of subcortical participation in language, more recently studies based on deep-brain stimulation have also indicated a possible role for the subthalamic nucleus in language processes (Whelan *et al.*, 2003, 2004).

Role of the cerebellum in language: historical perspective

Investigation of a possible role for the cerebellum in the mediation of cognitive processes, including language, has historically been overshadowed by research interest in cerebellar coordination of motor control. Over the past two decades, however, the question of a possible participation of the cerebellum in language processing itself has come to the forefront. In particular, recent advances in our understanding of the neuroanatomy of the cerebellum combined with evidence from functional neuroimaging, neurophysiological and neuropsychological research, has, however, extended our view of the cerebellum from that of a simple coordinator of autonomic and somatic motor function. Rather it is now more widely accepted that the cerebellum, and in particular the right cerebellar hemisphere, participates in modulation of cognitive functioning, especially to those parts of the brain to which it is reciprocally connected (Marien *et al.*, 2001). Indeed, the discovery of major reciprocal neural pathways between the cerebellum and the frontal areas of the language-dominant hemisphere, including Broca's area and the supplementary motor area, was a major impetus in the development of the concept of cerebellar involvement in non-motor linguistic processes.

Much of the credit for this development goes to Leiner, Leiner and Dow, who wrote a series of articles reviewing the potential role of the cerebellum in cognition. In their first publication (Leiner *et al.*, 1986) they reviewed long-neglected evidence that portions of the lateral cerebellar hemispheres and dentate nuclei were greatly expanded in humans. They hypothesized that these cerebellar regions project to prefrontal and other association cortices in humans and higher primates, forming cortical-cerebellar loops used for certain types of cognitive skill. In support of this hypothesis non-motor behavioural deficits associated with cerebellar damage or abnormalities were reported by several investigators and functional neuroanatomical studies using PET during the late 1980s demonstrated the selective activation of some cerebellar structures during language tasks (Petersen *et al.*, 1989). In the early 1990s, Fiez *et al.* (1992) described a patient with an extensive right-cerebellar lesion who presented with language disturbances. Since that time numerous studies have identified the presence of disturbed language processing in association with primary lesions of various aetiologies involving both the right (Marien *et al.*, 2001) and left (Murdoch and Whelan, 2007) cerebellar hemispheres. A comprehensive review of the evidence supporting a role for the cerebellum in language is presented in Chapter 7.

Functional neuroimaging

Further clarification of the role of subcortical structures in language is likely to come through the use of functional neuroimaging techniques and neurophysiological methods such as electrical and magnetic evoked responses. Functional neuroimaging techniques such as fMRI and PET enable brain images to be collected while the patient is performing various language-production tasks (e.g. picture naming, generating nouns) or during language comprehension (e.g. listening to stories). These techniques therefore enable visualization of the brain regions involved in a language task, with a spatial resolution as low as a few millimetres. Although functional neuroimaging does therefore offer promise of a tool to unravel the role of subcortical structures in language, results from functional neuroimaging studies to date have proven less than definitive (Cabeza and Nyberg, 2000). These studies have, however, revealed a number of cortical and subcortical structures beyond the perisylvian cortex to be active during linguistic processing (Petersen *et al.*, 1989; Warburton *et al.*, 1996; Crosson *et al.*, 1999), providing support for a distributed network model of language organization (Mesulam, 2000). In particular, word-generation studies have shown consistent activation of the medial frontal cortex, usually near the boundary of the pre-supplementary motor area and the rostral cingulate zone. Although the supplementary motor area is known to have extensive subcortical connections, including projections to the striatal grey matter spanning the internal capsule and to the caudate nucleus and putamen as well as receiving connections from the ventral anterior and dorsal medial thalamus, in the majority of functional neuroimaging studies these subcortical components have not shown consistent activity in studies of word generation. This reported inconsistency in activation of the basal ganglia and thalamus may be the product of limitations in numbers of subjects studied, number of trials during functional neuroimaging and experimental design. Recently, Crosson *et al.* (2003) using fMRI observed significant activity in the subcortical structures during lexical generation tasks but not during nonsense syllable generation. They inferred the existence of a left pre-supplementary motor area-dorsal caudate-ventral anterior thalamic loop involved in lexical retrieval. Further, Crosson *et al.* (2003) hypothesized 'that activity in this loop was related to maintaining a bias toward the retrieval of one lexical item versus competing alternatives for each response during word generation blocks' (p. 1075). Several PET studies have also demonstrated activation of the thalamus and basal ganglia during completion of language tasks such as picture naming (Price *et al.*, 1996a) and word repetition (Price *et al.*, 1996b).

In relation to the role of the cerebellum in language, functional neuroimaging studies have provided a possible explanation for the occurrence of language problems subsequent to cerebellar pathology. Specifically, studies based on functional neuroimaging techniques such as single-photon emission computed tomography (SPECT), PET and fMRI have consistently revealed regions of contralateral cortical hypoperfusion in relation to the orientation of the cerebellar lesion (Silveri *et al.*, 1994; Beldarrain *et al.*, 1997), a phenomenon called crossed cerebello-cerebral diaschisis. Several authors have proposed that this phenomenon, reflecting a functional depression of supratentorial language areas due to reduced input via cerebello-cortical pathways, may represent the neuropathological mechanism responsible for language problems associated with cerebellar pathology (Broich *et al.*, 1987; Marien *et al.*, 2001).

Summary

Although it has been recognized that lesions involving subcortical structures such as the basal ganglia and cerebellum are associated with motor impairments, including motor speech disorders, for more than a century, it is only relatively recently that attention has been directed at the potential role of these subcortical structures in language processing. Although controversy still exists as to whether the structures of the striatocapsular region and the cerebellum participate directly in language processing or play a role as supporting structures for language, contemporary theories suggest that, as in the case of motor functions, the role of subcortical structures in language is essentially neuroregulatory. Evidence based on neuroanatomical, clinical and functional neuroimaging studies indicate that speech and language functions are mediated by complex, segregated neural circuits that comprise networks linking activity in many parts of the brain at both the cortical and subcortical level, with subcortical structures such as the basal ganglia and cerebellum representing important relays in these complex pathways. Subsequent chapters of this volume will explore this concept further as part of discussion of specific aspects of subcortical mechanisms in speech and language function.

References

Alexander, M.P. (1989). Clinico-anatomical correlations of aphasia following predominantly subcortical lesions. In F. Boller and J. Grafman (eds), *Handbook of Neuropsychology* (pp. 47–67). Amsterdam: Elsevier.

Alexander, G.E., DeLong, M.R. and Strick, P.L. (1986). Parallel organization of functionally segregated circuits linking basal ganglia and cortex. *Annual Review of Neuroscience* 9, 357–81.

Alexander, G.E., Naeser, M.A. and Palumbo, C.L. (1987). Correlations of subcortical CT lesion sites and aphasia profiles. *Brain* 110, 961–91.

Babinski, J. (1913). *Exposé des travaux scientifiques: syndrome céerebelleux*. Paris: Masson.

Beldarrain, M.G., Garcia-Monco, J.C., Quintana, J.M., Llorens, V. and Rodeno, E. (1997). Diaschisis and neuropsychological performance after cerebellar stroke. *European Neurology* 37, 82–9.

Broadbent, G. (1872). *On the Cerebral Mechanism of Speech and Thought*. London: Longman.

Broca, P. (1861). Remarques sur le siège de la faculté de la parole articulée, suivies d'une observation d'aphemie (perte de parole). *Bulletins-Société Anthropologie (Paris)* 2, 235–8.

Broich, K., Hartmann, A., Biersack, H.J. and Horn, R. (1987). Crossed cerebello-cerebral diaschisis in a patient with cerebellar infarction. *Neuroscience Letters* 83, 7–12.

Cabeza, R. and Nyberg, L. (2000). Imagine cognition II: an empirical review of 275 PET and fMRI studies. *Journal of Cognitive Neuroscience* 12, 1–47.

Cappa, S.F. and Vallar, G. (1992). Neuropsychological disorders after subcortical lesions: implications for neural models of language and spatial attention. In G. Vallar, S.F. Cappa and C.-W. Wallesch (eds), *Neuropsychological Disorders Associated with Subcortical Lesions* (pp. 7–41). Oxford: Oxford University Press.

Cappa, S.F. and Wallesch, C.-W. (1994). Subcortical lesions and cognitive deficits. In A. Kertesz (ed.), *Localization and Neuroimaging in Neuropsychology* (pp. 545–66). San Diego: Academic Press.

Crosson, B. (1985). Subcortical function in language: a working model. *Brain and Language* 25, 257–92.

Crosson, B., Sadek, J.R., Bobholz, J.A., Gökçay, D., Mohr, C.M. *et al.* (1999). Activity in the parasingulate and singulate sulci during word generation: an fMRI study of functional anatomy. *Cerebral Cortex* 9, 307–16.

Crosson, B., Benefield, H., Cato, M.A., Sadek, J.R., Moore, A.B. *et al.* (2003). Left and right basal ganglia and frontal activity during language generation: contributions to lexical, semantic and phonological processes. *Journal of the International Neuropsychological Society* 9, 1061–77.

Darley, F.L., Aronson, A.E. and Brown, J.R. (1975). *Motor Speech Disorders*. Philadelphia: W.B. Saunders.

Delong, M.R. and Georgopoulos, A.P. (1981). Motor function of the basal ganglia. In J.M. Brookhart and V.B. Mountcastle (eds), *Handbook of Physiology*, section 1, vol. II, part 2 (pp. 1017–61). Bethesda: American Physiological Society.

D'Esposito, M. and Alexander, M.P. (1995). Subcortical aphasia: Distinct profiles following left putaminal hemorrhage. *Neurology* 45, 38–41.

Dronkers, N.F., Shapiro, J.K., Redfern, B. and Knight, R.T. (1992). The role of Broca's area in Broca's aphasia. *Journal of Clinical and Experimental Neuropsychology* 14, 198.

Fabbro, F. (2000). Introduction to language and cerebellum. *Journal of Neurolinguistics* 13, 83–94.

Fiez, J.A., Petersen, S.E., Cheny, M.K. and Raichle, M.E. (1992). Impaired non-motor learning and error detection associated with cerebellar damage. *Brain* 115, 155–78.

Fisher, C.M. (1959). The pathologic and clinical aspects of thalamic hemorrhage. *Transactions of the American Neurological Association* 84, 56–9.

Flourens, P. (1824). Recherches expérimentales sur les fonctions du système nerveux dans les animaux vertébrés. Paris: Crevot.

Gall, F.J. (1809). *Recherches sur le système nerveux*. Paris: B. Bailliere.

Graybiel, A.M. and Kimura, M. (1995). Adaptive neural networks in the basal ganglia. In J.C. Houk, J.L. Davis and D.G. Beiser (eds), *Models of Information Processing in the Basal Ganglia* (pp. 103–16). Cambridge: MIT Press.

Henschen, S.E. (1922). *Klinische und anatomishe beitrage zur pathologic des gehirns*. Stockholm: Almquist and Wiksell.

Holmes, G. (1917). The symptoms of acute cerebellar injuries due to gunshot injuries. *Brain* 40, 401–534.

Holmes, G. (1922). Clinical symptoms of cerebellar disease and their interpretation. *Lancet* 2, 59–65.

Hunt, R. (1917). Progressive atrophy of the globus pallidus: a contribution to functions of the corpus striatum. *Brain* 40, 58–148.

Hunt, R. (1933). Primary paralysis agitans (primary atrophy of the efferent striatal and pallidal systems. *Archives of Neurology and Psychiatry* 30, 1332–49.

Jackson, J.H. (1868) Observations on the physiology and pathology of hemichorea. *Edinburgh Medical Journal* 14, 294–303.

Leiner, H.C., Leiner, A.L. and Dow, R.S. (1986). Does the cerebellum contribute to mental skills? *Behavioral Neuroscience* 100, 443–54.

Leiner, H.C., Leiner, A.L. and Dow, R.S. (1993). Cognitive and language functions of the cerebellum. *Trends in Neurosciences* 16, 444–7.

Lichtheim, L. (1885). On aphasia. *Brain* 7, 433–84.

Lieberman, P. (2000). *Human Language and Our Reptilian Brain: the Subcortical Bases of Speech, Syntax and Thought*. Cambridge, MA: Harvard University Press.

Marie, P. (1906) The third left frontal convolution plays no special role in the function of language. In M.F. Cole and M. Cole (eds), *Pierre Marie's Papers on Speech Disorders*. New York: Hafner 1971.

Marien, P., Engelborghs, S., Fabbro, F. and DeDeyn, P.P. (2001). The lateralized linguistic cerebellum: a review and a new hypothesis. *Brain and Language* 79, 580–600.

Mega, M.S. and Alexander, M.P. (1994). Subcortical aphasia. The core profile of capsulostriatal infarction. *Neurology* 44, 1824–9.

Mesulam, M.M. (1990). Large-scale neurocognitive networks and distributed processing for attention, language and memory. *Annals of Neurology* 28, 597–613.

Mesulam, M.M. (2000). Behavioural neuroanatomy: Large scale networks, association cortex, frontal syndromes, the limbic system and hemispheric specializations. In M. Mesulam (ed.), *Principles of Behavioural and Cognitive Neurology* (pp. 1–120). Oxford: Oxford University Press.

Middleton, F.A. and Strick, P.L. (1994). Anatomical evidence for cerebellar and basal ganglia involvement in higher cognitive function. *Science* 266, 458–61.

Middleton, F.A. and Strick, P.L. (1997). Dentate output channels: motor and cognitive components. *Progress in Brain Research* 114, 555–68.

Middleton, F.A. and Strick, P.L. (2000). Basal ganglia output and cognition: evidence from anatomical, behavioural and clinical studies. *Brain and Cognition* 42, 183–200.

Monokow, C. (1914). *Die lokalisation in grosshirn*. Wiesbaden: Bergmann.

Moutier, F. (1908). *L'aphasie de Broca*. Doctoral dissertation, Paris.

Murdoch, B.E. (1996). The role of subcortical structures in language: cliniconeuroradiological studies of brain damaged subjects. In B. Dodd, R. Campbell and L. Worrall (eds), *Evaluating Theories of Language: Evidence from Disordered Communication* (pp. 137–60). London: Whurr Publishers.

Murdoch, B.E. (1998). *Dysarthria: a Physiological Approach to Assessment and Treatment*. Cheltenham: Stanley Thornes Publishers.

Murdoch, B.E. and Theodoros, D.G. (1998). Ataxic dysarthria. In B.E. Murdoch (ed.), *Dysarthria: a Physiological Approach to Assessment and Treatment* (pp. 242–65). Cheltenham: Stanley Thornes Publishers.

Murdoch, B.E. and Whelan, B.-M. (2007). Language disorders subsequent to left cerebellar lesions: a case for bilateral cerebellar involvement in language? *Folia Phoniatrica et Logopaedica* 59, 184–9.

Nadeau, S.E. and Crosson, B. (1997). Subcortical aphasia. *Brain and Language* 58, 355–402.

Nauta, W.J.H. and Mehler, W.H. (1966). Projections of the lentiform nucleus in the monkey. *Brain Research* 1, 3–42.

Nielsen, J.M. (1946). *Agnosia, Apraxia, Aphasia*. New York: Hoeber.

Penfield, W. and Roberts, L. (1959). *Speech and Brain Mechanisms*. Princeton: Princeton University Press.

Petersen, S.E., Fox, P.T., Posner, M.I., Mintum, M. and Raichle, M.E. (1989). Positron mission tomographic studies of the processing of single words. *Journal of Cognitive Neuroscience* 1, 153–70.

Price, C.J., Moore, C., Humphreys, G.W., Frackowiak, R.S. and Friston, K.J. (1996a). The neural signs sustaining object recognition and naming. *Proceedings of the Royal Society of London Series B Biological Sciences* 263, 1501–7.

Price, C.J., Wise, R.J., Warburton, E.A., Moore, C.J., Howard, D. *et al.* (1996b). Hearing and saying: the functional neuroanatomy of auditory word processing. *Brain* 119, 919–31.

Schmahmann, J.D. (1997). Rediscovery of an early concept. *International Review of Neurobiology* 41, 3–27.

Silveri, M.C., Leggio, M.G. and Molinari, M. (1994). The cerebellum contributes to linguistic production: a case of agrammatic speech following a right cerebellar lesion. *Neurology* 44, 2047–50.

Stuss, D.T. and Benson, D.F. (1986). *The Frontal Lobes*. New York: Raven.

Theodoros, D.G. and Murdoch, B.E. (1998). Hypokinetic dysarthria. In B.E. Murdoch (ed.), *Dysarthria: a Physiological Approach to Assessment and Treatment* (pp. 266–313). Cheltenham: Stanley Thornes Publishers.

Trouillas, P., Takayanagi, T., Hallett, M., Currier, R.D., Subramony, S.H. *et al.* (1997). International cooperative ataxia rating scale for pharmacological assessment of the cerebellar syndrome. *Journal of Neurological Sciences* 145, 205–11.

Wallesch, C.-W. and Papagno, C. (1988). Subcortical aphasia. In F.C. Rose, R. Whurr and M.A. Wyke (eds), *Aphasia* (pp. 256–87). London: Whurr Publishers.

Warburton, E., Wise, R.J.S., Price, C.J., Weiller, C., Hadar, U. *et al.* (1996). Noun and verb retrieval by normal subjects: studies with PET. *Brain* 119, 159–79.

Wernicke, C. (1874). *Der aphasische symtomencomplex: Eine psychologische studie auf anatomischer basis.* Breslau: Cohn and Weigert.

Whelan, B.-M., Murdoch, B.E. and Theodoros, D.G. (2003). Defining a role for the subthalamic nucleus with operative theoretical models of subcortical participation in language. *Journal of Neurology, Neurosurgery and Psychiatry* 74, 1543–50.

Whelan, B.-M., Murdoch, B.E., Theodoros, D.G., Silburn, P.A. and Hall, B. (2004). Re- appraising contemporary theories of subcortical participation in language: proposing an interhemispheric regulatory function for the subthalamic nucleus in the mediation of high level linguistic processing. *Neurocase* 10, 345–52.

Wilson, S.A.K. (1912). Progressive lenticular degeneration: a familial nervous system disease associated with cirrhosis of the liver. *Brain* 34, 295–507.

Wilson, S.A.K. (1928). *Modern Problems in Neurology.* London: Arnold.

2 Neuroanatomy and functional neurology of the subcortical region

Introduction

The subcortical region refers to structures positioned deep within each cerebral hemisphere, beneath the level of the cortical mantle. Descriptions of this region conventionally refer to a number of grey nuclear masses termed the subcortical nuclei, as well as white matter pathways which facilitate communication between these nuclei and the cerebral cortex. The subcortical structures of interest in the current chapter specifically include the basal ganglia, internal capsule, thalamus, brain stem and cerebellum. As such, this chapter attempts to orient the reader to the gross and functional neuroanatomy of the above structures, relevant blood supply, underlying subcortical circuits and neurotransmitter systems, as well as major pathologies of the subcortical region and associated behavioural ramifications.

The basal ganglia and connections

Clinically, the basal ganglia represent a functional system of interconnected grey matter components which typically include the corpus striatum (i.e. caudate nucleus, putamen and globus pallidus), amygdaloid nucleus and claustrum. Although not considered part of the basal ganglia, the subthalamic nucleus (STN), substantia nigra and red nucleus are functionally related to the basal nuclei, and are therefore also considered within this section.

Corpus striatum

Situated in a lateral position to the thalamus, the corpus striatum is divided into two nuclear bodies, namely the caudate and lentiform nuclei, by a band of white matter fibres known as the internal capsule. As its name implies, this region is frequently referred to as the striatocapsular region.

Caudate nucleus

The caudate nucleus may be further subdivided into three parts: a head, body and tail (see Figure 2.1). The nuclear head constitutes a component of the wall of the anterior horn of the lateral ventrical (see Figure 2.2), and is continuous inferiorly with the putamen; a segment of the lentiform nucleus. Within the region of the intraventricular foramen, the body of the caudate nucleus is continuous with the head of the

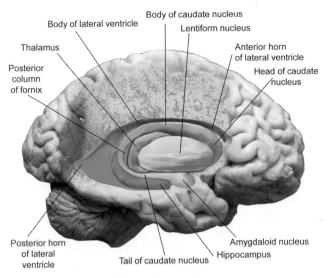

Figure 2.1 Lateral view of the right cerebral hemisphere dissected to show the position of the different basal ganglia.

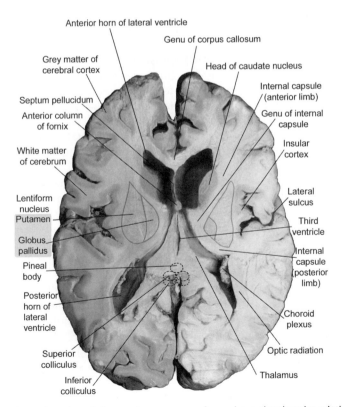

Figure 2.2 Horizontal section of the cerebrum as seen from above showing the relationship of the different basal ganglia.

caudate nucleus and constitutes a portion of the floor of the lateral ventricle. The tail terminates as the amygdaloid nucleus (see Figure 2.1) after following the course of the lateral ventricle.

Lentiform nucleus

The lentiform nucleus has been described as a bilateral wedge-shaped mass of grey matter situated deep within the white matter of each cerebral hemisphere, separated from the caudate nucleus and thalamus by the anterior and posterior limbs of the internal capsule (see Figure 2.2). The lentiform nucleus is laterally bounded by an additional layer of white matter known as the external capsule, dividing it from a further body of grey matter called the claustrum. The lentiform nucleus itself is further subdiveded by a band of white matter into two components known as the putamen and globus pallidus.

The putamen and caudate nucleus have been described as the major input-receiving structures of the basal ganglia and the globus pallidus as the primary output structure of the same system. The cerebral cortex, thalamus and substantia nigra represent the origin of striatal afferents (Crossman and Neary, 1995). The entire cortical mantle has been reported to somatotopically innervate the striatum (Snell, 1997); however, motor and associative projections synapse within differential striatal regions. Typically, corticostriatal motor fibres project to the putamen (Tanridag and Kirshner, 1987) and associative fibres to the caudate nucleus (Goldman-Rakic, 1984) and are glutamatergic and excitatory in nature (Snell, 2006). With respect to language cortices, Broca's and Wernicke's projection fibres have been documented to innervate the same location in the head of the caudate nucleus (Damasio *et al.*, 1982). Thalamostriatal projections originate in the centromedian and parafascicular nuclei of the ipsilateral thalamus (Crossman and Neary, 1995). Nigrostriatal fibres originate in the substantia nigra pars compacta (SNc) and serve to influence striatal and consequently pallidal activity by way of inhibitory dopamine-regulated neurotransmission (Snell, 1997). Ascending fibres from the brain stem also terminate in the striatum and use serotonin to exert inhibitory influences. Striatonigral fibres and striatal outputs to the globus pallidus represent the primary efferent projections of striatal neurones (Snell, 1997), and utilize γ-aminobutyric acid (GABA) and/or acetylcholine, dynorphin or substance P as their neurotransmitter agent (Mink, 2007).

The globus pallidus lies in a medial position to the striatum (i.e. caudate nucleus and putamen), and consists of internal (globus pallidus internus, GPi) and external (globus pallidus externus, GPe) segments which are separated by a white matter partition known as the medial medullary lamina (Crossman and Neary, 1995). Each pallidal segment receives afferents from the striatum and subthalamic nucleus. Despite morphological and phenotypic regularities among pallidal neurones, however, stark differences relative to efferent terminations have served to categorize the GPi and GPe as distinct functional entities (Parent *et al.*, 1991). The GPe is typically considered an integral control structure within basal ganglia circuitry, and the GPi as a principal gateway for basal ganglion output (Parent and Hazrati, 1995). Furthermore, the GPi and substantia nigra pars reticulata (SNr) of the midbrain are generally considered in conjunction (i.e. GPi-SNr complex), given evidence of cytological and connective commonalties between these two structures (Crossman and Neary, 1995).

By way of the aforementioned external and internal divisions, the globus pallidus provides both indirect and direct channels for striatal influences upon basal ganglia output. The GPe has reciprocal links with the subthalamic nucleus in addition to projecting output neurones to the GPi-SNr complex and the reticular nucleus of the thalamus (Parent and Hazrati, 1995). Concentrated GPe projections to neurones within the GPi and SNr (Hazrati *et al.*, 1990; Kincaid *et al.*, 1991) reportedly place the GPe in a crucial position to regulate output stations of the basal ganglia. Current opinion supports the notion that robust GABAergic output from the GPe may in fact overrule distant striatal and glutamatergic subthalamic influences upon GPi-SNr efferents (Parent and Hazrati, 1993).

The internal segment of the globus pallidus, in tandem with the SNr, primarily projects neurones to the ventral lateral (VL), ventral anterior (VA) and centromedian nuclei of the thalamus (Crossman and Neary, 1995), which in turn regulate cortical activity. Cerebral cortex activation is achieved by way of potent glutamatergic thalamocortical projections (Parent and Hazrati, 1995). The thalamus and composite nuclei subserving language function will be discussed in detail in Chapter 3.

Amygdaloid nucleus

Situated within the temporal lobe (see Figure 2.1), the amygdaloid nucleus is classified as a component of the limbic system.

Claustrum

As mentioned above, the claustrum is a thin body of grey matter positioned on the lateral surface of the lentiform nucleus but separated from it by the external capsule (see Figure 2.2). The function of the claustrum is essentially unknown.

Subthalamic nucleus

Positioned inferiorly to the thalamus, the STN has been shown to exert excitatory (i.e. glutamatergic) influences upon basal ganglia structures (Carpenter, 1991). The STN receives afferents from the GPe, motor, premotor and prefrontal cortices, centrum medianum and parafascicular nucleus of the thalamus, and the pedunculopontine nucleus (Carpenter, 1991). Subthalamic efferents are excitatory (i.e. glutamatergic) and include projections to both the internal and external segments of the globus pallidus as well as the substantia nigra (Carpenter, 1991).

Substantia nigra

The substantia nigra is a mass of grey matter located within the midbrain and is composed of two compartments: (1) compacta (SNc) and (2) reticulata (SNr) (Afifi and Bergman, 2005). Although a midbrain structure, it is considered functionally related to basal ganglia activity via connections with the corpus striatum, and contains dopaminergic neurones with inhibitory influences upon connected structures. It receives inputs from the cerebral cortex, globus pallidus, caudate nucleus, STN and other midbrain nuclei, and projects to the cerebral cortex, globus pallidus, red nucleus, STN, thalamus, amygdaloid nucleus, reticular formation and superior colliculus (Afifi and Bergman, 2005).

Red nucleus

The red nucleus is located within the tegmentum of the brain stem, positioned between the cerebral aquaduct and substantia nigra (Snell, 1992). Inputs to the red nucleus arise from the cerebral cortex via the corticospinal tracts, cerebellum via the superior cerebellar peduncle, lentiform, subthalamic and hypothalamic nuclei, substantia nigra and spinal cord. Outputs from the red nucleus terminate in the spinal cord via the rubrospinal tract, reticular formation via the rubroreticular tract, thalamus and substantia nigra.

Basal ganglia circuitry and associated neurotransmission mechanisms

The basal ganglia constitute a group of nuclei integrally involved in linking cortical and subcortical regions via the formation of complex neural circuits which regulate motor and non-motor behaviour. Simply, five parallel yet functionally segregated basal ganglia circuits have been identified on the basis of their cortical origin (DeLong and Wichmann, 2007), which play a role in the regulation of skeletomotor and occulomotor control, cognition and emotional functioning (Alexander et al., 1990; Mink, 2007). In more detail, each circuit shares a similar loop-like configuration in that it commences within a specific area of the frontal cortex, projects to related regions within the basal ganglia followed by the thalamus, and then back to the same cortical area of origin (Alexander et al., 1986). The motor loop focuses on the precentral motor fields, the occulomotor loop on frontal and supplementary eye fields, the cognitive loops on dorsolateral prefrontal and lateral orbitofrontal cortices, and the limbic loop on anterior cingulate and medial orbitofrontal cortex (Alexander et al., 1990).

Each circuit may be generally divided into principle input and output structures. The primary input area of the basal ganglia is represented by the striatum, which receives excitatory glutamatergic projections from the entire cortical mantle, dopaminergic input from the SNc (see Figure 2.3) and serotonergic and noradrenergic input from the dorsal raphe and locus ceruleus nuclei of the brain stem, respectively (Alexander and Crutcher, 1990; Sohn and Hallet, 2005). Central basal ganglia output structures include the GPi and SNr, which play a primary role in regulating thalamic (Alexander and Crutcher, 1990) and, to some extent, brain stem (DeLong and Wichmann, 2007) activity via the projection of inhibitory GABAergic outflow. The thalamus, in turn, influences cortical activity via the projection of excitatory glutamatergic outflow to specific cortical regions.

Within each circuit, inhibitory outflow from the GPi-SNr is largely dependent upon activity within two parallel yet opposing pathways which connect the striatum to these primary output structures (Alexander and Crutcher, 1990). Connections between the striatum and GPi-SNr are mediated via two pathways, a monosynaptic inhibitory (i.e. GABA, dynorphin and substance P) *direct pathway* and a polysynaptic net excitatory (i.e. glutamatergic) *indirect pathway* that incorporates the GPe and STN (Alexander and Crutcher, 1990; DeLong and Wichmann, 2007; Mink, 2007) (see Figure 2.3).

Neurotransmitters within the polysynaptic indirect pathway include inhibitory GABAergic and enkephalinergic outputs to the GPe, inhibitory GABAergic output from the GPe to STN and excitatory glutamatergic outflow from the STN to GPi-SNr. Activation of these individual pathways is importantly influenced by nigrostriatal

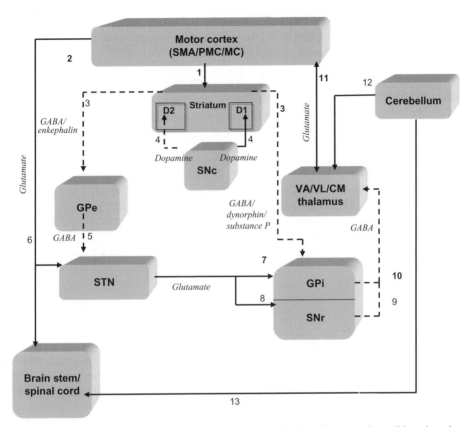

Figure 2.3 Modified schematic diagram of skeletomotor circuit under normal conditions based on DeLong (1990) and Mink (2007). Glutamate, GABA (γ-aminobutyric acid), enkephalin, dynorphin and substance P are active neurotransmitters. CM, centrum medianum; D1, striatal output neurone receptor type D1; D2, striatal output receptor type D2; GPe, globus pallidus externus; GPi, globus pallidus internus; MC, motor cortex; PMC, pre-motor cortex; SMA, supplementary motor area;; SNc, substantia nigra pars compacta; SNr, substantia nigra pars reticulata; STN, subthalamic nucleus; VA, ventral anterior nucleus of thalamus; VL, ventral lateral nucleus of thalamus; solid arrow, excitatory pathway; dashed arrow, inhibitory pathway; 1, cortico-striatal pathway; 2, cortico-bulbar and cortico-spinal pathways; 3, striato-pallidal pathways; 4, nigro-striatal pathways; 5, pallido-subthalamic pathway,; 6, cortico-subthalamic pathway; 7, subthalamo-pallidal pathway; 8, subthalamo-nigral pathway; 9, nigro-thalamic pathway; 10, pallido-thalamic pathway; 11, thalamo-cortical and cortico-thalamic pathways; 12, cerebello-thalamic pathway; 13, cerebello-rubral pathway.

dopaminergic projections (Mink, 2007). In more detail, striatal neurones contain dopamine-sensitive receptors classified as either D1 or D2 receptors, which dopamine affects in oppositional ways. Dopamine has been reported to have a net excitatory effect upon D1 striatal receptors, which initiate direct pathway activity, and a net inhibitory effect upon D2 receptors initiating indirect pathway activity (Alexander and Crutcher, 1990; Mink, 2007). These distinct striatal efferent systems impose oppositional effects upon basal ganglia output nuclei and hence thalamocortical activity (Alexander and Crutcher, 1990). In terms of functionality, striatal dopamine has been hypothesized to reinforce cortical activation of basal ganglia–thalamocortical loops by facilitating and suppressing activity within the direct and indirect pathways, respectively (Alexander and Crutcher, 1990). In this way, activity within the indirect pathway may serve to smooth or brake cortically generated activity reinforced by direct pathway activity (Alexander and Crutcher, 1990).

Connecting white matter pathways

Association, commissural and projection fibres constitute the white matter pathways of the cerebral hemispheres, which originate and/or terminate within the cerebral cortex (Crossman and Neary, 1995). The white matter pathways are comprised of myelinated nerve fibres classified according to their relative connections: (1) association fibres connect ipsilateral cortical centres; (2) commissural fibres connect contralateral, yet functionally related, cortical areas and (3) projection fibres link cortical and subcortical structures (Crossman and Neary, 1995; Snell, 1997). Projection fibres provide a means of neural communication between the brain stem and cerebral cortex. By way of their anatomical configuration, projection fibres traverse the subcortical grey matter and, as such, constitute the focus of the ensuing summary.

The internal capsule

The internal capsule has been defined as a concentration of white matter projection fibres (Barr and Kiernan, 1993) located in the upper region of the brain stem, bordered by the caudate and lenticular nuclei (i.e. putamen and globus pallidus) as well as the thalamus. This structure provides a dedicated pathway through which cortical afferents and efferents may travel (Nolte, 1993). The projection fibres of the internal capsule funnel inferiorly into the cerebral peduncle and expand superiorly to form the corona radiata, whereby they merge with the cerebral white matter, prior to reaching their cortical terminations or origins (Nolte, 1993).

Anatomically, the internal capsule is bowed in appearance and consists of an anterior limb, genu, posterior limb, retrolentiform and sublentiform components (Barr and Kiernan, 1993; Snell, 1997, 2006) (see Figure 2.4). The lentiform nucleus and head of the caudate nucleus border the anterior limb of the internal capsule and the posterior limb provides a division between the thalamus and lentiform nucleus. The apex of the lentiform nucleus is positioned laterally to the genu of the internal capsule. The retrolentiform and sublentiform portions occupy the area posterior to the lentiform nucleus and the area ventral to the posterior portion of the lentiform nucleus, respectively.

The internal capsule houses thalamic radiations, consisting of a variety of reciprocal thalamocortical projection fibres, in addition to corticofugal or motor projection fibres (Barr and Kiernan, 1993). The anterior limb of the internal capsule contains the anterior thalamic radiation (Barr and Kiernan, 1993), which is comprised of projection fibres connecting the dorsomedial nucleus of the thalamus with the prefrontal cortex, the anterior nucleus with the cingulate gyrus and the frontal lobe with pontine nuclei (Nolte, 1993). The genu of the internal capsule has been described as a transition zone between the anterior limb and posterior limb, and reportedly contains frontopontine fibres in addition to projections linking the VA and VL thalamic nuclei with the motor and premotor cortices (Nolte, 1993). The posterior limb of the internal capsule contains the middle thalamic radiation which links the ventral posterior thalamus with the somesthetic and association areas of the parietal lobe (Barr and Kiernan, 1993). In

Anterior limb
1. Anterior thalamic peduncle
2. Frontopontine tract

Genu

Posterior limb
Lenticulothalamic part
3. Superior thalamic peduncle
4. Pyramidal tract

Sublenticular part
5. Ansa peduncularis
6. Thalamotemporal radiations
7. Auditory radiations
8. Optic radiations

Retrolenticular part
9. Posterior thalamic peduncle
10. Temporoparietopontine tract
11. Corticotectotegmental tract

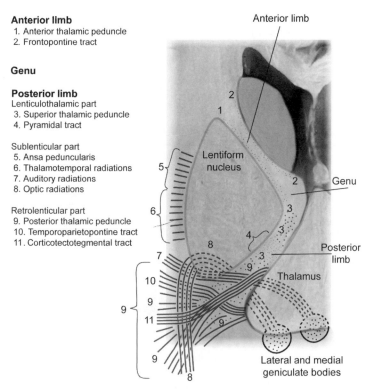

Figure 2.4 Horizontal section of the left internal capsule, as seen from above. Dots represent pathways that run in the vertical axis of the capsule or that run radially. Lines, solid or interrupted, represent pathways that run transversely across the vertical axis of the capsule.

addition, the posterior limb also consists of corticobulbar and corticospinal fibres as well as projections linking the VA and VL thalamic nuclei with the premotor and motor cortices. The retrolentiform component of the internal capsule contains the pulvinar-parieto-occipito-temporal association and parieto-pontine and lateral geniculate-occipital projection fibres and the sublentiform portion houses medial geniculate-temporal lobe projections (Nolte, 1993). Additional motor projection pathways have also been reported to traverse the internal capsule, including: (1) corticostriate fibres primarily linking sensorimotor cortices with the striatum; (2) corticorubral fibres connecting premotor and motor areas of the frontal lobe with the red nucleus; (3) corticoreticular fibres linking motor and parietal cortices to the reticular nuclei and (4) cortico-olivary fibres connecting motor areas of the cerebral cortex with the inferior olivary complex (Barr and Kiernan, 1993).

Blood supply to the basal ganglia and internal capsule

The main blood supply to the brain arises from two arterial pairs: two internal carotid arteries and two vertebral arteries. These arteries lie within the subarachnoid space of the brain and meet on the inferior surface of the brain to form the Circle of Willis (see Figure 2.5), branches from which provide blood to each cerebral hemisphere.

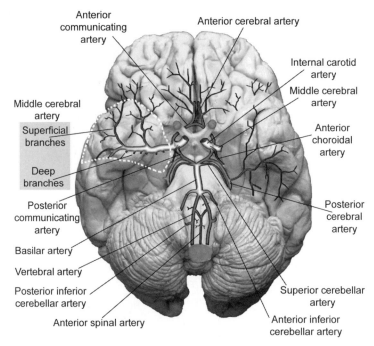

Anterior
communicating
artery

Anterior cerebral artery

Internal carotid
artery

Middle cerebral
artery

Middle cerebral
artery

Superficial
branches

Anterior
choroidal
artery

Deep
branches

Posterior
communicating
artery

Posterior
cerebral
artery

Basilar artery

Vertebral artery

Posterior inferior
cerebellar artery

Superior cerebellar
artery

Anterior spinal artery

Anterior inferior
cerebellar artery

Figure 2.5 Diagram of the ventral surface of the brain and cerebral hemispheres illustrating the key components of the anterior (carotid) circulation and the posterior (vertebral-basilar) circulation. The anterior portion of the temporal lobe of the right hemisphere has been removed to illustrate the course of the middle cerebral artery through the lateral (sylvian) fissure.

Specific vascular components of this formation include the anterior communicating, anterior cerebral, internal carotid, posterior communicating, posterior cerebral and basilar arteries, each of which will be discussed in detail below.

The internal carotid artery is a branch of the common carotid artery. Ascending through the neck, it enters the skull via the carotid canal of the temporal bone and later subdivides further into the anterior and middle cerebral arteries. Contralateral anterior cerebral arteries are linked by the anterior communicating artery, and supply blood to the entire medial surface of cerebral cortex. The middle cerebral artery represents the largest branch of the internal carotid artery, and supplies blood to the majority of the lateral surface of the cerebral hemispheres. Other branches of the internal carotid artery include ophthalmic artery, posterior communicating artery and choroidal artery.

The vertebral artery is a branch of the subclavian artery that enters the skull through the foramen magnum to eventually lie within the subarachnoid space. From there it travels upward where it rests upon the medial medulla oblongata. Branches of the vertebral artery include meningeal, posterior spinal, anterior spinal, posterior inferior cerbellar and medullary arteries. At the level of the lower pons, contralateral vertebral arteries join to form the basilar artery. Branches of the basilar artery include pontine, labyrinthine, anterior inferior cerebellar, superior cerebellar and posterior cerebral arteries.

The basal ganglia and internal capsule receive their blood supply from both anterior and posterior circulations originating in the cerebral arteries or internal carotid artery

(Martin, 2003). Arterial supply of the basal ganglia is provided by the anterior and middle cerebral arteries, otherwise known as the lenticulostriate arteries, as well as the anterior choroidal artery. The upper halves of the anterior and posterior limbs of the internal capsule and the genu are supplied by middle cerebral artery branches and the lower or more inferior half of the internal capsule is supplied by the anterior cerebral and anterior choroidal arteries.

Functional role of the basal ganglia and internal capsule in movement and cognition

The basal ganglia are interconnected with each other and linked to additional areas of the nervous system by a complex network of neurones. In general, the striatum typically receives input from the cerebral cortex, thalamus, STN and brain stem, incorporating the substantia nigra. Incoming information is hypothetically processed within the striatum and then relayed back to the aforementioned areas of efferentation.

Traditionally, a motor function has been well established for the basal ganglia. For example, the initiation of activity within the basal ganglia is thought to occur as a consequence of premotor, supplementary motor and primary sensory cortex, thalamus and brain-stem input. After processing this information, the basal ganglia direct output to the globus pallidus, which has the capacity to regulate the motor cortex and motor areas of the brain stem via connections with these structures. In this way, the basal ganglia are thought to play a role in the execution of learned motor plans as well as in the preparation of movement (Afifi and Bergman, 2005), via direct influences on the cerebral cortex, as opposed to control via descending pathways to the brain stem and spinal cord.

Most recently, the basal ganglia have been implicated in the scaling and focusing of movement, via focused facilitation and surround inhibition of thalamocortical targets (Mink, 2007). In more detail, the indirect basal ganglia pathway provides fast, widespread divergent excitation of the GPi-SNr via the STN, and the direct pathway focused inhibition of the GPi-SNr via the striatum. Within a normal neurological system, basal ganglia inhibitory output functions as a 'brake' in relation to motor pattern generators in the cerebal cortex, via the thalamus and brain stem. In the event of movement initiation, mediated via motor pattern generators within the cerebral cortex, increased firing rates occur in basal ganglia neurones which project to competing motor pattern generators, resulting in increased thalamic inhibition and subsequent braking of these generators. Basal ganglia neurones projecting to motor pattern generators required to execute a desired movement subsequently reduce their firing rates, resulting in the release of braking relative to desired motor output. As a consequence, the desired movement is executed and competing movement patterns are extinguished.

Although the motor circuit represents the most widely researched and discussed basal ganglia circuit in the literature (DeLong and Wichmann, 2007), it has been postulated that the fundamental principles of function will also apply to non-motor circuits. Indeed, the basal ganglia have also been linked to deficits in cognitive set shifting or the ability to change from one mental set that guides behaviour to another (Hayes *et al.*, 1998), akin to movement disorders resulting from an impaired ability to scale and focus competing motor acts.

Basal ganglia and internal capsule pathology and behavioural manifestations

Pathology of the basal ganglia is typically associated with involuntary movement disorders (Afifi and Bergman, 2005), which are generally divided into hyperkinetic and hypokinetic categories. Hyperkinetic disorders (i.e. excessive abnormal movements) and hypokinetic disorders (i.e. abnormal poverty of movement) arise as a consequence of damage to the basal ganglia. Hyperkinetic disorders encompass conditions such as chorea and ballismus and athetosis. Hypokinetic disorders typically include Parkinson's disease.

Chorea is classified as a syndrome whereby patients present with fast involuntary movements that are jerky, irregular and non-repetitive in nature. Huntington's disease is a form of chorea that presents in adulthood, and is acquired as an autosomal dominant inherited condition. Symptoms include choreiform movements (i.e. facial grimacing and involuntary movements of the limbs with progressive deterioration over time, producing immobility, dysarthria and dysphagia) and progressive dementia. The syndrome occurs due to overactivation of dopamine-secreting neurones within the substantia nigra, resulting in inhibition of the striatum and abnormal movements, and is commonly associated with degeneration of the caudate nuclei. (The effect of Huntington's disease on speech and language function is discussed in Chapters 11 and 8 respectively.) In contrast, Syndenham's chorea (i.e. St Vitus' dance) presents in childhood and involves involuntary irregular movements of the limbs, trunk and face. This form of chorea is thought to occur as a result of rheumatic fever, whereby host antibodies attack basal ganglia neurones producing choreiform movements. However, the condition is not progressive and full recovery occurs over time.

Hemiballismus is another form of hyperkinetic movement disorder typically involving unilateral involuntary movements. The condition usually arises as a result of lesions to the STN or related pathways, and patients usually present with flailing limbs. Athetosis is a condition which arises as a result of degeneration within the globus pallidus, causing the production of slow writhing movements of the limbs. (Motor speech impairments associated with various hyperkinetic disorders are described and discussed in Chapter 11.)

Parkinson's disease is commonly classified as a hypokinetic movement disorder resulting from neuronal degeneration within the substantia nigra, which in turn causes a reduction in the amount of dopamine released within the striatum. Symptoms commonly include resting tremor, rigidity, bradykinesia (i.e. difficulty initiating movements and executing novel movements) and postural disturbances. (Speech and language disorders associated with Parkinson's disease are described and discussed in Chapters 11 and 8 respectively.)

In addition to their role in regulating motor functions, the basal ganglia have also been hypothesized to play a role in the mediation of cognitive functions. In particular, lesions of the dorsolateral prefrontal basal ganglia circuit have been reported to result in cognitive deficits including impaired spatial, episodic and semantic memory, commonly observed in patients with schizophrenia, Huntington's disease and Parkinson's disease (Afifi and Bergman, 2005). Lesions of the orbitofrontal basal ganglia circuit have been associated with the manifestation of obsessive compulsive disorder (Afifi and Bergman, 2005). Neurobehavioural disorders have also been described as a consequence of discrete lesions within cognitive-limbic territories of the basal ganglia; for example, following stroke (Levy, 2007). Lesions of the caudate nucleus and ventral striatum have been reported to rarely produce motor deficits, but to evoke cognitive disturbances similar to prefrontal lesions such as confusion, apathy, impaired executive function, aphasia and disinhibition (Levy, 2007). In contrast, lesions of the putamen are rarely linked to neurobehavioural disorders, but apraxia and visual neglect are commonly reported deficits. Discrete lesions of the GPe may elicit attention deficits, hyperactivity, compulsive behaviour and/or dyskinesia. Lesions of the GPi have been associated with psychic akinesia/self-activation deficit primarily involving cognitive intertia (i.e. reduced ability to generate and activate cognitive strategies, slowness, delayed response initiation and reduced mental flexibility) as part of a dysexecutive syndrome (Levy, 2007).

The majority of fibres within the internal capsule belong to two possible systems: (1) cortical efferents travelling to the brain stem and spinal cord and (2) thalamic peduncles accommodating thalamocortical and corticothalamic circuits (DeMyer, 1998). Isolated lesions of the internal capsule have been significantly associated with pure motor hemiparesis, dysarthria-clumsy hand syndrome, as well as general sensory motor deficits (Arboix et al., 2005). In more detail, lesions at the level of the genu have been associated with cranial nerve signs; lesions within the posterior limb of the internal capsule have been associated with contralateral hemisensory loss and hemiplegia; and lesions within terminal posterior zones of the internal capsule have been known to produce contralateral visual and hearing loss (Afifi and Bergman, 2005).

The thalamus and connections

The thalamus has been identified as the largest nuclear mass in the nervous system (Fitzgerald et al., 2007), comprising more than 30 anatomically and functionally distinct nuclei (Wallesch and Papagno, 1988). Represented in each hemisphere, the bilateral egg-shaped mass of grey matter lies at the centre of the brain (Fitzgerald et al., 2007). From a medial aspect the two bodies of grey matter are positioned opposite to one another, each facing the third ventricle, and are joined by an interthalamic adhesion (see Figures 2.6 and 2.7). Laterally the thalamus is bordered by the posterior limb of the internal capsule which separates it from the globus pallidus. The anterior segment of the thalamus constitutes the posterior boundary of the interventricular foramen and the posterior aspect is comprised of a large nucleus known as the pulvinar, which projects over the superior colliculus and superior brachium (Snell, 1997). Inferiorly, the thalamus is continuous with the midbrain and superiorly it constitutes a portion of the floor of the lateral ventricle.

A y-shaped body of white matter, the internal medullary lamina, serves to divide the grey matter of the thalamus into three separate nuclear groups namely, anterior, medial and lateral nuclei (Crossman and Neary, 1995) (see Figure 2.7). The internal medullary lamina also contains its own nuclear complex, referred to as the intralaminar nuclei, which contains nerve fibres allowing communication between thalamic nuclei. The external medullary lamina and stratum zonale represent additional layers of white matter encasing the thalamus on its lateral and superior borders, respectively. Medial and lateral geniculate nuclei lie on the posterior surface of the thalamus, depicted by small swellings (Fitzgerald, 1996). A further nuclear mass, the reticular nucleus, lies between the posterior limb of the internal capsule and the external medullary lamina (Barr and Kiernan, 1993; Crossman and Neary, 1995). With the exception of the reticular nucleus, each of the thalamic nuclei demonstrate reciprocal connections with the cerebral cortex (Crossman and Neary, 1995; Fitzgerald, 1996). On the

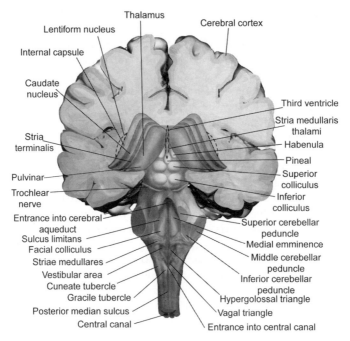

Figure 2.6 Posterior view of the brain stem showing the thalamus and tectum of the midbrain.

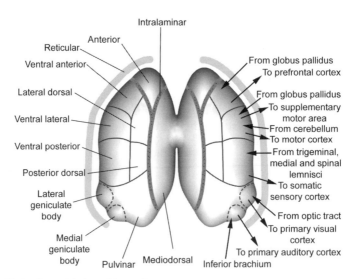

Figure 2.7 Thalamic nuclei viewed from above.

basis of this configuration, it has been hypothesized that the thalamus and cerebral cortex are compelled to share information, and that each is capable of influencing activity in the other. The ventral aspect of the thalamus also receives inputs from the cerebellum, spinal cord and globus pallidus (Fitzgerald *et al.*, 2007). In fact the thalamus has been identified as a significant relay station for two major sensory-motor circuits: (1) cerebellar-rubro-thalamic-cortico-ponto-cerebellar circuit and (2) cortico-striatal-pallidal-thalamic-cortical circuit.

The thalamus has been hailed as the primary integrating and regulating component of the neuroaxis (Carpenter, 1991). Thalamocortical fibre terminations determine the functional nature of thalamic nuclei, which are classified within three possible groups, including specific, non-specific and association nuclei (Fitzgerald et al., 2007). Specific thalamic nuclei are described as having distinct reciprocal connections with areas of the cerebral cortex that have been designated an exclusive motor or sensory function (Crossman and Neary, 1995; Fitzgerald, 1996; Fitzgerald et al., 2007). The ventral tier of the lateral nuclear group and the geniculate nuclei belong to this functional category, including the VA, VL , ventral posterior, lateral geniculate and medial geniculate nuclei (Crossman and Neary, 1995; Fitzgerald, 1996). Non-specific nuclei reportedly have a more generic function on the basis that they lack exclusive reciprocal connections with distinctive motor and sensory cortical areas (Fitzgerald et al., 2007). They project to a wider range of cortical areas than do specific thalamic nuclei; however, their main output projections are to non-cortical targets, including the basal ganglia (Nolte, 1993). The intralaminar and reticular nuclei are grouped within this functional category (Fitzgerald et al., 2007). Thalamic association nuclei share reciprocal connections with association areas of the cerebral cortex (Fitzgerald, 1996; Fitzgerald et al., 2007; Nolte, 1993). Nuclei belonging to this functional category include the anterior nucleus, mediodorsal nucleus and the lateral posterior nuclear complex which includes the pulvinar (Fitzgerald, 1996). Afferent and efferent connections of primary thalamic nuclei are listed in Table 2.1.

Blood supply to the thalamus

Although the striatocapsular region is supplied by branches of the middle and anterior cerebral arteries, branches of the posterior cerebral artery provide the major blood supply to the thalamus. Part of the thalamic blood supply depends on branches of the middle cerebral artery known as lenticulo-striate arteries. These branches circulate blood to the majority of internal hemispheric structures including the thalamus, and basal ganglia (Hendelman, 2000) (see Figure 2.8). The thalamus also receives blood supply from some of the branches within the Circle of Willis, including the posterior communicating artery, the basilar artery and posterior cerebral artery (Snell, 1992) (see Figure 2.5). In more detail, the medial thalamus is supplied by the paramedian branches of the basilar root of the posterior cerebral artery (Afifi and Bergman, 2005). The antero-lateral aspect of the thalamus is supplied by the tuberothalamic branch of the posterior communicating artery, the posterolateral aspect of the thalamus is supplied by the geniculothalamic branch of the posterior cerebral artery and the lateral aspect of the thalamus receives blood supply from the anterior choroidal branch of the internal carotid artery (Afifi and Bergman, 2005).

Functional role of the thalamus in movement and cognition

As mentioned previously the thalamus has been described as the primary integrating and regulating component of the neuroaxis (Carpenter, 1991). An enormous amount of information is received by the thalamus, and potentially integrated via thalamic internuclear connections. The thalamus and cerebral cortex are closely linked from an

Table 2.1 Primary thalamic nuclei and their afferent and efferent connections and designated function (adapted from Snell, 2006).

Type	Nucleus	Afferents	Efferents	Function
Specific	Anterior	Mammillary body, cingulated gyrus and hypothalamus	Cingulate gyrus, hypothalamus	Recent memory and regulation of emotional tone
	VA	Reticular formation, substantia nigra, striatum, premotor cortex, other thalamic nuclei	Reticular formation, substantia nigra, corpus striatum, premotor cortex, other thalamic nuclei	Regulation of motor cortex activity
	VL	As per VA nucleus but includes input from cerebellum and red nucleus	As per VA nucleus	Influences activity within motor cortex
	Ventral posterior medial	Trigeminal lemniscus, gustatory fibres	Primary somatosensory cortex	Relays sensations to consciousness
	Ventral posterior lateral	Medial and spinal lemnisci	Primary somatosensory cortex	Relays sensations to consciousness
	Medial geniculate	Inferior colliculus, lateral lemniscus	Superior temporal gyrus	Hearing
	Lateral geniculate	Optic tract	Visual cortex of occipital lobe	Vision
Association	Lateral dorsal, lateral posterior and pulvinar	Cerebral cortex and other thalamic nuclei	Cerebral cortex and other thalamic nuclei	Unknown
Non-specific	Intralaminar	Reticular formation, spinothalamic and trigeminothalamic tracts	Cerebral cortex via other thalamic nuclei, striatum	Consciousness and alertness
	Reticular	Reticular formation, cerebral cortex	Other thalamic nuclei	Cerebral cortex regulates thalamus

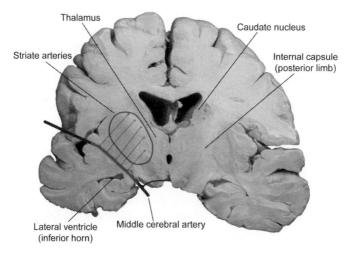

Thalamus

Caudate nucleus

Striate arteries

Internal capsule
(posterior limb)

Lateral ventricle   Middle cerebral artery
(inferior horn)

Figure 2.8 Blood supply to the internal capsule and basal ganglia.

anatomical and functional perspective. With evidence of reciprocal connections, the thalamus and cerebral cortex share information with each other and have the ability to mutually influence activity. Specific thalamic nuclei have been assigned defined motor and sensory functions. Receiving input from the globus pallidus and relaying fibres to the prefrontal, premotor and supplementary motor areas of the cerebral cortex, the ventroanterior and ventrolateral nuclei have been assigned a role in the regulation of voluntary movements (Snell, 2006). In addition, the VL thalamus has been postulated to accommodate a tremorogenic centre (Afifi and Bergman, 2005). The medial thalamus has been hypothesized to participate in the mediation of emotional states and executive function via connections with the prefrontal cortex (Afifi and Bergman, 2005). The anterior thalamus has been reported to play a role in the regulation of memory, organ function and emotion given connections with the cingulated gyrus and hypothalamus (Afifi and Bergman, 2005). The intralaminar nuclei have been assigned a role in regulating levels of consciousness and alertness, given their connections with the reticular formation and associated links to the regulation of cerebral cortex activity (Snell, 2006).

Thalamocortical neurones have been described as anatomically and physiologically expedient in relation to the transfer of afferent information to the cerebral cortex (Steriade *et al.*, 1990). Hypotheses pertaining to thalamic participation in language have primarily attributed roles to the VA and VL nuclei, pulvinar (Wallesch and Papagno, 1988) and more recently, non-specific nuclei, including the centrum medianum, parafascicular nucleus and nucleus reticularis (Nadeau and Crosson, 1997).

The VA (Crosson, 1985; Wallesch and Papagno, 1988) and VL (Wallesch and Papagno, 1988) thalamic nuclei have been postulated to participate in a fundamental language-processing circuit, involving a cortico-striato-pallido-thalamo-cortical loop. Cortico-striatal inputs to this circuit were reported to arise from the entire cortical mantle, and terminal VA- and VL-cortical projections to innervate the dorsolateral frontal language area (Wallesch and Papagno, 1988). The pulvinar has also been hypothesized to contribute to language functions by way of its reciprocal connections with the parietal, temporal and occipital association cortices (Jones, 1985). The direct role of the aforementioned nuclei in linking cortical language centres has served to fortify the notion of their potential involvement in the mediation of linguistic processes. Wallesch and Papagno (1988), however, highlighted the need to consider the potentially complex nature of interactions between thalamic nuclei and the possible role of nuclei that are not reciprocally linked to the cerebral cortex in influencing language processes. Indeed, non-specific thalamic nuclei have been described as well-suited to the role of regulating cortical excitability on the basis of their extensive connections with the cerebral cortex, and their relationship with the reticular activating system, which modulates non-specific nuclei output, indirectly regulating cortical activity (Nolte, 1993). Penfield and Roberts (1959) supported this functional hypothesis with the proposal that the centrum medianum, the largest of the non-specific nuclei, was involved in a complex circuit dedicated to the transference of linguistic information, between the posterior language area, thalamus and anterior language area. More recently, Nadeau and Crosson (1997) proposed a role for the centrum medianum and nucleus reticularis in the selective engagement of cortical nets dedicated to linguistic functions.

Thalamic pathology and behavioural manifestations

Pathological processes within the thalamus commonly involve neoplasms, degeneration due to disease of arterial supply or damage as a consequence of haemorrhage. Regardless of aetiology, thalamic damage may have catastrophic effects on nervous system functioning, given the profound integrative and relay-station roles of this nuclear mass. Lesions of the thalamus have been documented to result in an array of possible outcomes, including memory disturbances, language disorders, affective disorders, pain, hemiparesis, dyskinesia, disturbed consciousness and sensory disturbances (Afifi and Bergman, 2005).

Vascular lesions of the thalamus have enabled the most accurate correlation of signs and symptoms with specific thalamic territories (Afifi and Bergman, 2005). For example, infarcts within the posterolateral territory of the thalamus (i.e. ventralposterolateral, ventralposteromedial and medial geniculate nuclei, pulvinar and centrum medianum) have been commonly associated with a global sensory loss, parasthesia and pain. Other potential symptoms may also include contralateral hemiataxia, tremor, choreiform movements, spatial neglect, hemiparesis and homonymous hemianopsia. Lesions within the anterolateral thalamus (i.e. ventral anterior, ventral lateral, dorsomedial and anterior nuclei) have been observed to produce contralateral facial paresis, visual field deficits, hemiparesis, hemisensory loss, abulia, reduced spontaneity and non-fluent speech. In addition, impaired intelligence, language and memory are more commonly associated with left-sided anterolateral thalamic lesions and reduced visuospatial functioning with right-sided lesions. Lesions within the medial thalamic territory (i.e. intralaminar and dorsomedial nuclei, as well as ventral lateral, ventral anterior and ventral posterior nuclei) have been reported to produce drowsiness as well as short-term memory deficits, reduced attention, hemiparesis and hemiataxia. Lesions within the lateral thalamic territory (i.e. lateral geniculate, ventralposterolateral, pulvinar and reticular nuclei), which also typically involve the posterior limb of the internal capsule as well as the temporal lobe, have been associated with contralateral hemiparesis and dysarthria. Other symptoms may also include sensory loss, visual field deficits, reduced memory and visuospatial functioning. Finally, posterior thalamic territory infarcts (i.e. lateral geniculate, pulvinar and dorsolateral nuclei) have been reported to produce homonymous quadrantanopsia, hemihypesthesia, reduced memory, transcortical aphasia and possibly contralateral hemiparesis and choreoathetosis.

Specific clinical syndromes reported to arise following thalamic damage include thalamic pain syndromes (i.e. abnormalities in perception of pain and sensation), memory deficits, reduced cortical arousal, cheiro-oral syndrome (i.e. sensory disturbance within a hand and ipsilateral oral region), alien hand syndrome (i.e. uncontrollable upper limb movement and failure to recognize the limb), thalamic acalculia and aphasia (i.e. typically anomic or transcortical subtypes) (Afifi and Bergman, 2005).

The brain stem and connections

The brain stem is stalk-like in appearance, providing a conduit between the spinal cord and forebrain. It consists of three primary subdivisions (the midbrain, the pons and the medulla oblongata) and provides an input and output channel for 10 of the 12 cranial nerves (Martin, 2003).

The midbrain

The midbrain serves to connect the forebrain with the pons and cerebellum, and contains a narrow opening containing cerebrospinal fluid known as the cerebral aqueduct, which connects the third and fourth ventricles. Posteriorly, the midbrain may be distinguished by the presence of four colliculi: an inferior and superior pair (see Figure 2.6). Below the inferior colliculi, the trochlear nerve emerges. Anteriorly, the occulomotor nerve emerges from the midbrain.

Internally, the midbrain may be viewed as two lateral halves termed the cerebral peduncles, divided anteriorly as the crus cerebri and posteriorly as the tegmentum by a band of grey matter called the substantia nigra (see Figure 2.9). Posterior to the cerebral aquaduct is an additional portion of the midbrain known as the tectum. The tectum accommodates the two pairs of swellings known as the superior and inferior colliculi.

The red nucleus is an important mass of grey matter located between the substantia nigra and cerebral aquaduct, at the level of the superior colliculus (see Figure 2.10). Red nucleus afferents include cerebral cortex via corticospinal tracts, cerebellum via the superior cerebellar peduncle, lentiform, subthalamic and hypothalamic nuclei, substantia nigra and spinal cord. Red nucleus efferents include spinal cord via the rubrospinal tract, reticular formation via the rubroreticular tract, thalamus and substantia nigra. Posterior to the red nucleus within the tegmentum lies the reticular formation. At the level of the inferior colliculus, the crus cerebri contains the corticospinal, corticonuclear and corticopontine tracts.

The pons

The pons sits in an anterior position to the cerebellum, connecting the medulla oblongata to the midbrain. The anterior surface is convex in shape, converging laterally to form the middle cerebellar peduncle. A medial groove, known as the basilar groove, houses the basilar artery. The trigeminal nerve emerges bilaterally from the pons on the anterolateral surface. Emerging between the junction of the pons

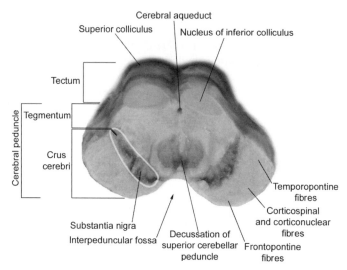

Figure 2.9 Transverse section of the midbrain through the inferior colliculi showing the division of the midbrain into the tectum and the cerebral peduncles. The cerebral peduncles are subdivided by the substantia nigra into the tegmentum and the crus cerebri.

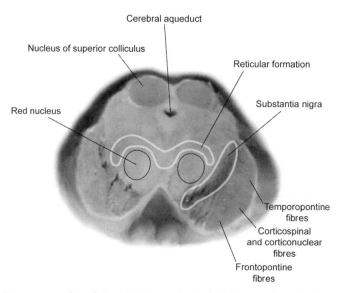

Figure 2.10 Transverse section of the midbrain at the level of the superior colliculus.

and medulla oblongata are the abducens, facial and vestibulocochlear cranial nerves (see Figure 2.11).

The posterior pons is covered by the cerebellum, and forms a portion of the floor of the fourth ventricle. It is divided into symmetrical halves by the median sulcus and is bordered laterally by the superior cerebellar peduncles (see Figure 2.12). A medial elevation emerges laterally to the median sulcus known as the medial eminence,

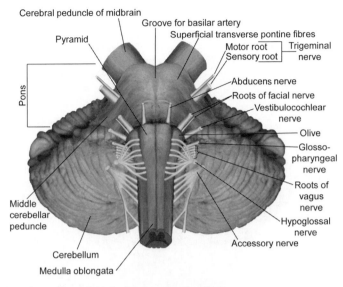

Figure 2.11 Anterior surface of the brain stem showing the pons.

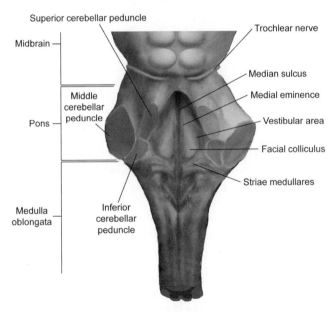

Figure 2.12 Posterior surface of the brain stem showing the pons. (Note: the cerebellum has been removed.)

forming an additional sulcus known as the sulcus limitans. The tail of the medial eminence terminates in a rounded swelling known as the facial colliculus, formed by the facial nerve wrapping around the nucleus of the abducens nerve.

Internally, the pons is typically studied at two transverse levels: (1) the caudal level through the facial colliculus and (2) the cranial level through the trigeminal nuclei.

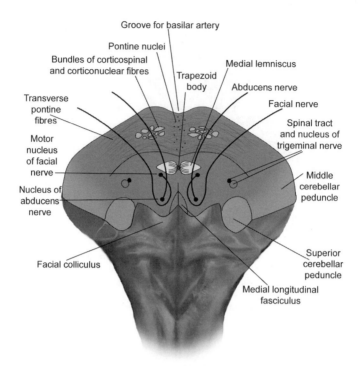

Figure 2.13 Transverse section through the caudal part of the pons at the level of the facial colliculus.

Caudal level

Accompanied by the spinal and lateral lemnisci, the medial lemniscus is observable at the caudal level of the pons, in the most anterior segment of the tegmentum (see Figure 2.13). The facial nucleus lies in a posterolateral position to the medial lemniscus. The facial colliculus forms as a result of the facial nerve winding around the nucleus of the abducens nerve. Facial nerve fibres then traverse anteriorly between the nucleus of the spinal tract of the trigeminal nerve and the facial nucleus. The medial longitudinal fasciculus is positioned bilaterally beneath the floor of the fourth ventricle, providing the primary pathway connecting vestibular, cochlear, occulomotor, trochlear and abducens nuclei. Lateral to the abducens nucleus lies the medial vestibular nucleus. The anterior and posterior cochlear nuclei may also be observed at the caudal level of the pons.

On the anteromedial aspect of the inferior cerebellar peduncle lies the spinal nucleus of the trigeminal nerve. Traversing the anterior part of the tegmentum are fibres of the cochlear nuclei and trapezoid body. At this level, the basilar portion of the pons contains pontine nuclei, which provide the termination point for corticopontine fibres of the midbrain, and also produce transverse fibres that decussate at the midline, intersecting with and dividing corticospinal and corticonuclear tracts. From there, the transverse fibres enter the cerebellum via the middle cerebellar peduncle.

Cranial level

The internal constituents of the cranial level of the pons are similar to those seen at the caudal level; however, they also include the motor and sensory nuclei of the tri-

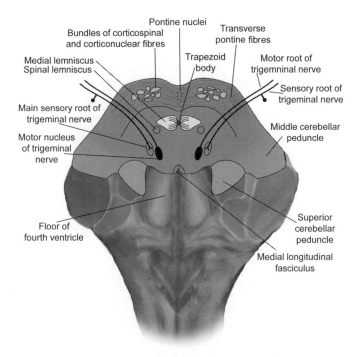

Figure 2.14 Transverse section through the pons at the level of the trigeminal nuclei.

geminal nerve (see Figure 2.14). In a posterolateral position to the motor nucleus of the trigeminal nerve are the superior cerebellar peduncle and the anterior spinocerebellar tract. The trapezoid body and medial lemniscus are evident as per the caudal level, and the lateral and spinal lemnisci are positioned at the lateral borders of the medial lemniscus.

The medulla oblongata

The medulla oblongata is cone-shaped and connects the pons and spinal cord (see Figure 2.15). The spine and medulla oblongata merge at the level of the foramen magnum, encompassing the anterior and posterior roots of the first cervical spinal nerve. In the upper half of the medulla oblongata the central canal of the spinal cord expands to form the cavity of the fourth ventricle. The anterior median fissure sits on the anterior surface of the medulla oblongata, which is continuous with the anterior median fissure of the spinal cord (see Figure 2.15). Bilateral swellings known as the pyramids, which taper inferiorly, are located on either side of the anterior median fissure. The pyramids are made up of bundles of corticospinal fibres originating in the precentral gyrus of the cerebral cortex. The narrowing of the pyramids is referred to as the decussation of the pyramids, a region in the neural axis where the majority of descending fibres cross to the contralateral side of the nervous system. In a posterolateral position to the pyramids lie additional swellings known as the olives, which are formed by internal inferior olivary nuclei. Hypoglossal cranial nerve roots emerge from a furrow between the pyramids and olives. The inferior cerebellar peduncles lie posteriorly to the olives, providing a conduit between the medulla

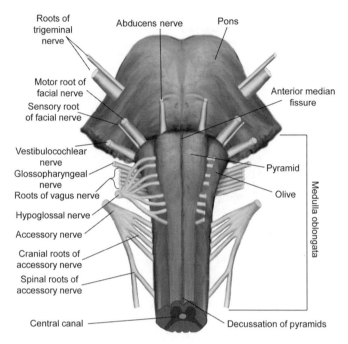

Figure 2.15 Anterior view of the medulla oblongata.

oblongata and cerebellum. Glossopharyngeal, vagus and accessory canial nerve roots arise from the furrow between the olives and inferior cerebellar peduncle.

The floor of the fourth ventricle is formed by the posterior surface of the upper half of the medulla oblongata (see Figure 2.16). The lower half is again continous with the spinal cord and accommodates a posterior median sulcus. Bilateral swellings known as the gracile tubercles are located on either side of the posterior median sulcus, formed by the underlying gracile nucleus. An additional swelling, the cuneate tubercle, lies laterally to the gracile tubercle, formed by the internal cuneate nucleus.

Internally, the medulla oblongata is typically studied at four levels: (1) the decussation of pyramids, (2) decussation of lemnisci, (3) level of the olives and (4) level inferior to the pons.

Decussation of pyramids

The decussation of the pyramids is also referred to as the great motor decussation, and may be viewed via a transverse section of the inferior half of the medulla oblongata (see Figure 2.17). Corticospinal fibres form the pyramids in the superior half of the medulla oblongata, but the majority of fibres cross over at the decussation to form the lateral cortical spinal tract within the contralateral white column of the spinal cord. Cunate and gracile nuclei and their associated fasciculi are represented at this level, as is the spinal nucleus of the trigeminal nerve and the nuclei of the accessory and hypoglossal nerves. The lateral and anterior white columns of the spinal cord are easily viewed at this level.

Decussation of lemnisci

A further transverse section anterior to the decussation of the pyramids passes through the great sensory decussation, or the decussation of lemnisci. The lemnisci are pro-

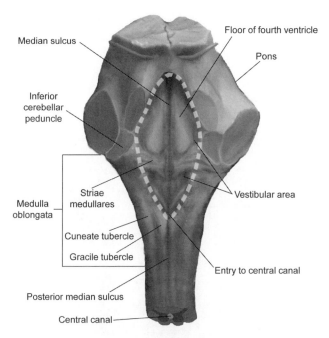

Figure 2.16 Posterior view of the medulla oblongata (cerebellum removed).

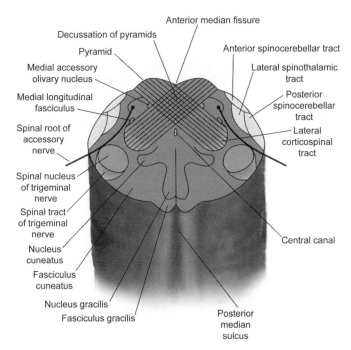

Figure 2.17 Transverse section of the medulla oblongata at the level of the decussation of the pyramids.

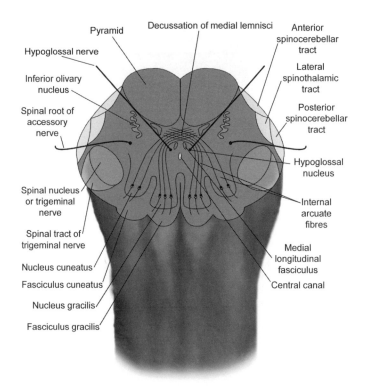

Pyramid
Decussation of medial lemnisci
Anterior spinocerebellar tract
Hypoglossal nerve
Inferior olivary nucleus
Lateral spinothalamic tract
Spinal root of accessory nerve
Posterior spinocerebellar tract
Hypoglossal nucleus
Spinal nucleus or trigeminal nerve
Internal arcuate fibres
Spinal tract of trigeminal nerve
Medial longitudinal fasciculus
Nucleus cuneatus
Central canal
Fasciculus cuneatus
Nucleus gracilis
Fasciculus gracilis

Figure 2.18   Transverse section of the medulla oblongata at the level of the decussation of the medial lemnisci.

duced from internal arcuate fibres, which originate in the gracile and cuneate nuclei. The internal arcuate fibres bilaterally traverse in an anterolateral direction through central grey matter, and then curve medially toward the midline where they cross over to the contralateral side (see Figure 2.18). The nucleus and spinal tract of the trigeminal nerve lie in a lateral position to the internal arcuate fibres. Lateral to the decussation of the lemnisci lie the lateral and anterior spinothalamic tracts and the spinotectal tracts. In the anterolateral medulla oblongata lie the spinocerebellar, vestibulospinal, and rubrospinal tracts. The nuclei of the hypoglossal and accessory nerves are also visible at this level.

Level of the olives
A further transverse section through the medulla oblongata at the level of the olives encompasses the inferior aspect of the fourth ventricle (see Figure 2.19). At this level the volume of grey matter increases to accommodate the olivary nuclear complex and the vestibulocochlear, glossopharyngeal, vagus, accessory, hypoglossal and arcuate nuclei.

The olivary complex is comprised of inferior olivary nucleus, as well as dorsal and medial accessory olivary nuclei. The inferior olivary nucleus is the largest within the complex. Fibres from this nucleus are projected across the midline to enter the cerebellum via the inferior cerebellar peduncle. Afferent fibres to this nucleus arise from the spinal cord, cerebellum and cerebral cortex.

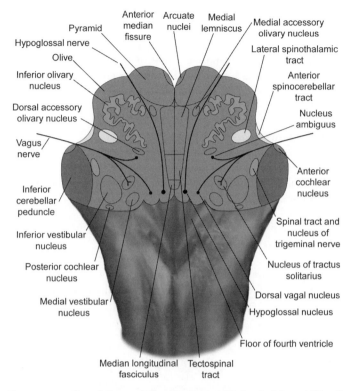

Figure 2.19 Transverse section of the medulla oblongata at the level of the middle olivary nuclei.

The vestibular nuclear complex consists of the medial, inferior, lateral and superior vestibular nuclei; however, only the medial and inferior components are visible at this level. The inferior cerebellar peduncle accommodates the two (i.e. anterior and posterior) cochlear nuclei. The nucleus ambiguus is located within the reticular formation, and consists of large motor neurones. Emerging nerve fibres from this nucleus join the glossopharyngeal, vagus and accessory nerves.

Beneath the floor of the fourth ventricle at this level lies the central grey matter, containing the hypoglossal, dorsal vagus, tractus solitarius, medial and inferior vestibular nuclei. Arcuate nuclei, which are thought to represent dislodged pontine nuclei, are positioned on the anterior aspect of the pyramids. These nuclei receive afferents from the cerebral cortex and project efferents to the cerebellum via the external arcuate fibres. The pyramids are positioned anteriorly, separated by the anterior median fissure. Corticospinal fibres descend via the pyramids to the spinal cord. Corticonuclear fibres within the pyramids synapse within motor nuclei of the cranial nerves located in the medulla oblongata. Posterior to the pyramids lie flattened tracts known as the medial lemnisci. Fibres within these tracts arise from the decussation of the lemnisci and transmit sensory information to the thalamus. Posterior to the medial lemnisci and anterior to the hypoglossal nucleus is another tract known as the medial longitudinal fasciculus. Lateral to the fourth ventricle is the inferior cerebellar peduncle, containing the spinal tract of the trigeminal nerve and its associated nucleus. Lying between the inferior olivary nucleus and nucleus of the spinal tract of the trigeminal nerve is the anterior spinocerbellar tract. The anterior and lateral spinothalamic tracts and spinotectal tracts are also visible at this level.

The reticular formation is positioned posteriorly to the olivary nucleus, and the glossopharyngeal, vagus and cranial segment of the accessory nerves traverse the lateral reticular formation in a forwards direction, to emerge between the olives and inferior cerebellar peduncles. The hypoglossal nerves emerge at this level between the pyramids and olives.

Level inferior to the pons

Grey and white matter distributions are equivalent at this level to those at the level of the olives. The cochlear nuclei are now visible on the anterior and posterior aspects of the inferior cerebellar peduncle and the lateral vestibular nucleus is replaced by the inferior vestibular nucleus.

Blood supply to the brain stem

Arterial blood supply to the three regions of the brain stem arise from the posterior circulation (Martin, 2003) (see Figure 2.20). In contrast to ventral and dorsal spinal

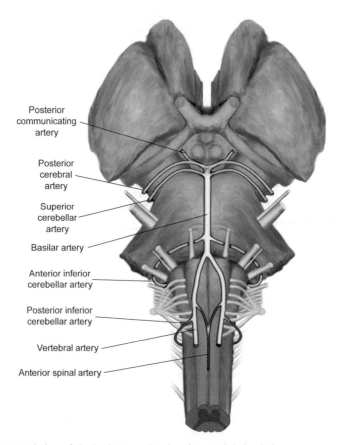

Posterior
communicating
artery

Posterior
cerebral
artery

Superior
cerebellar
artery

Basilar artery

Anterior inferior
cerebellar artery

Posterior inferior
cerebellar artery

Vertebral artery

Anterior spinal artery

Figure 2.20   Ventral view of the brain stem showing the arterial circulation.

blood supply, brain-stem blood supply is almost exclusively distributed along the ventral surface. Ventral arteries branch directly, or penetrate or circumscribe the brain stem in order to supply blood to dorsal brain-stem structures. The vertebral and basilar arteries produce three circulatory branches important to brain-stem blood supply – the paramedian, short circumferential and long circumferential branches – integral to the circulation of midline, lateral and dorsolateral brain-stem regions, respectively. The spinal arteries supply blood to a small region of the caudal medulla oblongata. Given that they are positioned in close proximity to the dorsal and ventral midline, they typically nourish the more medial region of the medulla oblongata. The more lateral regions are supplied by short circumferential branches of the vertebral arteries. The majority of the medulla's blood supply is derived from ventral vertebral arteries. The medial medulla is supplied by small unnamed branches of the main artery (e.g. paramedian and short circumferential), and the dorsolateral region is supplied by a major, laterally emerging long circumferential vertebral artery branch called the posterior inferior cerebellar artery.

At the pontomedullary junction, the vertebral arteries anastomose to form the basilar artery. The base of the pons is supplied by paramedian and short circumferential arteries. The dorsolateral regions of the caudal pons and the rostral pons are supplied by the anterior inferior and superior cerebellar arteries, respectively, each representing long circumferential branches of the basilar artery.

Midbrain circulation is almost exclusively supplied by the posterior cerebral artery. Short circumferential and paramedian branches of this artery supply the base of the midbrain and tegmentum, and long cirumferential branches supply the tectum. The most dorsal region of the tectum, accommodating the colliculi, also receives some blood supply from the superior cerebellar artery.

Venous drainage of the midbrain occurs via the basal and/or great cerebral veins (Snell, 1992). The pons is drained via veins which empty into the basal vein, cerebellar veins or adjacent venous sinuses and the medulla oblongata is drained via veins which open into the great cerebral vein or adjacent venous sinuses.

Functional role of the brain stem in movement and cognition

In general, the brain stem has been attributed three broad functions: (1) as a conduit for ascending and descending tracts connecting the spinal cord and forebrain, (2) in accommodating critical reflex centres involved in cardiovascular and respiratory control and (3) in accommodating nuclei of cranial nerves III–XII.

Brain-stem pathology and behavioural manifestations

Signs of brain-stem pathology are dependent upon the location of damage relative to longitudinal (e.g. midbrain, pons, medulla oblongata) and cross-sectional (e.g. basis or tegmentum) aspects of the brain stem (DeMyer, 1998).

Clinical significance of the midbrain

The midbrain may be susceptible to a range of injuries, including trauma, blockage of the cerebral aquaduct and vascular lesions. Given that the midbrain contains a number of important structures critical to motor functioning, including oculomotor and trochlear cranial nerve nuclei, reflex centres (i.e. colliculi), red nucleus and substantia nigra, in addition to providing a thoroughfare for a range of ascending and descending motor tracts, injury may generate a broad symptom complex.

Four special midbrain syndromes have been described in the literature: (1) decerebrate rigidity, (2) Parkinson's disease, (3) miscellaneous hyperkinesias and (4) coma plus occulomotor paralysis and pupilodilation (DeMyer, 1998). Decerebrate rigidity is a distinctive posture involving arching of the back with the arms and legs extended in rigid positions and flexion of the hands and feet. This condition arises as a consequence of midbrain disconnection from the cerebrum. The midbrain has been described as vulnerable to the effects of trauma, given that it is circumscribed by a rigid dural flap known as the tentorium cerebelli. Abrupt movements of the head, particularly in a lateral direction, may commonly result in damage to the cerebral peduncles. In addition, shearing of the midbrain may also result as a consequence of the larger forebrain and lower brain structures moving at different velocities during a traumatic brain injury.

Parkinson's disease, also known as paralysis agitans, develops as a result of damage to or degeneration of dopaminergic neurones within the substantia nigra, producing a syndrome of resting tremor as well as muscle rigidity and bradykinesia (DeMyer, 1998). Miscellaneous hyperkinesias occur as a consequence of damage to the rostral midbrain which disconnects brain-stem motor nuclei connections with the diencephalon (DeMyer, 1998). Resultant conditions may include contralateral tremor, hemichorea or hemiballismus. Coma may occur as a result of bilateral damage to the tegmentum of the midbrain accommodating the reticular activating system (DeMyer, 1998). Such lesions also commonly involve the occulomotor cranial nerve, resulting in paralysis of the eye muscles as well as pupilodilation (DeMyer, 1998). Damage to the oculomotor nucleus may produce ipsilateral paralysis in a range of muscles, including the levator paplebrae superioris, superior, inferior and medial rectus muscles and inferior oblique muscle (Snell, 2006). Damage to the trochlear nucleus within this region may also result in contralateral paralysis of the superior oblique muscle of the eye. A potentially fatal midbrain syndrome consisting of decerebrate rigidity, quadriparesis, coma, immobile eyes and dilated pupils may also arise when brain damage causes the cerebrum and diencephalon to herniate through the tentorium, compressing the midbrain (DeMyer, 1998).

The cerebral aqueduct within the midbrain is classified as part of the ventricular system. Cerebrospinal fluid produced within the third and lateral ventricles typically travels through this duct to the fourth ventricle and on to the subarachnoid space. Conditions such as congenital hydrocephalus may result from a blockage or abnormality of the cerebral aquaduct, preventing normal circulation of cerebrospinal fluid. Tumours of the midbrain and/or its surrounds may also result in compression of the cerebral aquaduct and resultant hydrocephalus. Blockage of the cerebral aquaduct may produce lesions within the midbrain.

Vascular lesions of the midbrain may also result from two primary syndromes. Weber's syndrome typically develops following occlusion of the posterior cerebral artery supplying the midbrain. Occlusion of this vessel commonly results in necrosis of brain tissue accommodating the oculomotor nerve and crus cerebri. Clinically, patients with this syndrome present ipsilateral ophthalmoplegia and contralateral paralysis of the lower face, tongue, arm and leg. The eyeball typically deviates in a lateral direction due to paralysis of the medial rectus muscle, and ptosis of the upper lid as well as fixed and dilated pupils are also evident. Benedikt's syndrome similarly results from occlusion of the posterior cerebral artery and with consequent necrosis of the medial lemniscus and red nucleus producing contralateral hemianaesthesia and involuntary movements of contralateral limbs.

Clinical significance of the pons

The pons is located beneath the tentorium cerebelli within the posterior cranial fossa. It forms a portion of the floor of the fourth ventricle and contains a number of important structures including nuclei of the trigeminal, abducens, facial and vestibulocochlear cranial nerves. It accommodates many ascending and descending neural pathways such as the corticonuclear, corticopontine and corticospinal tracts, as well as the medial longitudinal, medial, spinal and lateral lemnisci. Tumours and vascular disorders constitute the main pathological processes with implications for the pons.

Three primary pontine syndromes have been described: (1) locked-in syndrome of the pontine basis, (2) caudal pontine respiratory syndrome and (3) impaired hearing as a result of tegmental lesions (DeMyer, 1998). In more detail, locked-in syndrome typically occurs as a consequence of infarct, neoplasm, trauma or demyelination at the base of the pons and involves quadriplegia and facial and bulbar palsy as a result of disconnection of the pyramidal tracts. Exclusive maintenance of vertical eye movement is apparent. Caudal pontine respiratory syndrome results following damage to the tegmental region of the pons and/or damage to the abducens and facial cranial nerves (DeMyer, 1998). Disruption to hearing may result from lesions or damage to the tegmental pons implicating the superior olivary nuclei and trapezoid body (DeMyer, 1998).

The most commonly occurring tumour of the brain stem, an astrocytoma, has been reported to occur in the pons during childhood. Infiltration of the aforementioned cranial nerve nuclei and/or ascending and descending neural pathways may result in the following symptoms: ipsilateral facial nerve weakness, ipsilateral or bilateral weakness of the lateral rectus muscle, nystagmus, jaw muscle weakness, hearing impairment, contralateral hemiparesis, quadriparesis, distorted sensation and cerebellar signs.

Damage to the pons may also arise as a consequence of vascular infarction or haemorrhage. Infarctions typically occur following embolism or thrombosis of the basilar artery or its branches. Involvement of the paramedian aspect of the pons may have implications for the pontine nuclei, corticospinal tracts and cerebellar pathways traversing the middle cerebellar peduncle. Infarcts involving the lateral pons may implicate the trigeminal nerve, medial lemniscus, middle cerebellar peduncle and corticospinal tracts to the lower limbs. Haemorrhage of the basilar artery or anterior, inferior or superior cerebellar arteries supplying the pons may result in ipsilateral facial paralysis and contralateral limb paralysis if the lesion is unilateral. Bilateral lesions may be associated with pinpoint pupils, bilateral facial and limb paralysis and disruption to heat-regulation mechanisms.

Clinical significance of the medulla oblongata

Containing a range of cranial nerve nuclei serving critical functions, such as regulation of heart rate and respiration, as well as a number of ascending and descending tracts connecting the brain stem with the higher brain structures, damage to the medulla oblongata may result in catastrophic conditions, typically caused by demyelination, neoplasms and/or vascular disease.

Given its position in the posterior cranial fossa, tumours in this region commonly result in raised intracranial pressure, causing symptoms of headache, paralysis of the glossopharyngeal, vagus, accessory and/or hypoglossal nerves and neck stiffness. This occurs as a result of the medulla oblongata and cerebellum being pushed downward towards or through the foramen magnum, otherwise known as herniation.

Arnold–Chiari malformation is a type of congenital herniation of the cerebellum and medulla oblongata into the vertebral canal via the foramen magnum, often seen in patients with spina bifida or craniovertebral anomalies. Hydrocephalus results as a consequence of blockage of the fourth ventricle. Dysfunction of the glossopharyngeal, vagus, accessory and hypoglossal nerves may also be seen due to increased pressure on the cerebellum and medulla oblongata.

Vascular disorders of the medulla oblongata have been broadly classified into two syndromes: (1) lateral medullary syndrome and (2) medial medullary syndrome. Thrombosis of either the posterior inferior cerebellar artery or the vertebral artery, which supply blood to the lateral medulla, may result in ipsilateral palatal and laryngeal paralysis, manifesting as dysarthria and dysphagia (i.e. involvement of nucleus ambiguus), distortions in sensation to the ipsilateral side of the face (i.e. nucleus and spinal tract of trigeminal nerve), vertigo, nausea, vomiting, nystagmus (i.e. involvement of vestibular nuclei), ipsilateral cerebellar signs (i.e. involvement of cerebellum or inferior cerebellar peduncle) and contralateral loss of pain and temperature sensations in the limbs (i.e. involvement of spinal lemniscus/spinothalamic tract). The medial medulla receives its blood supply from the vertebral artery. Thrombosis of this vessel results in contralateral hemiparesis (i.e. involvement of pyramidal tract), ipsilateral paralysis of tongue muscles accompanied by deviation to the affected side on protrusion (i.e. involvement of hypoglossal nerve), impaired sensations of movement, tactile discrimination and positioning on the contralateral side (i.e. involvement of the medial lemniscus).

Bulbar and pseudobulbar palsy may also result as a consequence of damage to the medulla oblongata (DeMyer, 1998; Afifi and Bergman, 2005). Lesions to the glossopharyngeal, vagus and/or hypoglossal cranial nerve nuclei within this structure may result in bulbar palsy, which consists of paralysis of the tongue, palate, pharynx and/or larynx, presenting as dysphagia, dysarthria and dysphonia. Pseudobulbar palsy arises as a consequence of disruption to corticobulbar tracts resulting in weakness of voluntary facial and oropharyngeal muscle movements and associated dysarthria, dysphagia, dysphonia and emotional lability (DeMyer, 1998).

The cerebellum and connections

In terms of gross anatomy, the cerebellum is located in a dorsal position to the pons and medulla oblongata, and is kept separate from the cerebral cortex by a dural flap called the cerebellar tentorium (Martin, 2003). Similar to the cerebral cortex, it is comprised of two highly convoluted hemispheres connected at the midline by the vermis. The hemispheres are divided into three separate lobes: anterior, posterior and flocculonodular (see Figure 2.21). The external surface of the cerebellum comprises grey matter and the internal structure consists primarily of white matter. Within this internal white matter are embedded four bilaterally paired masses of grey matter known as intracerebellar (or deep) nuclei; namely, the dentate, emboliform, globose

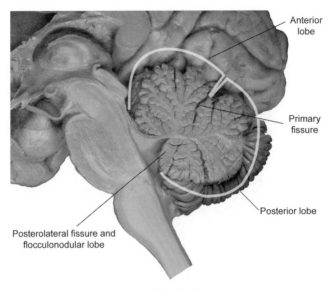

Figure 2.21 Mid-sagittal section through the brain stem and cerebellum.

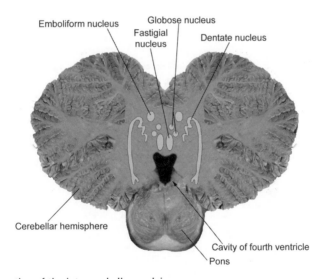

Figure 2.22 Location of the intracerebellar nuclei.

and fastigial nuclei (see Figure 2.22). Axonal inputs and outputs enter and exit the cerebellum via three fibre bundles or peduncles: superior, middle or inferior (see Figure 2.23).

Cerebellar grey matter is composed of three cell layers: the outer molecular layer, middle Purkinje layer and the inner granular layer (see Figure 2.24). Within these layers exist five neuronal classifications: the molecular layer consists of stellate cell and basket cell neurones, the Purkinje layer consists of Purkinje cell neurones and the granular layer consists of granule cell and Golgi cell neurones. Purkinje cells have

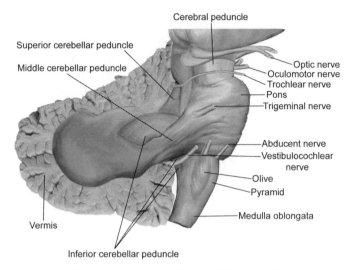

Figure 2.23   Lateral view of the brain stem (cerebellum partially removed) showing the three cerebellar peduncles connecting the cerebellum to the brain stem.

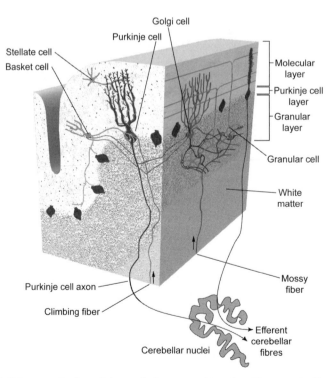

Figure 2.24   Cellular organization of the cerebellar cortex. Note the afferent and efferent fibres.

been recognized as the most important neuronal cell type in the cerebellum (Hendelman, 2000), and are the only axonal bodies to leave the cerebellum. Purkinje cells accommodate large dendrites which receive a range of excitatory afferent fibres from the spinal cord, brain stem, vestibular system and cerebral cortex. These inputs influence the activity of the deep cerebellar nuclei, and subsequently cerebral cortex activity. In more detail, excitatory cerebellar afferents innervate both the cerebellar cortex and deep nuclei. Afferent cerebellar input to inhibitory Purkinje cells result in either increased or decreased firing of these neurones, which in turn influence the deep cerebellar nuclei. Graded excitatory output from the cerebellar nuclei is then transmitted to the brain stem or cerebral cortex via the thalamus, resulting in the modulation of motor and/or sensory activity.

Afferent cerebellar tracts are typically composed of climbing and mossy fibres which exert excitatory effects upon Purkinje cells (Snell, 2006). The Purkinje cell is considered the primary functional unit of the cerebellar cortex, in that afferent pathway influences on these cells dictate cortical and brain-stem activity, and hence behaviour. Climbing and mossy fibres and there neuroregulatory influences upon cerebellar, brain-stem and cerebral cortex activity will be discussed in more detail in Chapter 7.

Blood supply to the cerebellum

Arterial blood supply to the cerebellum is provided by the superior cerebellar, anterior inferior cerebellar and posterior inferior cerebellar vessels. These arterial branches principally arise from the vertebro-basilar arterial system that supplies the brain stem, cerebellum and posterior part of the cerebral cortex (Hendelman, 2000). The vertebral arteries travel from the spinal cord to the brain, where they traverse the medial medulla oblongata and anastomose at the lower level of the pons, to form the basilar artery. Prior to anastomosis, each vertebral artery gives rise to a posterior inferior cerebellar artery which provides blood supply to the inferior surface of the vermis, cerebellar nuclei and medial surface of the cerebellar hemisphere (Snell, 1992). The basilar artery, in turn, gives off both the anterior inferior cerebellar artery which supplies the anterior and inferior aspects of the cerebellum, and the superior cerebellar artery which supplies the superior aspect of the cerebellum (see Figure 2.25). Venous drainage of the cerebellum occurs via the great cerebral vein and superior petrosal sinus (Martin, 2003).

Functional role of the cerebellum in movement and cognition

Cerebellar damage has been commonly associated with incoordinated movement as a result of disturbances in movement speed, timing, range and force, and as such the cerebellum is typically recognized as a central control unit involved in the coordination of movement. It has been hypothesized to have the ability to compare outputs from motor areas of the cerebral cortex with proprioceptive input from muscles of action, and to subsequently execute changes or necessary alterations in motor behaviour by regulating firing modes within lower motor neurones. In more detail, the cerebral cortex provides information to the cerebellum, via cerebrocerebellar pathways, regarding intended movements. During movement execution, the cerebellum is informed of movement progress via peripheral receptors (e.g. muscle spindles), and

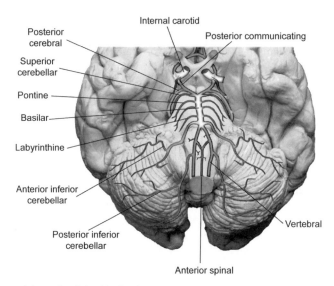

Figure 2.25 Arterial supply of the hindbrain.

has the ability to then compare peripheral feedback with central (i.e. intended movement pattern) information, and to make error corrections accordingly. In addition, the cerebellum has also been attributed a role in movement initiation and motor learning (Afifi and Bergman, 2005).

In more recent times, the cerebellum has also been assigned a role in the regulation of cognitive processes. Analgous to the overshooting and undershooting of ataxic limb movements commonly associated with cerebellar damage, incoordination or dysmmetria of thought, entailing the inadequate or overly elaborate planning or misinterpretation of stimuli, has also been observed in cerebellar lesion patients (Schmahmann and Sherman, 1998). The intact cerebellum has been described as capable of detecting, preventing and correcting mismatches between intended outcomes and perceived outcomes; therefore, in the same way that the cerebellum regulates the rate, force, rhythm and accuracy of movement, it may also control the speed, capacity, consistency and appropriateness of cognitive processing.

Three functional subdivisions of the cerebellum have been described, named according to their predominant sources of information: spinocerebellum, cerebrocerebellum and vestibulocerebellum (Martin, 2003) (see Figure 2.26). As its name suggests the spinocerebellum primarily receives somatic sensory input from the spinal cord and has been assigned a role in posture, trunk and limb movements. It is comprised of the vermis and intermediate cerebellar hemisphere of the anterior and posterior lobes, as well as the fastigial, globose and emboliform nuclei. The cerebrocerebellum receives its primary input from the cerebral cortex and has been postulated to be involved in the planning of movement. The cerebrocerebellum has also been implicated in non-motor functions, given its connections with association areas of the cerebral cortex (Martin, 2003). The cerebrocerebellum consists of the anterior and posterior lobes of the lateral cerebellar hemisphere, and the dentate nucleus. The vestibulocerebellum is involved in maintaining balance, head control and eye movements, and receives its major input from the vestibular labyrinth. It is comprised of the flocculonodular lobe.

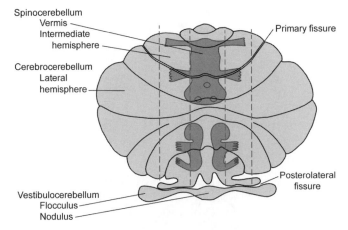

Figure 2.26   Schematic view of the three functional divisions of the cerebellum.

In terms of functional organization, the cerebellar cortex receives two primary types of input (i.e. from spinal cord or cerebral cortex) which are typically forward fed to intracerebellar nuclei and the cerebral cortex (Martin, 2003). Cerebellar outputs are generally derived from the intracerebellar nuclei. Afferent and efferent fibres enter and leave the cerebellum via three peduncles. The superior cerbellar peduncle adjoins the midbrain and cerebellum, the inferior peduncle connects the medulla oblongata and cerebellum and the medial peduncle joins the pons and cerebellum.

Cerebellar afferents from the spinal cord

The spinocerebellum accommodates three afferent tracts which transmit information from the spinal cord to the cerebellum, namely the anterior and posterior spinocerebellar tracts, and the cuneocerebellar tract (see Figure 2.27).

Anterior spinocerebellar tract
The anterior spinocerebellar tract is represented at all levels of the spinal cord. It has been assigned a role in transmitting information from the skin and superficial fascia, as well as the muscles, tendons and joints of the upper and lower limbs, to the cerebellum. Spinal cord axons from the posterior root ganglion project to neurones of the nucleus dorsalis in the posterior grey column. In turn, the majority of these axons cross over to the contralateral white column and ascend to the cerebellar cortex as the anterior spinocerebellar tract. A smaller number of axons, however, ascend as the anterior spinocerbellar tract within the ipsilateral white column. All fibres terminate within the cerebellum as mossy fibres, and are received from the spinal cord via the superior cerebellar peduncle.

Posterior spinocerebellar tract
The posterior spinocerebellar tract transfers information from the muscles, tendons and joints of the lower limbs to the cerebellum. Again, spinal cord axons from the posterior root ganglion innervate the nucleus dorsalis within the posterior grey column. In turn, these neurones then project to the ipsilateral posterolateral portion of the lateral grey column, where they ascend as the posterior spinocerebellar tract,

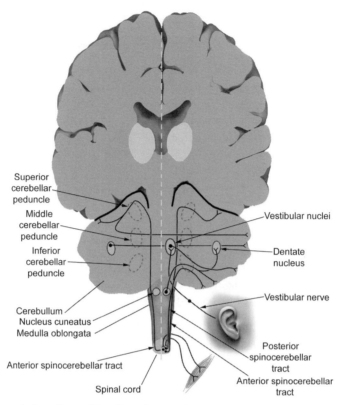

Figure 2.27   Cerebellar afferent fibres from the spinal cord and internal ear.

to the medulla oblongata. The tract then innervates the cerebellum via the inferior cerebellar peduncle and again terminates as mossy fibres.

Cuneocerebellar tract
The cuneocerebellar tract transfers information from the muscles, tendons and joints of the upper limbs and thorax to the cerebellum. Originating in the nucleus cuneatus of the medulla oblongata, fibres of the cuneocerebellar tract enter the ipsilateral cerebellum via the inferior cerebellar peduncle, where they terminate as mossy fibres.

Cerebellar afferents from the cerebral cortex

The cerebrocerebellum also accommodates three afferent tracts which siphon information from the cerebral cortex to the cerebellum, namely the corticopontocerebellar tract, cerebro-olivocerebellar tract and cerebroreticulocerebellar tract (see Figure 2.28).

Corticopontocerebellar tract
The corticopontocerebellar tract transmits information from nerve cells across all lobes of the cerebral cortex, via the corona radiata and internal capsule, to terminate within pontine nuclei of the brain stem. Transverse fibres of the pons, in turn, cross

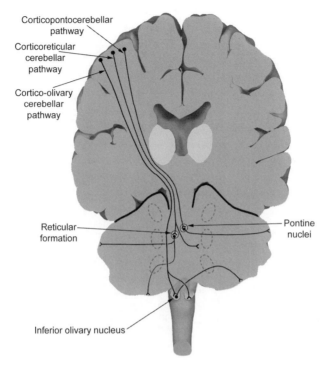

Figure 2.28 Cerebellar afferent fibres from the cerebral cortex.

the midline and enter the contralateral cerebellum via the middle cerebellar peduncle.

Cerebro-olivocerebellar tract
The cerebro-olivocerebellar tract also transmits information from an array of cortical areas, traversing a descending pathway which incorporates the corona radiata and internal capsule, terminating bilaterally in the inferior olivary nuclei of the brain stem. The inferior olivary nuclei subsequently give rise to fibres which cross the midline and terminate as climbing fibres within the contralateral cerebellar hemisphere, after entry via the inferior cerebellar peduncle.

Cerebroreticulocerebellar tract
The cerebroreticulocerebellar tract has been implicated in the regulation of voluntary movement, specifically the cerebellar monitoring and adjustment of muscle activity as a consequence of cortical input. This tract principally transmits information from sensorimotor areas of the cerebral cortex to the cerebellum, by synapsing within the ipsilateral reticular formation and contralateral pons and medulla of the brain stem. Reticulocerebellar fibres subsequently arise from the reticular formation and enter the ipsilateral cerebellar hemisphere via the middle and inferior cerebellar peduncles.

Cerebellar efferents

The majority of outflow from the cerebellum originates within the intracerebellar nuclei. Cerebellar efferents principally intersect with the red nucleus, thalamus,

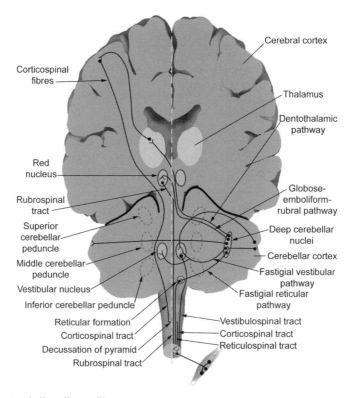

Figure 2.29 Cerebellar efferent fibres.

vestibular system or reticular formation, via four common pathways, namely the globose-emboliform-rubral pathway, dentothalamic pathway, fastigial vestibular pathway and fastigial reticular pathway (see Figure 2.29).

Globose-emboliform-rubral pathway
The globose-emboliform-rubral pathway regulates ipsilateral motor functions. Axons originating in the globose and emboliform intracerebellar nuclei exit the cerebellum via the superior cerebellar peduncle, crossing the midline at the decussation of the superior peduncles and terminating in the red nucleus, contralateral to the side of origin. The rubrospinal tract then arises from the red nucleus, feeding information to the spinal cord, ipsilateral to the side of origin.

Dentothalamic pathway
The dentothalamic pathway has been attributed a role in the regulation of ipsilateral muscle activity. Axons originating in the dentate nucleus again exit the cerebellum via the superior cerebellar peduncle, crossing the midline at the decussation of the cerebellar peduncles, and terminate within the ventrolateral thalamic nucleus. From the thalamus, neurones travel up through the internal capsule and corona radiata to the cerebral cortex, namely the primary motor area. Information from the motor cortex is then transmitted to the spinal cord via the corticospinal tract, which descends from the cortex to cross the midline at the decussation of the pyramids or spinal segments.

Fastigial vestibular pathway

The fastigial vestibular pathway has been assigned a role in influencing ipsilateral extensor muscle tone. Axons exit the fastigial nucleus via the inferior cerebellar peduncle and project bilaterally to the lateral vestibular nuclei of the brain stem. The vestibular nuclei subsequently give rise to neurones of the vestibulospinal tract.

Fastigial reticular pathway

The fastigial reticular pathway has been hypothesized to be involved in regulating ipsilateral muscle tone. Fastigial nucleus axons again exit the cerebellum via the inferior cerebellar peduncle and terminate within the reticular formation of the brain stem. The reticular formation then gives rise to the reticulospinal tract, which influences ipsilateral spinal motor activity.

Cerebellar circuitry and neurochemical correlates/neuroregulation

The cerebellum has been attributed unique neuroregulatory characteristics on the basis of its cellular organization. As mentioned previously, mossy and climbing fibres represent the two primary fibre types relating to cerebellar input, and each exert excitatory (i.e. glutmatergic) influences upon Purkinje cell neurones. Climbing fibres originate in the inferior olivary nucleus of the brain stem, and terminate in the molecular layer of the cerebellar cortex, after repeated division. Climbing fibres embrace and make contact with a large number of Purkinje cell dendrites, involving up to 10 Purkinje neurones. Some climbing fibre branches also synapse with stellate and basket cells.

Mossy fibres represent all other cerebellar afferent fibres (i.e. from spinal cord and brain-stem nuclei) and exert greater excitatory effects than climbing fibres, due to their branching configuration. An individual mossy fibre is capable of stimulating thousands of Purkinje cells via synapses with excitatory granule cells. All other cell types (i.e. stellate, Golgi and basket) are considered inhibitory cerebellar interneurones, with the capacity to influence endpoint cerebral cortex activity via their interactions with Purkinje cells. In more detail, differential inhibitory impulses from Purkinje cells, containing GABAergic neurones (Afifi and Bergman, 2005; Mizuno, 2005), influence cerebral cortex activity via the deep intracerebellar nuclei, which project excitatory outputs to the brain stem and thalamus (Valls-Sole, 2007).

Cerebellar pathology and behavioural manifestations

Clinically, disorders of the cerebellum have been reported to arise as a result of multiple conditions, including inherited conditions and congenital abnormalities as well as neoplastic, vascular, demyelinating, metabolic, infectious and toxic disease processes. The following clinical characteristics are, however, shared: ipsilateral signs, limb ataxia associated with lateral hemisphere lesions, truncal ataxia related to midline/vermal lesions, less severe symptoms resulting from lesions of the cerebellar hemisphere when compared to effects of lesions in deep nuclei or superior peduncle, and evidence of improvement over time.

Acute cerebellar conditions (e.g. vascular infarct) have been reported to produce more severe and disabling symptoms when compared to more chronic conditions such as space-occupying lesions/tumours. This has been attributed to the fact that in the case of chronic lesions the central nervous system is afforded time to compensate for the loss of cerebellar function over time. Despite these differences in symptom severity, however, seven main symptoms have typically been described to result as a consequence of cerebellar damage, including (1) hypotonia (i.e. reduction of resistance to passive movements of joints), (2) postural and gait changes (i.e. wide-based gait evident on standing and perhaps stiff-legged to accommodate lost muscle tone as well as staggering gait towards affected side; rotation and flexion of head, and on side of lesion shoulder in lower position), (3) ataxia (i.e. intention tremor and incoordinated movement/decomposition of movement), (4) dysdiadochokinesia (i.e. inability to repeatedly perform rapid alternating movements; slow and jerky movements evident on side of lesion), (5) reflex disturbances (i.e. prolonged tendon reflexes), (6) nystagmus (i.e. rhythmical oscillations of the eyes) and (7) dysarthria (i.e. incoordination and reduced muscle tone of the speech musculature resulting in pronounced deficits of articulation and prosody; Murdoch and Theodoros, 1998). As discussed in Chapter 7, in addition to the disturbance of motor functions, cerebellar damage has also been more recently associated with the manifestation of cerebellar cognitive affective syndrome (Schmahmann, 1991, 1996). This non-motor syndrome is characterized by impaired executive function, spatial cognition, language processing and affective regulation; operationally defined as 'dysmetria of thought'.

Major syndromes of the cerebellum are typically divided into two groups: cerebellar hemisphere syndromes and vermis syndromes. Cerebellar hemisphere syndrome has been reported to result as a consequence of tumours or infarcts of the cerebellar hemispheres (DeMyer, 1998; Snell, 2006). Symptoms are typically unilateral in presentation, implicating muscles on the same side of the body as the damaged cerebellar hemisphere. Limb movements, particularly arm movements, are disrupted. Unsteady gait involving swaying or falling towards the side of the damaged cerebellar hemisphere, as well as dysarthria and nystagmus, are also common.

Vermis syndrome may be divided into two subtypes: caudal and rostral. Caudal vermis syndrome has been reported to generally occur as a result of tumours of the vermis, and is very common in children resulting from medulloblastomas of the vermal region. Symptoms include incoordination of the head and trunk, such as difficulty holding the head in a steady upright position or difficulty holding the trunk erect, as well as a tendency to fall forward or backward. Nystagmus may also be a presenting symptom (DeMyer, 1998). Rostral vermis syndrome may involve disproportionate incoordination of the lower limbs in comparison to relatively intact upper limb, speech and eye muscle function, and is frequently diagnosed in chronic alcoholic patients (DeMyer, 1998).

An additional syndrome, pancerebellar syndrome, arises as a result of damage to the entire cerebellum as a consequence of degenerative disease including multiple sclerosis or acute alcoholic intoxication (DeMyer, 1998). Symptoms include bilateral incoordination of axial and limb muscles, dysarthria, nystagmus and voluntary muscle hypotonia. Furthermore, damage to dentothalamic or dentorubral pathways within the cerebellum may also manifest as terminal tremor (i.e. tremor of the extremities).

Summary

This chapter has provided a summary of subcortical neuroanatomy and functional neurology. Taking a component-by-component approach, the subcortical axis, consisting of the basal ganglia, thalamus, brain stem and cerebellum, was described in terms of gross anatomy, connectivity, neurotransmission systems, blood supply, proposed functions, recognized pathologies and associated behavioural syndromes.

References

Afifi, A.K. and Bergman, R.A. (2005). *Functional Neuroanatomy: Text and Atlas*. New York: Lange Medical Books/McGraw-Hill.

Alexander, G.E. and Crutcher, M.D. (1990). Functional architecture of basal ganglia circuits: neural substrates of parallel processing. *Trends in Neuroscience* 13, 266–71.

Alexander, G.E., DeLong, M.R. and Strick, P.L. (1986). Parallel organisation of functionally segregated circuits linking basal ganglia and cortex. *Annual Review of Neuroscience* 9, 357–81.

Alexander, G.E., Crutcher, M.D. and DeLong, M.R. (1990). Basal ganglia-thalamocortical circuits: parallel substrates for motor, oculomotor, "prefrontal" and "limbic" functions. *Progress in Brain Research* 85, 119–46.

Arboix, A., Martinez-Rebollar, M., Oliveres, M., Garcia-Eroles, L., Massons, J. and Targa, C. (2005). Acute isolated capsular stroke: a clinical study of 148 cases. *Clinical Neurology and Neurosurgery* 107, 88–94.

Barr, M.L. and Kiernan, J.A. (1993). *The Human Nervous System: an Anatomical Viewpoint*, 6th edn. Philadelphia: J.B. Lippincott Company.

Carpenter, M.B. (1991). *Core Text of Neuroanatomy*, 4th edn. Baltimore: Williams and Wilkins.

Crossman, A.R. and Neary, D. (1995). *Neuroanatomy: an Illustrated Colour Text*. Edinburgh: Churchill Livingstone.

Crosson, B. (1985). Subcortical functions in language: a working model. *Brain and Language* 25, 257–92.

Damasio, A.R., Damasio, H., Rizzo, M., Varney, N. and Gersh, F. (1982). Aphasia with non-hemorrhagic lesions in the basal ganglia and internal capsule. *Archives of Neurology* 29, 15–20.

Delong, M.R. (1990). Primate models of movement disorders of basal ganglia origin. *Trends in Neuroscience* 13, 281–5.

DeLong, M.R. and Wichmann, T. (2007). Circuits and circuit disorders of the basal ganglia. *Archives of Neurology* 64, 20–4.

DeMyer, W. (1998). *Neuroanatomy*, 2nd edn. Baltimore: Williams and Wilkins.

Fitzgerald, M.J.T. (1996). Neuroanatomy: basic and clinical. London: W.B. Saunders.

Fitzgerald, M.J.T., Gruener, G. and Mtui, E. (eds) (2007). *Clinical Neuroanatomy and Neuroscience*, 5th edn. Edinburgh: Elsevier Saunders.

Goldman-Rakic, P.S. (1984). Modular organisation of the prefrontal cortex. *Trends in Neuroscience* 7, 419–24.

Hayes, A.E., Davidson, M.C., Keele, S.W. and Rafal, R.D. (1998). Toward a functional analysis of the basal ganglia. *Journal of Cognitive Neuroscience* 10(2), 178–98.

Hazrati, L.-N., Parent, A., Mitchell, S. and Haber, S.N. (1990). Evidence for interconnections between the two segments of the globus pallidus in primates: a pha-l anterograde tracing study. *Brain Research* 533, 171–5.

Hendelman, W.J. (2000). *Atlas of Funtional Neuroanatomy*. London: CRC Press.

Jones, E. (1985). *The Thalamus*. New York: Plenum Press.

Kincaid, A.E., Penny, J.B., Young, A.B. and Newman, S.W. (1991). Evidence for a projection from the globus pallidus to the endopeduncular nucleus in the rat. *Neuroscience Letters* 128, 121–5.

Levy, R. (2007). Neurobehavioural disorders associated with basal ganglia lesions. In J. Jankovic and E. Tolosa (eds), *Parkinson's Disease and Movement Disorders* (pp. 23–32). Philadelphia: Lippincott Williams and Wilkins.

Martin, J.H. (2003). *Neuroanatomy Text and Atlas*, 3rd edn. New York: McGraw-Hill.

Mink, J.W. (2007). Functional organisation of the basal ganglia. In J. Jankovic and E. Tolosa (eds), *Parkinson's Disease and Movement Disorders* (pp. 1–6). Philadelphia: Lippincott Williams and Wilkins.

Mizuno, Y. (2005). Pathophysiology of Parkinson's disease, neurochemical pathology: other neurotransmitters. In M. Ebadi and R.F. Pfeiffer (eds), *Parkinson's Disease* (pp. 443–77). Boca Raton: CRC Press.

Murdoch, B.E. and Theodoros, D.G. (1998). Ataxic dysarthria. In B.E. Murdoch (ed.), *Dysarthria: a Physiological Approach to Assessment and Treatment*. Cheltenham: Stanley Thornes.

Nadeau, S.E. and Crosson, B. (1997). Subcortical aphasia. *Brain and Language* 58, 355–402.

Nolte, J. (1993). *The Human Brain: an Introduction to its Functional Anatomy*, 3rd edn. St Louis: Mosby-Year Book.

Parent, A. and Hazrati, L.-N. (1993). Anatomical aspects of information processing in primate basal ganglia. *Trends in Neuroscience* 16, 111–16.

Parent, A. and Hazrati, L.-N. (1995). Functional anatomy of the basal ganglia. I. The cortico-basal ganglia-thalamo-cortical loop. *Brain Research Reviews* 20, 91–127.

Parent, A., Hazrati, L.-N. and Lavoie, B. (1991). The pallidum as a duel structure in primates. In G. Bernadi, M.B. Carpenter, G. DiChiara, M. Morelli and P. Stanzione (eds), *The Basal Ganglia III* (pp. 81–8). New York: Plenum Press.

Penfield, W. and Roberts, L. (1959). *Speech and Brain Mechanisms*. Princeton: Princeton University Press.

Schmahmann, J.D. (1991). An emerging concept: the cerebellar contribution to higher function. *Archives of Neurology* 48, 1178–87.

Schmahmann, J.D. (1996). From movement to thought: anatomic substrates of the cerebellar contribution to cognitive processing. *Human Brain Mapping* 4, 174–98.

Schmahmann, J.D. and Sherman, J.C. (1998). The cerebellar cogitive affective syndrome. *Brain* 121, 561–79.

Snell, R.S. (1992). *Neuroanatomy: a Review with Questions and Answers*. London: Little, Brown and Company.

Snell, R.S. (1997). *Clinical Neuroanatomy for Medical Students*. Philadelphia: Lippincott Raven Publishers.

Snell, R.S. (2006). *Clinical Neuroanatomy*. Philadelphia: Lippincott, Williams and Wilkins.

Sohn, Y.H. and Hallet, M. (2005). Basal ganglia, motor control and Parkinsonism. In N. Galvez-Jimenez (ed.), *Scientific Basis for the Treatment of Parkinson's Disease* (pp. 33–51). London: Taylor and Francis.

Steriade, M., Jones, E. and Llinas, R.R. (1990). *Thalamic Oscillations and Signaling*. New York: Wiley.

Tanridag, O. and Kirshner, H.S. (1987). Language disorders in stroke syndromes of the dominant capsulostriatum: a clinical review. *Aphasiology* 1, 107–17.

Valls-Sole, J. (2007). Neurophysiology of motor control and movement disorders. In J. Jankovic and E. Tolosa (eds), *Parkinson's Disease and Movement Disorders* (pp. 7–22). Philadelphia: Lippincott Williams and Wilkins.

Wallesch, C.-W. and Papagno, C. (1988). Subcortical aphasia. In F.C. Rose, R. Whurr and M.A. Wyke (eds), *Aphasia* (pp. 256–87). London: Whurr Publishers.

Section B   Subcortical language disorders

3 Models of subcortical participation in language

Introduction

Within the compendium of historical literature investigating brain–language relationships, the cerebral cortex has been well established as the neural substrate responsible for sustaining language-processing abilities. This postulatum was derived from time-honoured observations of aphasia subsequent to cortical lesions, most characteristically confined to the left hemisphere (Goodglass, 1993). However, the evolution of neuroimaging over the past 30 years has served to ardently challenge this localizationist paradigm (Murdoch, 1996). More specifically, spontaneous vascular subcortical lesions (i.e. typically within the thalamus, periventricular white matter (PVWM) and striatocapsular region), identified via techniques such as computed tomography (CT) and magnetic resonance imaging (MRI), associated with manifestations of aphasia, suggested a potential contribution from these structures to the mediation of language processes.

This phenomenon subsequently catalysed the development of contemporary language theories which proffer functional roles for the subcortical nuclei; principally the striatum, globus pallidus and thalamus (Crosson, 1985; Wallesch and Papagno, 1988; Nadeau and Crosson, 1997a). These theoretical constructs specifically promote a network model of language organization (Cappa and Vallar, 1992), whereby cortico-subcortical-cortical pathways represent the neural basis of linguistic processing, in preference to exclusive cortico-cortical connections.

Classical language theory in relation to subcortical aphasia

Aphasia has been traditionally defined as the impairment or loss of language subsequent to brain injury (Murdoch, 1990). Throughout the literature, two main doctrines of thought exist pertaining to neural mechanisms underlying aphasia, and brain–language relationships in general. Localizationists theorized that specific cortical areas within the brain were responsible for the production of various linguistic behaviours (Lecours et al., 1988). Aphasic behaviours were considered to reflect damage to a circumscribed area of the cerebral cortex, previously dedicated to performing a specialized linguistic function.

Wernicke (1874) and Lichtheim (1885) developed perhaps the most widely acknowledged systems of aphasia classification (Lecours et al., 1988), based on localizationist theory. Specifically, anterior cortical lesions (i.e. lesions within the third frontal convolution of the left hemisphere) produced expressive (i.e. motor) or more typically

Broca's aphasia, resulting in difficulty formulating or producing speech and/or language. Posterior lesions (i.e. lesions within the first temporal convolution of the left hemisphere) typically produced receptive (i.e. sensory) language disturbances, resulting in auditory comprehension deficits, characteristic of Wernicke's aphasia. In addition, lesions of the association pathways between the motor and sensory cortical regions, between these regions and concept centres, or other input and output areas including the subcortical region, produced commissural aphasias (i.e. conduction aphasia, transcortical motor and transcortical sensory aphasia, and subcortical aphasias). Localizationist theory did not consider the subcortical nuclei to be directly involved in mediating language processes.

In contrast, however, holists proposed that it was the interaction of the brain as a unit that galvanized language, as opposed to isolated cortical regions (Jackson, 1932), supporting a potential role for the subcortical nuclei. Jackson (1932), a renowned holist, postulated that language was the result of a dynamic psychological operation, rather than the by-product of an isolated physiological mechanism. Aphasic individuals reportedly demonstrated impairment at the 'intellectual' level of speech, whereas 'automatic' or 'emotional' speech (e.g. recurrent utterances and interjections) was perceived to remain intact. These behaviours were considered to reflect a disruption to language orchestration mechanisms, wherein the brain was rendered incapable of operating as a functional unit. Dedicated proponents of this school of thought ardently avoided clinico-anatomical classification (Lecours *et al.*, 1988).

Despite this historical taxonomic debate, consensus abounds as to a mutual relationship between the left hemisphere and language function, following consistent observations of aphasia in individuals with left hemisphere damage (Goodglass, 1993). Holists reportedly acknowledged that damage to a number of distinct areas of the cerebral cortex more consistently produced language disturbances; however, dysfunction of isolated lesion sites was not held completely accountable for the behaviours observed (Murdoch, 1990). Furthermore, although localizationist theory has been largely successful in accurately indexing clinical manifestations of aphasia (Murdoch, 1990), there remains a heterogeneous clinical assembly of aphasic syndromes that are unable to be classified according to contemporary taxonomies such as the Bostonian system (e.g. Broca's, Wernicke's, anomic, etc.), given their atypical presentation. Subcortical aphasia is a prominent member of this constituency, with some studies reporting comparable subcortical lesions to produce disparate aphasia severity levels and language characteristics, with no evidence of a consistently demonstrable language syndrome (Nadeau and Crosson, 1997a).

Despite these irregularities, advancements in neuroimaging techniques (i.e. CT and MRI) over the last three decades have allowed more precise identification and localization of subcortical lesion parameters (Alexander *et al.*, 1987; Cappa and Wallesch, 1994), and hence the ability to evaluate the influence of specific lesions in producing motor and cognitive anomalies. Indeed, language disturbances subsequent to thalamic (Mohr *et al.*, 1975; Cappa and Vignolo, 1979; Alexander and LoVerme, 1980; Cohen *et al.*, 1980; McFarling *et al.*, 1982; Graff-Radford *et al.*, 1984; Murdoch, 1987; Bogousslavsky *et al.*, 1988), striatocapsular (Alexander and LoVerme, 1980; Brunner *et al.*, 1982; Damasio *et al.*, 1982; Naeser *et al.*, 1982; Wallesch *et al.*, 1983; Wallesch, 1985; Murdoch *et al.*, 1986, 1991; Kennedy and Murdoch, 1989) and PVWM lesions (Naeser *et al.*, 1982, 1989; Alexander *et al.*, 1987) have been well documented, lending support to holist doctrines. Consequently, the thalamus, basal ganglia and subcortical white matter pathways represent the anatomical structures that have received the most attention in proposed models of subcortical participation in language.

Development of subcortical language theories: lending from models of motor control

As mentioned in Chapter 2 the work of Alexander and colleagues (1986, 1990) provides the basis for our understanding of the anatomical and functional organization of cortico-subcortical-cortical circuits. Seminal schemas propose parallel yet functionally segregated basal ganglia–thalamocortical pathways to underlie skeletomotor, occulomotor, cognitive and limbic functions. Current knowledge pertaining to the functional characteristics of subcortical motor circuits, however, greatly overshadows our understanding of the way in which non-motor circuits influence behaviour. This disparity may be rationalized by the more 'measurable' nature of motor activity in comparison to cognition and an incapacity to empirically investigate many higher-order behaviours (including language) in human homologues. As such, contemporary models of subcortical participation in language have largely evolved from theories of motor control, the foundations of which were established within studies of basal ganglia dysfunction and related movement disorders in primates, with experimentally induced 1-methyl-4-phenyl-1,2,3,6-tetrahydropyridine (MPTP) toxicity (Starr et al., 1998).

Basal ganglia–thalamocortical skeletomotor circuit

Simian research promotes skeletomotor basal ganglia–thalamocortical circuits to play a pivotal role in modulating motor behaviour by way of feedback loops which link the motor, premotor and somatosensory cortices, sensorimotor components of various basal ganglia (including the putamen, globus pallidus internus (GPi), globus pallidus externus (GPe), subthalamic nucleus (STN) and substantia nigra pars reticulata (SNr)) and the motor thalamus (ventralis lateralis pars oralis, ventralis anterior parvocellularis and centrum medianum) (Alexander et al., 1990; Starr et al., 1998) (see Figure 2.3, p. 23). Motor activity is essentially orchestrated via the two dopamine-regulated pathways discussed in Chapter 2, which indirectly and directly influence the primary output nuclei of the basal ganglia (DeLong, 1990). In essence, cortical motor efferents project somatotopically to the striatum (i.e. putamen and caudate nucleus), which is comprised of output neurones containing distinct dopamine-sensitive receptors, specifically D1 and D2 receptors, influenced by dopaminergic input from the substantia nigra pars compacta (Lang and Lozano, 1998a, 1998b; Starr et al., 1998). The striatum then projects to the GPi-SNr directly, and via an indirect route incorporating the GPe and STN. The GPi-SNr then projects to motor nuclei of the thalamus, which in turn complete the motor circuit by sending outputs back to the supplementary motor area and premotor and primary motor cortices (Afifi and Bergman, 2005), which are subsequently responsible for the execution of motor acts.

Contemporary research has revealed the basal ganglia to exhibit a complex and intricate pattern of neuronal organization and functional specificity, comparable to that of the cerebral cortex (Alexander et al., 1986). Within the skeletomotor circuit, cortical somatotopy is maintained within the putamen and globus pallidus relevant to lower-limb, upper-limb and orofacial representations (Alexander and DeLong, 1985a, 1985b). This elaborate neural architecture subserves a range of locomotive functions, including motor planning and sequencing, in addition to the modulation and monitoring of movement parameters such as amplitude and velocity (Wichmann and DeLong, 1998).

Within a patent neurological system (i.e. non-dopamine-deficient state), homeostatic activity is maintained between the direct and indirect pathways, modulating basal ganglia outputs (Lang and Lozano, 1998a) (see Figure 2.3). In MPTP-treated primates and individuals with Parkinson's disease, dopamine deficiency within the substantia nigra pars compacta results in hyperactivity of the indirect pathway and the subsequent over-excitation (by way of STN glutamatergic output) of GPi and SNr inhibitory outputs to the motor thalamus (Lang and Lozano, 1998a) (see Figure 10.2, p. 224). Furthermore, dopamine deficiency also serves to reduce activity within the direct pathway, resulting in additional disinhibition of the GPi and SNr. Enhanced inhibitory GPi-SNr outflow by way of GABAergic neurotransmission results in the excessive inhibition of thalamic and brainstem nuclei (Alexander *et al.*, 1990; Lang and Lozano, 1998a). As discussed more fully in Chapter 10, thalamocortical inhibition has been identified as the precursor to manifestations of hypokinetic Parkinsonian motor signs such as akinesia, rigidity, tremor, gait and postural anomalies (Lang and Lozano, 1998a).

Extending theories of motor control to cognitive domains

As mentioned previously, in addition to their role in skeletomotor activity basal ganglia–thalamocortical circuits have also been hypothesized to orchestrate occulo-motor movements and a range of non-motor behaviours including limbic and higher-order cognitive functions, by way of structurally and functionally segregated, yet parallel, pathways (Alexander *et al.*, 1990). Specified non-motor pathways include (1) the dorsolateral prefrontal circuit subserving executive cognitive function (e.g. learning new concepts, accessing memory, manipulating environmental contingencies, shifting behavioural set, formulating motor programmes and verbal-manual association skills) (Cummings, 1993), (2) the lateral orbitofrontal circuit responsible for the regulation of socially appropriate behaviour and (3) the anterior cingulate circuit involved in the mediation of motivated behaviour (Mega and Cummings, 1994).

Current opinion supports analogous neural mechanisms within motor and non-motor basal ganglia–thalamocortical circuits (Alexander *et al.*, 1986), based on the premise that within subcortico-cortical pathways circuits run in parallel and at concurring levels, so synaptic organization is homologous (Nauta, 1979; DeLong and Georgopoulos, 1981). The generalized schema subserving classical cortico-striato-pallido-thalamo-cortical circuits proposes manifold yet functionally related cortico-striatal inputs which converge within the basal ganglia to re-emerge as highly specified cortical projections (i.e. typically targeting cortical areas that contributed cortico-striatal inputs to the relevant circuit), relayed through the thalamus (Alexander *et al.*, 1986). The extrapolation of linguistic circuitry on the basis of this schema has been proven to be well-founded, with the recent identification of functional neurophysiological links between motor and language systems (Pulvermuller *et al.*, 2005).

Contemporary theories of subcortical participation in language

Although simian research has provided the foundation for theories of basal ganglia–thalamocortical organization and function, the evolutionary proliferation of the frontal lobes and the concomitant cortical specificity of basal ganglia projections in *Homo sapiens* suggest that the utilization of simian cohorts in studies dedicated to the investigation of higher-order behaviours exclusive to humans may be somewhat unavailing (Alexander *et al.*, 1986). Indeed, language and the subsequent ability to engage in complex symbolic communication has been defined as our most human of attributes (Kirshner, 1991), rivaled by no other species. Given this inherent limitation of animal studies, contemporary thinking pertaining to the role of subcortical nuclei in language processing has relied primarily upon investigations of the behaviour of human populations with vascular lesions of the subcortical region.

Based on clinico-anatomical evidence thus far, three major basal ganglia–thalamo-cortical circuits have been speculated to participate in the mediation of language processes (Cappa and Vallar, 1992): (1) the anterior 'complex' loop (i.e. dorsolateral prefrontal and lateral orbitofrontal circuits; Alexander *et al.*, 1986): frontal association cortex-caudate nucleus-globus pallidus-ventral anterior thalamus-frontal association cortex; (2) the anterior 'motor' loop (i.e. skeletomotor circuit; Alexander *et al.*, 1986): sensory motor cortex-putamen-globus pallidus-ventral lateral thalamus-sensory motor cortex and (3) the posterior loop (Van Buren and Borke, 1969): temporoparietal cortex-pulvinar-temporoparietal cortex. The anterior 'complex' and 'motor' pathways were hypothesized to mediate lexical-semantic expression and articulation, respectively, and the posterior loop to facilitate auditory comprehension (Cappa and Vallar, 1992). Additional subcortico-cortical pathways have also been postulated to participate in the regulation of language (Cappa and Vallar, 1992), including the temporal auditory cortex-caudate nucleus pathway facilitating auditory comprehension (Van Hoesen *et al.*, 1981; Damasio *et al.*, 1982), and amygdala-temporal neocortex-dorsomedial thalamus (Cappa and Sterzi, 1990) and caudate nucleus-supplementary motor area-anterior cingulate (Naeser *et al.*, 1989), regulating speech production. The functional specificity of language-dedicated subcortical circuits to date has been largely restricted to the elementary linguistic faculties of auditory comprehension and verbal expression (Alexander *et al.*, 1986). It is anticipated, however, that contemporary research may serve to expose functional subdivisions in non-motor basal ganglia thalamocortical circuits, which reflect a similar level of organizational complexity to that of the somatotopic channels identified within subcortical motor circuitry (Alexander *et al.*, 1986). Indeed, this disclosure may potentially involve the elucidation of the neural substrates underpinning language at both single word and sentential levels of processing.

A number of theories have attempted to explicate the subcortical neural mechanisms underlying receptive and expressive linguistic abilities. The Subcortical White Matter Pathways (Alexander *et al.*, 1987), Response-Release Semantic Feedback (RRSF; Crosson, 1985), Lexical Decision Making (LDM; Wallesch and Papagno, 1988) and Selective Engagement (Nadeau and Crosson, 1997a) models represent the theoretical tenets which have served to heavily influence contemporary thinking.

Subcortical White Matter Pathways model

Presumably based on the precepts of classical language theory, the Subcortical White Matter Pathways model (Crosson, 1992), proposed by Alexander *et al.* (1987), dismisses a role for the subcortical nuclei in language and advocates cortico-cortical, cortico-striatal, thalamo-cortical and cortico-bulbar white matter pathways as critical to the facilitation of auditory comprehension and verbal expression. The fulcrum of this theoretical schema developed from a series of clinical-neuroradiological studies which highlighted an array of receptive and expressive language deficits in individuals with large striatal lesions, extending into the surrounding white matter pathways (Alexander *et al.*, 1987). This profile was in stark contrast to that observed in patients

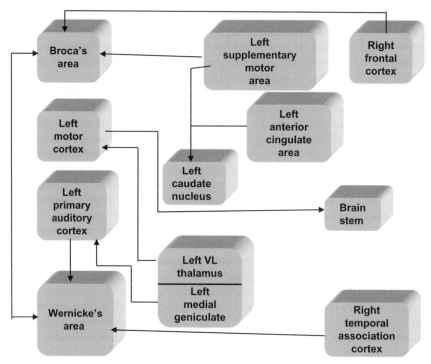

Figure 3.1 Schematic diagram of the Subcortical White Matter Pathways model (Alexander *et al.*, 1987) adapted from Crosson (1992). Left VL thalamus, left ventral lateral thalamus.

with relatively circumscribed lesions of the putamen and caudate nucleus, which resulted in covert or nominal disturbances to language such as mild word-finding difficulties and hesitant verbal output. This finding consequently supported a minimal function hypothesis for basal ganglia participation in language and directed discussion towards the white matter pathways linking cortico-cortical and subcortico-cortical regions (see Figure 3.1).

Vascular lesions of the striatum that extended beyond the lateral boundary of the anterior limb of the internal capsule, incorporating the anterior, extra anterior, anterior superior, superior or posterior PVWM, temporal isthmus, insular cortex and/or external capsule, were documented to produce a range of expressive and receptive language deficits (Alexander *et al.*, 1987). More specifically, non-thalamic lesions with extensions into the anterior-superior PVWM were reported to result in transcortical motor aphasia, largely evidenced as sparse verbal output and difficulty initiating speech. This symptom complex was hypothesized to result from damage to the fibre pathways connecting the supplementary motor area and Broca's area (see Figure 3.1).

Anterior-superior PVWM pathway disconnection was postulated to restrict limbic inputs to cortical language centres, resulting in reduced speech drive. Repetition deficits were reported to arise from lateral and/or superior lesion extensions relative to the putamen, which implicate the external and extreme capsules and, potentially, the arcuate fasciculus. In relation to speech motor control, corticobulbar fibres within the superior PVWM and genu of the internal capsule, in addition to cortico-cerebellar and thalamo-cortical fibres in the anterior portion of the superior PVWM and anterior limb of the internal capsule, were implicated. The temporal isthmus, linking the medial geniculate nucleus of the thalamus to the primary auditory association cortex and the auditory association callosal pathway connecting Wernicke's area and the right temporal association cortex (see Figure 3.1), were identified as the subcortical white matter pathways integral to auditory comprehension. Posterior striatal lesion extension incorporating these structures typically resulted in comprehension deficits and neologistic output. Furthermore, wide-ranging lesion extension relative to the putamen, including the anterior limb of the internal capsule, extra-anterior PVWM, anterior PVWM, anterior-superior PVWM and temporal isthmus, was reported to result in global language impairment.

In concert with the basal ganglia, Alexander *et al.* (1987) eluded to attribute a role in language functioning to the thalamus on the basis that language deficits resulting from thalamic and putaminal lesions are subserved by disparate pathophysiological mechanisms. Vascular lesions of the thalamus were postulated to result from disease of the posterior circulation, and as such were precluded from involving the critical nuclei and white matter pathways considered within the aforementioned schema of subcortical participation in language.

Indeed, white matter pathways have been defined as integral to the transfer of patterned or quantitative neuronal activity between brain structures (Crosson *et al.*, 1997b), including those involved in the mediation of linguistic processes. Current evidence, however, empirically and theoretically refutes that disconnection of white matter pathways provides a valid datum for clinical manifestations of subcortical damage (Cappa and Vallar, 1992). Given the postulate that white matter-pathway lesions may interrupt subcortical innervations and efferent projections, and that current neuroradiological techniques fail to strictly define the parameters of lesion extension, a role for the subcortical nuclei in language cannot be plausibly dismissed. As such, the remaining focus of this chapter will be directed towards the discussion of operative models of subcortical participation in language, which propose functionally distinct roles for the striatum, globus pallidus and thalamus.

Response-Release Semantic Feedback model

A postulated thalamocortical alerting system (Ojemann, 1976) represents the platform of the RRSF (Crosson, 1985) model of subcortical participation in language. Based on the results of neurostimulation studies, the dominant ventral lateral (VL) thalamus has been hypothesized to facilitate activation of cortical areas dedicated to verbal expression, via a highly specific focal alerting mechanism (Ojemann, 1976). Distinctive characteristics of this alerting mechanism will be discussed in further detail in the ensuing section.

In relation to cortical organization, the RRSF model proposes the encoding of language – including concept formation, word finding and syntactic processes – to take place in the anterior language cortex (ALC), together with motor speech programming. Given that verbal expression is considered to be the product of a complex motor act, the physical and temporal interaction of the neural substrates underlying language formulation and motor speech programming was deemed a tenable hypothesis. Sensory functions are assigned to the posterior cortex, including the comprehension of language. The temporoparietal cortex or posterior language centre (PLC) was postulated to phonologically and semantically decode language, from single sounds to a simple syntactic level. The comprehension of complex grammatical structures, however, was considered a function of the ALC.

With regard to subcortical participation in language, the RRSF model proposes a cortico-striato-pallido-thalamo-cortical loop as the purveyor of preverbal semantic feedback, response-release and tonic arousal mechanisms (Crosson, 1985). These operations and their underlying neural substrates will be discussed in detail in the following sections, relevant to proposed roles for the thalamus and basal ganglia.

Proposed role of the thalamus in the Response-Release Semantic Feedback model

Crosson (1985) proposed two distinct functions for the thalamus in language which primarily pertain to the regulation of cortical processes, including as a facilitator of preverbal semantic feedback and as a tonic arousal/activating center. The thalamus, by way of bi-directional connections with the anterior and posterior language areas of the cerebral cortex, was postulated to serve as a relay station for cortical information (see Figure 3.2). More specifically, language segments in phrasal or short-clause form which are formulated in the ALC are hypothetically relayed to the PLC for monitoring of semantic content, via a cortico-thalamo-cortical loop. Postulated

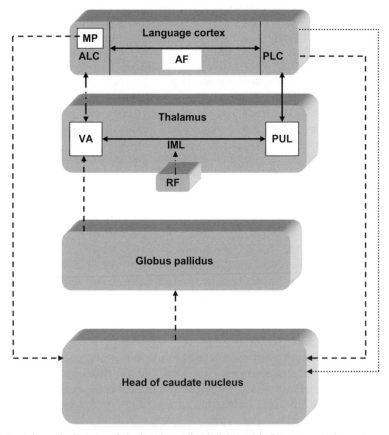

Figure 3.2 Schematic diagram of the basal ganglia–thalamocortical Response-Release Semantic Feedback model (adapted from Crosson, 1985, 1992). ALC, anterior language centre; AF, arcuate fasciculus; IML, internal medullary lamina; MP, motor programming cortex; PLC, posterior language centre; PUL, pulvinar; RF, reticular formation; VA, ventral anterior thalamic nucleus; dotted and dashed arrows, excitatory pathway; dashed arrows, inhibitory pathway; dotted arrows, disinhibitory pathway.

thalamic components within this cortico-subcortico-cortical circuit include the ventral anterior (VA) thalamus, internal medullary lamina and pulvinar (Crosson, 1992).

The PLC monitors and identifies semantic errors/inadequacies within conveyed language segments and communicates essential refinement commands to the ALC in preparation for motor speech programming, via the same cortico-thalamo-cortical loop. Semantic refinement commands, however, traverse the aforementioned circuit in the converse direction (i.e. pulvinar-internal medullary lamina-VA) to formulated language segments from the ALC. The process of language segment transfer, involving monitoring and refinement, has been defined as preverbal semantic feedback.

The RRSF model also proposes a requisite level of ALC arousal for efficient language production. Given that the VA thalamus represents the nexus of reticular formation efferents (by way of the intralaminar nuclei (ILN)) and frontal cortex afferents (see Figure 3.2), the VA nucleus was assigned an explicit cortical arousal function. Specifically, the VA nucleus was hypothesized to activate the ALC by selectively dispensing excitatory input from the reticular activating system. Of note, the globus pallidus was postulated to indirectly regulate the level of cortical arousal achieved, via inhibitory projections to the thalamus. In addition to the regulation of ALC arousal, the mechanism subserving the release of semantically verified language segments for verbal production was also considered to be largely under control of the basal ganglia. The proposed contribution of basal ganglia substrates relative to cortical arousal and response-release mechanisms has been summarized in the ensuing section.

Proposed role of the basal ganglia in the Response-Release Semantic Feedback model

The RRSF model proposes that the basal ganglia integrate linguistic information from the cerebral cortex, and consequently influence ALC activity by indirectly regulating thalamic outputs (Crosson, 1985). This regulatory role includes maintaining an appropriate level of thalamocortical arousal for efficient language production and facilitating the appropriate temporal release of semantically verified language segments for verbal production, via a response-release mechanism.

The regulation of basal ganglia-mediated thalamocortical activity is accomplished by way of a complex neural system, involving striato-pallidal and pallido-thalamic projections with inherent inhibitory properties. The caudate nucleus and putamen receive a vast array of cortical efferents; however, they fail to directly project outputs to the cerebral cortex (Crosson, 1985). Despite this organization, the anatomical orientation of the striatum and globus pallidus within a proposed cortico-striato-pallido-thalamo-cortical loop promotes the basal ganglia as a potentially potent group of counterbalancing nuclei, with the ability to integrate cortical inputs and indirectly influence cortical outputs, by way of a striato-pallido-thalamo feed-forward mechanism.

Within the RRSF model, proposed tonic cortical arousal and response-release mechanisms are considered closely related by way of shared neural constituents, namely the caudate nucleus and globus pallidus (Crosson, 1985). The head of the caudate nucleus was identified as the locus of the response-release mechanism. By way of ALC and PLC inputs, in addition to pallidal outputs, the caudate nucleus was hypothesized to govern the temporally constrained release of semantically verified language segments for motor speech production. At rest (i.e. no verbal output) or awaiting semantic verification, the PLC exercises inhibitory control over the caudate nucleus, permitting the globus pallidus to inhibit thalamocortical outputs to the ALC, which consequently impedes verbal production. Verbal output is a consequence of semantic verification. When the semantic content of a language segment has been verified as suitable, the PLC releases inhibitory control over the caudate nucleus, which in turn inhibits pallidal mechanisms, permitting thalamic excitation of the anterior cortex and the release of the semantically verified language segment for motor speech programming. At the completion of motor programming, the anterior cortex deactivates inhibitory caudate influences upon the globus pallidus, via fronto-caudate pathways, allowing the temporoparietal cortex to recommence over-riding inhibitory control of caudate mechanisms. Motor execution, although not the focus of this discussion, was hypothesized to eventuate as a consequence of PLC-determined compatibility of motor speech programmes with appropriate phonological patterns (Crosson, 1985). This phonological monitoring process is potentially mediated via the arcuate fasciculus.

Finally, an axiom of RRSF theory dictates that language processes (i.e. segment formulation, semantic monitoring, motor programming, phonological monitoring and motor execution) are managed in succession, within segments. In contrast, parallel processing was predicted between segments, whereby the motor execution of an individual language segment is undertaken simultaneously with the motor programming, phonological monitoring, semantic verification and formulation of successive language segments.

Testing the strength of the Response-Release Semantic Feedback model: does clinical evidence support theoretical predictions?

The RRSF model dictates that subcortical nuclei lesions result in a forfeiture of function, including the output of inherent excitatory or inhibitory influences upon surrounding structures (Crosson, 1992). Based on this postulate, lesions of the VA thalamus or thalamo-cortical pathways were predicted to result in non-fluent verbal output as a consequence of disturbed tonic arousal and response-release mechanisms (Crosson, 1992). Indeed, reduced spontaneous speech output has been documented subsequent to lesions of the dominant thalamus (Jonas, 1982). Furthermore, the production of inappropriate semantic content was also predicted subsequent to thalamic or thalamo-cortical pathway lesions, which impact upon preverbal semantic feedback mechanisms. Supporting this prediction, paraphasic output of a semantic nature has been documented following lesions of the dominant thalamus (Cappa and Vignolo, 1979; Alexander and LoVerme, 1980; Bogousslavsky et al., 1988; Kennedy and Murdoch, 1989).

Pallidal lesions (Crosson, 1992) or damage to pallido-thalamic pathways (Murdoch, 1996) were hypothesized to result in fluent language pathology as a consequence of thalamic disinhibition and hyperexcitation of the ALC. Increased cortical activation was hypothesized to generate extraneous verbal output, such as semantic paraphasias. Indeed, fluent language pathology including the production of semantic paraphasias has been reported subsequent to surgically induced lesions of the globus pallidus (Svennilson et al., 1960) and vascular capsular-putaminal lesions with anterior white matter extensions (Naeser et al., 1982).

Lesions of the caudate nucleus or striato-pallidal pathways were postulated to disinhibit pallidal mechanisms, thereby inhibiting the VA thalamus and reducing cortical activation of the ALC (Crosson, 1985). Evidence of non-fluent language disturbances has been reported in cases subsequent to vascular capsular-putaminal lesions with posterior white matter extension (Naeser et al., 1982).

Temporoparietal-caudate lesions were postulated to produce characteristics of fluent aphasia through disinhibition of the caudate nucleus, inhibition of the globus pallidus and thalamic hyperarousal of the ALC (Crosson, 1992). Fronto-caudate lesions were hypothesized to produce non-fluent language disturbances (e.g. perseveration), subsequent to disconnection of the ALC and pathways used to terminate utterances following the completion of motor programming (Crosson, 1992). Indeed, the arrest of ongoing speech has been documented subsequent to neurostimulation of fronto-caudate pathways in the vicinity of the caudate head (Van Buren, 1963, 1966), supporting the hypothesis that these pathways may serve to terminate caudate nucleus activity (Crosson, 1985).

Revised precepts of Response-Release Semantic Feedback model
Following the inception of the RRSF model of subcortical participation in language, several criticisms with respect to the verity of proposed neuroanatomical substrates emerged (Crosson and Early, 1990; Wallesch and Papagno, 1988), prompting a review of the seminal theory. Theoretical revisions addressed three pertinent polemics, including (1) the implausibility of two disparate linguistic functions (i.e. tonic arousal and response-release) for a single subcortical nucleus (i.e. VA thalamus) (Wallesch and Papagno, 1988; Crosson and Early, 1990), (2) evidence of glutamatergic cortico-striatal projections in opposition to hypothesized inhibitory cortical control of striatal mechanisms (Spencer, 1976; Kocsis et al., 1977) and (3) reports of adjacent versus overlapping cortico-striatal terminal fields with respect to ALC and PLC striatal afferents (Goldman-Rakic and Selemon, 1986). Relative to the revised model (see Figure 3.3) the neural substrates subserving the aforementioned semantic feedback, response-release and tonic arousal mechanisms were afforded a re-conceptualization (Crosson and Early, 1990), proffering direct implications for thalamic and basal ganglia organization.

With respect to the thalamus, the pulvinar was postulated to represent the solitary nucleus involved in semantic feedback processes (Crosson and Early, 1990), given evidence of morphologically distinct yet interactive neurones subserving pulvinar projection fibres which innervate the frontal and parietal cortices (Asanuma et al., 1985). Additional theoretical extensions to thalamic structure and function involved the dissociation of the integrated response-release and tonic arousal functions of the VA nucleus proposed in the original model. The ascending limb of the reticular formation has been reported to principally innervate the hypothalamus and ILN of the thalamus (Matzke and Foltz, 1983). Despite the fact that ILN relay fibres through the VA thalamus to the ALC, they do not project collaterals to the VA nucleus (Jones, 1985). As such, the ILN were assigned the authentic cortical arousal function, and the VA nucleus a role in facilitating the release of semantically refined language for verbal production, via the proposed cortico-striato-pallido-thalamo-cortical loop. Tonic cortical arousal, by way of the ILN, was hypothesized to involve slow-acting but extended neuromodulation of ALC activity (Crosson, 1992). The primary objective of tonic cortical arousal is to prepare the ALC to respond to internal and external linguistic cues. In contrast, VA-mediated response-release mechanisms were described as phasic, facilitating the efficient yet time-constrained release of semantically verified language segments for motor speech programming (Crosson, 1992). In relation to the original RRSF model, dominant VA thalamic lesions were largely hypothesized to produce non-fluent aphasia by way of deactivating cortical arousal mechanisms (Crosson, 1985). VA tuberothalamic infarcts, however, have been reported to produce both fluent and non-fluent language pathology (Graff-Radford et al., 1984; Bogousslavsky et al., 1988). The revised RRSF precepts lend support to this observation.

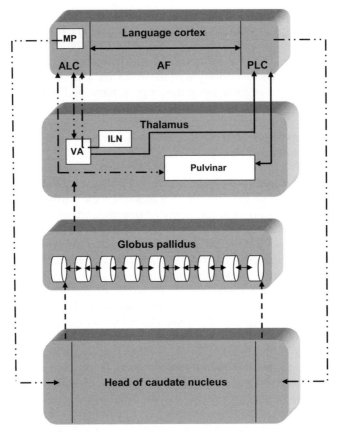

Figure 3.3 Schematic diagram of the revised basal ganglia–thalamocortical Response-Release Semantic Feedback model (adapted from Crosson, 1985, 1992). AF, arcuate fasciculus; ALC, anterior language centre; ILN, intralaminar nuclei; MP, motor programming cortex; PLC, posterior language centre; VA, ventral anterior thalamic nucleus; dotted and dashed arrows, excitatory pathway; dashed arrows, inhibitory pathway; discs, disc-shaped dendritic fields; double-headed arrows, spatial summation properties.

According to Crosson (1992), differentiating between the effects of isolated lesions of the VA thalamic nucleus and the ILN is complex, given their close anatomical association. As such, elements of both reduced spontaneous speech and paraphasic verbal output may be observed as a consequence of isolated or combined lesions of the VA and intralaminar thalamic nuclei. More specifically, damage to the VA nucleus will render it unable to exert excitatory influences upon the ALC, resulting in an inability to release formulated language segments for motor programming, evidenced as difficulties in initiating spontaneous speech. Lesions of the ILN or intralaminar nuclear pathways traversing the VA nucleus towards the anterior language area, however, were predicted to result in disorganized language, manifesting as paraphasic or jargonistic output. This hypothesis was formulated following observations of disorganized cognition subsequent to lesions of posterior intralaminar nuclear groups (Gentilini *et al.*, 1987).

Evidence of glutamatergic versus GABAergic cortico-striatal neurotransmission, in addition to postulated adjacent versus overlapping cortico-striatal terminal fields, also instigated a review of functional basal ganglia organization within the RRSF model. Upon revision, the caudate nucleus was assigned an integrative function with the capacity to transform patterned cortical input into quantitative striatal output (Crosson and Early, 1990). In more detail, the ALC and PLC were postulated to project to and terminate within adjacent regions of the caudate nucleus. Following the formulation of a language segment within the ALC, associated fronto-caudate neurones were predicted to exert an excitatory affect on their affiliated terminations. Cortico-striatal excitation was hypothesized to destabilize a striatal lateral inhibition threshold, generally maintained by a resident GABAergic spiny I neuronal network (Crosson and Early, 1990). This destabilization effect was postulated to result in an increase in inhibitory striatal outputs to disc-shaped dendritic fields within the globus pallidus. When the language segment has been semantically verified, PLC projections were also hypothesized to excite specific terminations within the caudate nucleus. Cumulative striatal excitation, mediated via ALC and PLC projection fibres, results in over-shooting of the aforementioned lateral striatal inhibition threshold. According to the model, exceeding the lateral inhibition threshold results in a significant increase in inhibitory striatal output and the consequent inhibition of pallidal mechanisms. Quantitative or spatial summation (see Figure 3.3) of inhibitory caudate inputs within pallidal dendritic fields hinders inhibitory pallidal outflow. This, in turn, disinhibits the thalamus, permitting excitation of the ALC and consequently the release of the semantically verified language segment as speech.

Lexical Decision Making model

In line with the RRSF model, the LDM model (Crosson, 1992; Wallesch and Papagno, 1988) also proffers a cortico-striato-pallido-thalamo-cortical loop as the neural platform for linguistic operations, including a specific thalamocortical arousal mechanism, consistent with Ojemann's (1976) theorem. Despite evident parallelisms, however, distinct incongruities prevail between these theoretical constructs, from the viewpoint of functional cortical organization, and the nature of proposed subcortical mechanisms.

The LDM model concedes the formulation of certain aspects of language (i.e. generation of lexical units) to occur within the PLC, and verbal output to be a function of the ALC. For the most part, however, precepts of classical language theory were discounted. In opposition to language-dedicated cortical areas exclusively subserving the mediation of receptive and expressive linguistic operations, Wallesch and Papagno (1988) proposed information-processing capacities for the subcortical constituents of the aforementioned cortico-striato-pallido-thalamo-cortical circuit, with respect to cortically generated situational, goal-directed and lexical 'modules'. The caudate nucleus, globus pallidus, thalamus and ALC were defined as a 'frontal lobe system', capable of integrating and regulating cortical activity by way of the striatum- and basal ganglia-governed thalamocortical outputs, respectively. This subcortical information-processing postulate was in stark contrast to the neuroregulatory role of the subcortical nuclei proposed by Crosson (1985).

According to the LDM model, 'modules' represent the axiom of functional cortical organization (Phillips et al., 1984). Hypothetically processed in parallel, efferent cortical modules are terminally defined by their thalamic afferents (Szentagothai, 1975), subsequent to striatal and pallidal perpension. Indeed, studies of motor function have postulated the ventral thalamus to communicate 'central commands' to the frontal cortex for processing, via a proposed thalamic gating mechanism (Phillips and Porter, 1977). Competitive inhibition of parallel modules reportedly dictates responses produced by the survival-of-the-fittest module (i.e. continued processing), which presumably constitutes the 'central command' (Eccles, 1977).

Proposed role of the thalamus within the Lexical Decision Making model

According to the LDM model, the VA and VL thalamic nuclei collectively, under the influence of the basal ganglia, are responsible for the gating of superordinate lexical alternatives to the ALC for processing within output channels and subsequent production as speech. Proposed basal ganglia mechanisms relative to the LDM model will be discussed in detail later in the current chapter, but some immediate comment in the current section was deemed necessary, given the recognized potency of basal ganglia influences upon thalamic outputs. The LDM model proffers language formulation to entail striatal integration of temporoparietal and frontal cortex inputs relative to lexical, situational and goal-directed constraints (see Figure 3.4). Following striatal integration, the basal ganglia were hypothesized to mediate the selection of appropri-

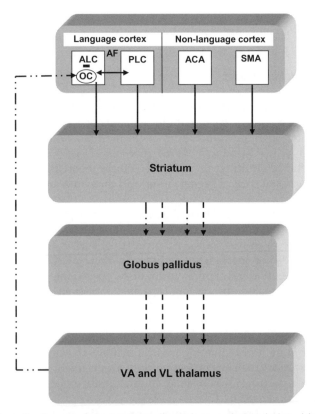

Figure 3.4 Schematic diagram of the basal ganglia–thalamocortical Lexical Decision Making model (adapted from Crosson, 1992). ACA, anterior cingulate area; AF, arcuate fasciculus; ALC, anterior language centre; OC, output channel; PLC, posterior language centre; SMA, supplementary motor area; VA, ventral anterior nucleus; VL, ventral lateral nucleus; black bar in ALC, inhibitory cortical interneurones; dashed arrows, inhibitory pathway; dotted and dashed arrows, excitatory pathway.

ate lexical alternatives with respect to external and internal constaints and to conse-quently govern thalamic gating of a central command to the frontal cortex, pertaining to the most suitable alternative. In essence, the striatum transmits the generated corpus of integrated lexical/situational/motivational alternatives to the thalamus, via the globus pallidus; however, only the 'central command' pertaining to the lexical alternative deemed most appropriate is successfully gated to the ALC for verbal pro-duction. Cortical processing of suitable alternatives is facilitated via gradational tha-lamic excitation of inhibitory cortical interneurones, presumably under pallidal control. Thus, thalamocortical inputs prohibit the expression of subordinate alterna-tives by disproportionately activating resident inhibitory cortical interneurones sub-serving the processing of inappropriate versus appropriate modules.

Furthermore, the LDM model dictates that the basal ganglia and thalamus represent functional units capable of manipulating multiple degrees of freedom within corti-cally defined contexts. The thalamic gating mechanism is hypothesized only to be effective when the required language production task has the potential to generate many degrees of freedom (i.e. a large number of responses) (Wallesch and Papagno, 1988). It was postulated that the thalamic gating mechanism would be ineffective during tasks that generate responses with restricted degrees of freedom. Gating of a 'central command' in this case is redundant, because all modules contain the same information.

Proposed role of the basal ganglia within the Lexical Decision Making model

The LDM model assigned to the striatum the role of information processor, involving the organization and integration of cortical information. Language formulation was hypothesized to entail striatal integration of cortical inputs from the PLC and retroro-landic, prefrontal and supplementary motor areas. In essence, the PLC was postulated to generate multiple lexical alternatives which are transmitted to the striatum in a modular fashion.

Retrorolandic-striatal projections communicate situational constraints relative to language output and the prefrontal and supplementary motor cortices provide goal-directed/motivational cues. Cortico-striatal inputs are then integrated within the striatum. Collectively, the basal ganglia then determine which among several poten-tial lexical alternatives is most appropriate for verbal production. Only the 'central command' pertaining to the most suitable lexical alternative is successfully gated by the thalamus to output channels within the ALC. Thalamic gating mechanisms sub-serving this function were discussed in the previous section.

The basal ganglia have been defined as a treasure trove of neural subsystems (Nolte, 1993). Consistent with this description, the LDM model proposes basal ganglia orga-nization to follow a highly complex schema. The striatum was hypothesized to have the capacity to exert both inhibitory and excitatory influences upon the globus palli-dus by way of internal and efferent excitatory and inhibitory mechanisms (Groves, 1983). In contrast, the pallidum was postulated to exclusively regulate thalamic gating by way of inherent inhibitory mechanisms.

Testing the strength of the Lexical Decision Making model: does clinical evidence support theoretical predictions?

Preserved morphosyntactic, repetition and naming abilities in the presence of dis-turbed spontaneous speech has been reported by a number of research bodies to characteristically represent the potential syndrome of subcortical aphasia (Alexander and LoVerme, 1980; Damasio *et al.*, 1982; Naeser *et al.*, 1982). This symptom complex lends support to the multiple-degrees-of-freedom postulate proposed by Wallesch and Papagno (1988).

Furthermore, according to the LDM model verbal output containing semantic paraphasias and/or inappropriate lexical content subsequent to lesions of the dominant thalamus and anterior limb of the internal capsule (Ojemann, 1976) supports the notion of thalamic gating, with respect to language production. Semantic paraphasias were hypothesized to result from ALC processing of subordinate alternatives subsequent to thalamic lesions which disrupt the mechanisms subserving graded thalamic excitation of inhibitory cortical interneurones (Crosson, 1992). Damaged thalamic gating mechanisms are hypothetically unresponsive to pallidal influences. Semantic paraphasias, therefore, represent cortical processing of subordinate response alternatives which failed to reach basal ganglia-determined specification requirements for verbal production.

In contrast, lesions of the globus pallidus were predicted to result in non-fluent language pathology as a consequence of thalamic disinhibition and unmitigated excitation of inhibitory cortical interneurones. Clinically, disinhibited thalamic gating was hypothesized to manifest as difficulty in initiating speech (Wallesch and Papagno, 1988). Indeed, reports of transcortical motor aphasia have been documented subsequent to lesions of the dominant pallidum (Brunner *et al.*, 1982; Damasio *et al.*, 1982).

Striatal lesions were hypothesized to produce a diverse range of potential language disturbances (Wallesch and Papagno, 1988), characteristic of both fluent and non-fluent aphasia. Potential internal and efferent excitatory and inhibitory striatal mechanisms (Groves, 1983) were postulated to exert both inhibitory and disinhibitory effects upon the globus pallidus, and hence, thalamocortical outputs (Wallesch and Papagno, 1988). The linguistic implications of striatal lesions therefore, may entail speech initiation difficulties and/or inappropriate lexical-semantic output. The authors acknowledged that the diverse nature of basal ganglia aphasia syndromes supports this organizational theory.

Murdoch (1996) extrapolated the theoretical constructs of Wallesch and Papagno's (1988) model with respect to the predicted impact of subcortical white matter pathway lesions on modular processing, specified within the LDM model. Lesions disconnecting the association areas of the prefrontal, temporal or parietal association cortices from the striatum were predicted to interrupt the transmission of lexical, goal-directed and situational constraints to the striatum, consequently disturbing language production. Striato-pallidal pathway lesions were hypothesized to disturb the transmission of parallel modules from the striatum to the globus pallidus, resulting in incomplete thalamic module definition. Pallido-thalamic fibre lesions were predicted to result in non-fluent language disturbances subsequent to thalamic disinhibition and overt excitation of inhibitory cortical interneurones, hindering language production. Thalamo-cortical pathway lesions were postulated to prohibit the thalamus from communicating central commands to output channels within the ALC. Reduced spontaneous speech was predicted following lesions of this type.

Revised precepts of the Lexical Decision Making model
Wallesch and Papagno (1988) acknowledged that the proposed cortico-striato-pallido-thalamo-cortical loop may not represent an exclusive subcortico-cortical linguistic circuit. Purportedly, the caudate nucleus, globus pallidus, thalamus and frontal cortex constitute a 'frontal lobe system', involved in language production. Fronto-frontal and

reciprocal connections between the thalamus and frontal cortex which bypass the basal ganglia have been identified as supplementary components of this system, which may also contribute to language processes. Indeed, the authors emphasized that the relative preservation of language in populations with extrapyramidal pathology supports potential involvement of these subsidiary pathways in the mediation of linguistic operations as well as the notion of functional plasticity, with respect to cortical and subcortical system components.

Furthermore, the LDM model proposed an integrative function for the striatum with respect to cortical inputs. This proposition violates the segregated pathway principle of basal ganglia–thalamocortical organization stipulated by Alexander *et al.* (1986). Despite acceptance of an information-processing hypothesis for the striatum by way of a patterned neuronal currency (Divac *et al.*, 1987), intrinsic basal ganglia organization schemas remain poorly understood (Wallesch, 1997). Current opinion supports a temporal co-ordination versus integration postulate for the basal ganglia, with respect to the parallel processing of multiple, segregated 'mini-loops' (Goldman-Rakic and Selemon, 1986, 1990), each dedicated to individual yet associated cortical modules (Wallesch, 1990). This theory is an extension of the original LDM model which proposed the integration and permutation of cortical modules within a solitary and unidirectional cortico-striato-pallido-thalamo-cortical loop.

The 'mini-loop' axiom operates upon the multiple-degrees-of-freedom premise. By way of disturbed basal ganglia-mediated cortical activation mechanisms, 'frontal lobe system' lesions were predicted to result in an array of possible language deficits, including inappropriate lexical output (i.e. semantic paraphasias), speech-initiation difficulties (i.e. transcortical motor aphasia) and/or increased dependency upon contextual constraints (i.e. propositional aphasia) (Wallesch, 1997). The authors acknowledged that such manifestations of language pathology have indeed been observed in cases of subcortical aphasia.

Selective Engagement model

Selective Engagement theory represents the most contemporary schema of subcortical participation in language and principally proposes a frontal-inferior thalamic peduncle (ITP)-nucleus reticularis (NR)-centrum medianum system (see Figure 3.5) to subserve the 'engagement' of cortical components which mediate attentional and behavioural processes, including language (Nadeau and Crosson, 1997a). This proposed linguistic 'frontal lobe system' complied with the tenets of the LDM model, with the exception of two distinct anomalies. In particular, selective engagement theory disputes a role for the basal ganglia in language (the rationale for which will be discussed later in this chapter), and redefines non-specific thalamic nuclei (i.e. NR, centrum medianum and parafascicular (PF) nucleus) as critical to the mediation of linguistic processes. Nadeau and Crosson (1997b) considered VA and VL thalamic participation in language an insolvent hypothesis. This postulate was largely fuelled by two lines of evidence: first, an observed decline in the incidence of aphasia following surgically induced lesions of the VA and VL thalamus, concomitant with enhanced stereotactic technique accuracy (Fox *et al.*, 1991); and second, the fact that aphasia resulting from tuberothalamic territory infarcts involving the VA nucleus typically resembles that following paramedian territory lesions, which spare the VA thalamus. Postulated thalamic engagement of the cortex, however, was in line with Ojemann's (1976) proposed ventral thalamic focal alerting mechanism in addition to Crosson's

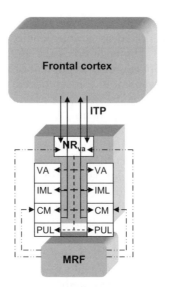

Figure 3.5 Schematic diagram of the frontal-inferior thalamic peduncle-nucleus reticularis-centrum medianum system subserving the proposed engagement of cortical language mechanisms (adapted from Nadeau and Crosson, 1997a). CM, centrum medianum; IML, internal medullary lamina; ITP, inferior thalamic peduncle; MRF, midbrain reticular formation; NR$_{va}$, ventral anterior nucleus reticularis; PUL, pulvinar; VA, ventral anterior thalamus; dotted and dashed arrows, excitatory pathway; dashed arrows, inhibitory pathway. Thalamocortical and corticothalamic pathways are largely unrepresented for the sake of clarity, with the exception of centrum medianum-frontal and frontal-ventral anterior nucleus reticularis projections.

(1985) VA response-release system, relative to the galvanization of verbal output channels. The expansion of these postulates to consider the activation of more extensive language-dedicated cortical mosaics (Ojemann, 1983), largely under NR control (Nadeau and Crosson, 1997a), accommodated manifestations of receptive as well as expressive language deficits observed subsequent to lesions of the thalamus.

The RRSF and LDM models previously discussed focused primarily on output versus input mechanisms, providing no discernible explanation for comprehension deficits. In contrast, the structural complexity of the neural system subserving Selective Engagement mechanisms accommodates the spectrum of aphasic characteristics observed following lesions of the dominant thalamus (Nadeau and Crosson, 1997b), perhaps approximating a more cogent axiom of subcortical participation in language than its antecedents.

Proposed role of the thalamus within the Selective Engagement Model

Selective Engagement theory proposed a role for the thalamus in language based on the observation of a relatively consistent aphasic syndrome subsequent to tuberothalamic and paramedian territory ischaemic infarcts (Nadeau and Crosson, 1997a). In a series of four cases, a relatively typical thalamic aphasia characterized by anomia in conversational speech, reduced word fluency, impaired confrontation naming, comparatively sound comprehension and normal repetition was reported. Anatomical regularities between subjects with respect to lesion parameters suggested damage to constituents of a frontal-ITP-NR-centrum medianum system, as the mainspring of the resultant language pathology.

As previously mentioned, the proposed frontal-ITP-NR-centrum medianum system hypothetically engages cortical nets subserving the mediation of attentional and behavioural processes. Attentional mechanisms in this sense reportedly involve a specialized form of neural convergence upon particular internal (i.e. thoughts) and external stimuli (Crosson, 1999). With respect to language, Selective Engagement has been reported to predominantly impact upon semantically driven lexical retrieval (Crosson, 1999) and access to declarative memory (Crosson, 1992). Non-declarative or implicit memory (Malamut et al., 1992), however, appears to be preserved following lesions which implicate the aforementioned frontal-ITP-NR-centrum medianum system. Declarative memory is defined as the conscious recollection of stored facts and events within association areas of the cortex (Nadeau and Crosson, 1997a). In contrast, non-declarative or implicit memory entails a range of skills, habits, priming and learned behaviours which are not consciously accessible. This lexical-semantic/ declarative versus non-declarative symptom dichotomy was interpreted in terms of attentional resource allocation. Lexical-semantic retrieval (Crosson, 1999) and access to declarative memory (Nadeau and Crosson, 1997a) are reportedly more dependent upon attentional and therefore Selective Engagement mechanisms than sublexical, lexical (Crosson, 1999) and non-declarative memory processes (Nadeau and Crosson, 1997a).

According to Selective Engagement theory, lexical-semantic retrieval entails the disproportionate activation of target versus semantically related lexical items represented within the cerebral cortex, as per parallel distributed processing models (Crosson and Nadeau, 1998). The production of semantic paraphasias during naming tasks has been interpreted as a failure of Selective Engagement mechanisms to sufficiently amplify target-item activation levels in preference to competing/semantically related lexical items (Nadeau and Crosson, 1997a). Furthermore, reported difficulty retrieving/engaging low- as opposed to high-frequency words during naming tasks (Raymer et al., 1997) following lesions of the frontal-ITP-NR-centrum medianum system supports the notion of graceful degradation within semantic networks (McClelland et al., 1986). Nadeau and Crosson (1997a) hypothesized that within a damaged or contaminated semantic network, weaker representations (i.e. those with fewer associations) are rendered redundant. Low-frequency lexical items were considered to characterize such representations.

Comparatively higher observed reaction times on tasks demanding semantically driven lexical retrieval (e.g. generation of a semantic associate) versus processing of a purely lexical nature (e.g. reading aloud) were postulated to indicate greater attentional resource allocation to lexical-semantic processes (Crosson, 1999). Naming and comprehension were also hypothesized to require conscious or attention-driven access to stored knowledge (i.e. declarative memory), in contrast to syntactic/ grammar-governed processes and repetition abilities which require no conscious awareness of constituent elements (i.e. non-declarative or implicit memory) for successful completion (Nadeau and Crosson, 1997b). The anatomical substrates subserving the aformentioned lexical-semantic and declarative memory mechanisms will be discussed below.

The NR has been hypothesized to largely control frontal-ITP-NR-centrum medianum mechanisms by way of its inherent ability to manipulate the firing mode of thalamic output nuclei (Nadeau and Crosson, 1997a). The NR represents a collection of inhibitory GABAergic neurones circumscribing the thalamus, which project to the majority of thalamic nuclei, with the exclusion of the anterior group (Nadeau and Crosson, 1997a). Projection neurones of the thalamus reportedly exist in either a hyperpolarized or partly depolarized state (McCormick and Feeser, 1990; Steriade *et al.*, 1990). Hyperpolarization (i.e. burst-firing mode) involves minimal correspondence between thalamic afferent and efferent projections. In contrast, the partly depolarized state (i.e. single-spike firing mode) entails strong correlations between thalamic inputs and outputs. The NR has been hypothesized to mediate thalamic depolarization (Nadeau and Crosson, 1997b). Depolarization reportedly facilitates the appositioning of thalamic afferents and efferents by way of reducing the firing rate of thalamic projection neurones. This transfiguration enables meaningful communication between the thalamus and cortex, considered to represent the basis of selective engagement. According to Nadeau and Crosson (1997a), two neural mechanisms influence NR activity: the midbrain reticular formation (Steriade and Llinas, 1988) and frontal-ITP-NR-centrum medianum system (Skinner and Yingling, 1977).

The NR receives ascending fibres from the midbrain reticular formation (Scheibel and Scheibel, 1972). Midbrain reticular formation activation of thalamic nuclei via direct and indirect (i.e. by way of the NR) pathways has been reported to facilitate depolarization of the entire gamut of thalamic projection neurones (Nadeau and Crosson, 1997a). The midbrain reticular formation-NR system was hypothesized to specifically mediate tonic, non-selective thalamocortical gating associated with arousal-driven or reflexive behaviour (Skinner and Yingling, 1977; Livingstone and Hubel, 1981). Nadeau and Crosson (1997a) proposed the frontal-ITP-NR-centrum medianum system to have a less flagrant yet more definitive influence over the thalamus than the midbrain reticular formation, involving the phasic engagement of thalamocortical outputs relative to intentionally guided attention and behaviour, including language.

In addition to midbrain reticular formation efferents, the NR also receives inputs from the descending fibres of the frontal cortex, via the ITP (Steriade *et al.*, 1984) and collaterals from thalamocortical axons (DeMyer, 1998). The ventral anterior portion of the NR (NR_{va}) represents a mortise for the ITP, via which fronto-thalamic and thalamo-frontal projections exit, enter and synapse within the thalamic complex (Campos-Ortega and Cluver, 1969). Furthermore, NR cells reportedly synapse upon thalamocortical neurones in addition to inhibitory thalamic interneurones, especially within the ILN (Steriade *et al.*, 1984). Despite knowledge of the anatomical substrates constituting the frontal-ITP-NR-centrum medianum system, however, the precise nature of thalamic Selective Engagement mechanisms remains largely unknown. Indeed, the evident neural complexity of the frontal-ITP-NR-centrum medianum system vindicates a currently abridged conceptualization of Selective Engagement mechanisms (Nadeau and Crosson, 1997a).

Current opinion dictates that the NR principally regulates selective cortical engagement by manipulating the firing mode of thalamic nuclei. Nadeau and Crosson (1997a) postulated the pulvinar to be the most likely thalamic nucleus to be involved in the selective engagement of language mechanisms, given its extensive connections with the temporoparietal cortex (Jones, 1985). In line with Crosson's (1985) model, Selective Engagement theory also proposes the ILN to potentially mediate language processes. Given its considerable size in humans, evidence of NR_{va} innervations (Steriade *et al.*, 1984), and diffuse outputs to the full extent of the cortical mantle (Jones, 1985), the centrum medianum-PF complex was considered a viable intralaminar contributor to the selective engagement of language production and comprehension mechanisms (Nadeau and Crosson, 1997a). The Selective Engagement of language-dedicated cortical nets, therefore, was hypothesized to result from three potential mechanisms: first, NR-regulated pulvinar-cortical engagement; second, NR-regulated centrum medianum-/PF-cortical engagement, and third, centrum medianum-/PF-frontal lobe-NR-thalamus (e.g. pulvinar)-cortical engagement (Nadeau and Crosson, 1997a). Defective Selective Engagement mechanisms were postulated to result in the erroneous recruitment of cortical nets via pulvinar and/or centrum medianum projections, culminating in lexical-semantic field and declarative memory disturbances.

Proposed role of the basal ganglia within the Selective Engagement model
The Selective Engagement theory discounts a role for the basal ganglia in language. A variable symptom complex with respect to observed manifestations of language pathology in the presence of classically defined striatocapsular lesions formed the basis of this postulate. In more detail, Nadeau and Crosson (1997a) analysed the linguistic profiles of 50 cases subsequent to relatively uniform striatocapsular infarctions, including the caudate head, putamen, anterior limb of the internal capsule and portions of the globus pallidus. Vast heterogeneity relative to the severity and incidence of language deficits, including fluency, articulation, comprehension, repetition and naming, was reported. Nadeau and Crosson (1997a) hypothesized that an integral role for the basal ganglia in language would be fortified by a coherent aphasic syndrome, in the event of uniform damage. Based on the above evidence, therefore, a minimal function hypothesis with respect to the contribution of the basal ganglia to language functions was promoted.

Nadeau and Crosson (1997a) largely attributed language disturbances subsequent to lesions of the basal ganglia to cortical hypoperfusion. Thrombotic or embolic occlusions primarily of the middle cerebral artery, or less commonly the internal carotid artery, were identified as precursors to striatocapsular infarction (Weiller *et al.*, 1990). More importantly, circulatory dynamics pertaining to the rate of arterial recanalization and the efficiency of anastomotic circulation following basal ganglia infarction were considered integral factors in determining the presence or absence of aphasia. Perisylvian cortex ischaemia by way of middle cerebral artery occlusion-induced cystic infarction, neuronal drop-out or generalized tissue dysfunction (Nadeau and Crosson, 1997a) provided a tenable explanation for the variable array of expressive and receptive language deficits associated with striatocapsular infarcts. Furthermore, haemorrhagic basal ganglia lesions were also postulated to disturb cortical circulatory dynamics relevant to language functions. Pressure effects inducing cortical ischaemia were held responsible for consequent manifestations of aphasia.

Testing the strength of the Selective Engagement model: does clinical evidence support theoretical predictions?
Relative to language abilities, vascular lesions which encroach upon the frontal-ITP-NR- centrum medianum system have been affiliated with lexical-semantic and declarative memory deficits (Nadeau and Crosson, 1997a). Evaluating the specific contribution to language, relative to each of the constituents of the frontal-ITP-NR-centrum medianum system, has been made difficult by the infiltrative nature of spontaneous vascular lesions of the thalamus. Despite this limitation, some studies have attempted to explicate the underlying mechanisms subserving selective engagement. In support of the frontal lobe system, impaired spontaneous speech has been reported following paramedian territory infarcts (Goldenberg *et al.*, 1983; Lhermitte, 1984). Deficits in semantic concept generation evidenced by a disorganization of ideas, paucity of detail and vague conceptual markers have been observed (Nadeau and

Crosson, 1997a). Fronto-thalamic disconnection by way of deep ventral thalamic lesions in addition to more anterior lesions which infiltrate the ITP have been held accountable for this symptom complex (Nadeau and Crosson, 1997b).

Less convincingly, manifestations of lexical-semantic and declarative memory impairments have also been reported subsequent to lesions which fall outside the realm of the frontal-ITP-NR-centrum medianum system, serving to both obscure and consolidate our understanding of Selective Engagement mechanisms. Crosson (1984) reported an aphasic case subsequent to a haemorrhagic lesion of the left lateral nucleus extending to the superior pulvinar. The aphasic syndrome presented involved fluent output with evidence of semantic and neologistic paraphasias in addition to mildly impaired repetition and comprehension. This symptom complex was in concert with the language pathology previously associated with anterior thalamic lesions, which infiltrated the frontal-ITP-NR-centrum medianum system. This apparent viola-tion of the established Selective Engagement axiom has potential implications for schemas pertaining to functional thalamic organization. The current results lend support to a potential interrelationship between anterior (i.e. NR) and posterior (i.e. pulvinar) thalamic mechanisms (Crosson, 1999). This postulate is in support of NR-regulated Selective Engagement of language mechanisms by way of pulvinar-cortical projections.

Despite the fact that paraphasic output subsequent to lesions of the thalamus is typically semantic in nature, phonemic and neologistic elements have also been observed (Robin and Schienberg, 1990). This phenomenon was considered a violation of the operative Selective Engagement schema if morpho-phonemic conversion in the course of spontaneous speech is considered a function of non-declarative memory (Nadeau and Crosson, 1997a). Current evidence now suggests that sublexical ele-ments (e.g. phonemes, inflectional grammatic morphemes, derivational morphemes and syllables) may be represented within declarative memory during the acquisition of language, either as a sublexicon or juxtaposed with semantic representations (Buck-ingham, 1987). As a result, disturbed lexical access mechanisms as a consequence of thalamic infarction may affect the selection of lexical items independent of their meaning. Alternatively, Nadeau and Crosson (1997a) postulated that thalamic lesions may serve to disturb operational mechanisms within semantic networks. As a result, competing lexical entries have the capacity for mutual activation and consequently the amalgamation of relevant morphemic and phonological elements. Neologisms and phonemic paraphasias were considered to represent the end product of either mechanism.

Revised precepts of Selective Engagement model
Contemporary research involving functional magnetic resonance imaging (fMRI) and more in-depth linguistic analysis procedures has served to shed additional light on the role of the thalamus in language, including a proposed contribution to working memory and category-specific naming. More specifically, fMRI studies have revealed activation of the anterior thalamus during working memory tasks that demand semantic and phonological judgements, or the manipulation of 'complete' lexical items. In contrast, tasks that required the recruitment of sublexical processes (e.g. orthographic form judgements) failed to activate the anterior thalamus in a parallel fashion (Crosson et al., 1999). As such, Selective Engagement mechanisms have also been hypothesized to facilitate the on-line 'holding' of lexical information within working memory, in addition to the activation of pre-existing or 'complete' cortical representations relative to lexical content (Crosson, 1999).

Lesions of the posterior (i.e. including pulvinar and centrum medianum) as well as anterior (i.e. tuberothalamic territory) thalamus have been reported to result in category-specific anomia. Isolated case studies have revealed a specific anomia for medical terms following posterior thalamic lesion (Crosson *et al.*, 1997a) and proper noun anomia following a lesion of the anterior thalamus (Lucchelli and De Renzi, 1992). Currently it is thought that category-specific naming may be orchestrated via thalamic engagement of a broad array of distinct semantic networks distributed throughout the cortex (Crosson, 1999). Indeed, positron emission tomography (PET) studies have demonstrated temporal lobe activation during semantic fluency tasks (Boivin *et al.*, 1992) compared with dorsolateral prefrontal cortex activation during phonemic fluency tasks (Pujol *et al.*, 1996). Evidence of this dichotomy alone suggests that distinct brain regions accommodate semantically and phonologically constrained information. Future investigations of brain functioning during categorical naming tasks may serve to extricate the precise nature of semantic system and indeed language organization, and to potentially expand the frontiers of classical language theory.

The finial revision to Nadeau and Crosson's (1997a) Selective Engagement theory relates to the minimal function hypothesis for the basal ganglia in language. Certain bodies of research dispute the claim that language deficits resulting from lesions of the striatocapsular region fail to establish a homogenous aphasic syndrome. A coherent aphasic syndrome relative to generative aspects of language, including verbal fluency, sentence generation and extended discourse, has been reported (Mega and Alexander, 1994). This finding suggests a need to revisit the notion of basal ganglia aphasia paying particular attention to the scope and sensitivity of linguistic assessments utilized in addition to circulatory dynamics (Crosson *et al.*, 1997b). Indeed, this evidence supports a potential role for the basal ganglia in mediating linguistic processes. In all probability, this role may entail the regulation of thalamocortical engagement. Proposed mechanisms include the switching of engagement between neural nets (Malapani *et al.*, 1994).

Evident limitations with respect to operative theories of subcortical participation in language

The theories of subcortical participation in language previously discussed represent meritorious attempts to extricate the role of subcortical nuclei in the mediation of linguistic processes. Despite these efforts, however, the relevant models are ardently challenged by a foundation in studies of behaviour subsequent to subcortical lesions of vascular origin. The utilization of experimental cohorts with vascular lesions to evaluate the legitimacy of these models has been described as inexpedient (Murdoch, 1996), particularly when spontaneous lesions typically impact upon input as well as output mechanisms relative to critical subcortical structures, producing multiplex and potentially oppositional neuromodulatory effects (Crosson, 1992).

Nevertheless, over the course of the last 30 years the study of 'subcortical aphasia' as a consequence of spontaneous vascular lesions has gathered momentum, largely fuelled by the emergence of neuroimaging techniques which introduced the concept of *in vivo* lesion localization, such as CT and MRI (Alexander *et al.*, 1987; Cappa and Vallar, 1992; Murdoch, 1996). CT techniques have generated the largest corpus of data relative to cases of contained subcortical damage in the presence of aphasic characteristics (Murdoch, 1996). Despite these endeavors, however, the indeterminate and infiltrative nature of vascular lesions as well as the recognized failure of neuroimaging techniques to consistently reveal the true extent of resultant tissue damage has served to trammel the acceptance of operative theories of subcortical participation in language (Crosson, 1992).

The notion of subcortical aphasia has been irrefutably challenged by recognized limitations inherent to currently available neuroimaging techniques. CT and MRI techniques reportedly yield a 70–80% accuracy rating with respect to the identification of ischaemic damage (Nadeau *et al.*, 1993). Indeed, CT scanning has been documented to fail to detect small infarctions of less than 5 mm in diameter (Wodarz, 1980), and MRI has revealed cortical involvement in cases of subcortically defined lesions, determined by CT scanning (DeWitt *et al.*, 1985). Consequently, inaccurate lesion parameters may have served to contaminate our previous conceptualization of 'subcortical aphasia'.

In addition to the recognized shortcomings of current neuroimaging techniques, a number of physiological mechanisms have also been proposed which potentially attribute manifestations of subcortical aphasia to cortical dysfunction. Subcortical lesions have been reported to exert distance effects upon the cerebral cortex, including cortical hypoperfusion and hypometabolism (Perani *et al.*, 1987). Reduced cerebral blood flow has been reported to result in ischaemia-induced neuronal loss (Lassen *et al.*, 1983) and ischaemic penumbra (i.e. maintenance of tissue viability in the presence of neuronal dysfunction) (Astrup *et al.*, 1981), both mechanisms having the potential to disable cortical activity. Furthermore, blood flow is contingent upon the metabolic demands of appurtenant tissue and functional brain activity is directly linked to regional metabolism (Sokoloff, 1977).

Diaschisis has been defined as the loss of excitation, resulting in a cessation of function, in areas remote from yet connected to a primary site of brain damage (Von Monakow, 1969). Distance effects can be explained by this mechanism, given that changes in functional activity, as a result of deafferentation, have been linked to alterations in regional blood flow and glucose consumption (Reivich *et al.*, 1985). In general, distance effects have been translated to represent a reduction in neuronal activity as a result of afferent or efferent pathway disconnection (Martin and Raichle, 1983). Damage to the thalamus, striatum or internal capsule has been postulated to effect functional changes within remote yet interconnected brain regions, such as the temporoparietal cortex (Metter, 1987). Indeed, subcortico-cortical interactions have been postulated as integral to the facilitation of normal language processes (Kushner *et al.*, 1987).

Of note, Nadeau and Crosson (1997a) postulated that if subcortical nuclei play a legitimate role in the mediation of language processes, then direct or indirect effects of subcortical lesions should produce a relatively uniform aphasia symptom complex. At least in the case of non-thalamic subcortical lesions, a uniform aphasia symptom complex has not been able to be identified. In a study of 33 left striatocapsular infarct cases and associated aphasia, reported symptom profiles consisted of all severity types and possible language characteristics relative to the parameters of fluency, articulation, comprehension, naming, repetition and paraphasia. On the basis of these findings, Nadeau and Crosson (1997a) concluded that the most plausible neurophysiological explanation for the variety of language deficits associated with subcortical aphasia was stenosis or occlusion of large vessels resulting in cortical hypoperfusion. Postulates relating to (1) a direct role for the subcortical nuclei in mediating language, (2) cortical disconnection, (3) impaired subcortico-cortical interactions and (4) diaschisis were discounted, as these mechanisms were predicted to produce consistent aphasia symptoms. Hypoperfusion of a variety of cortical regions following occlusion or stenosis of vessels supplying the language cortex independent of striatocapsular infarcts, via occlusion of the lenticulostriate artery or the recurrent artery of Hubener, was hypothesized to produce a range of possible language deficits. Indeed, cortical hypoperfusion has been identified with blood-flow-imaging techniques in a variety of studies of aphasia associated with subcortical lesions (Metter *et al.*, 1983; Skyhoj Olsen *et al.*, 1986; Vallar *et al.*, 1988; Demonet *et al.*, 1992; Okuda *et al.*, 1994; Lim *et al.*, 1998; Hillis *et al.*, 2002, 2004; Radanovic and Scaff, 2003). Of particular interest, Hillis *et al.* (2002) revealed 100% (28/28) of patients with subcortical lesions and the presence of aphasia to demonstrate cortical hypoperfusion, using diffusion- and perfusion-weighted imaging techniques. In contrast, 0% (0/12) of patients in the same study with subcortical lesions and no aphasia demonstrated cortical hypoperfusion. Furthermore, in a follow-on study of 24 subjects with left caudate lesions subsequent to infarct, deficits in language and speech were associated with hypoperfusion in specific cortical regions (Hillis *et al.*, 2004). Four subjects were classified as having Broca's aphasia, four subjects with Wernicke's aphasia, two with global aphasia, two with anomic aphasia and the remainder of the sample (12) grouped with unclassifiable aphasia (i.e. mixture of fluent and non-fluent language deficits). Aphasia classifications were generally associated with areas of cortical hypoperfusion. For example, Broca's aphasia was associated with hypoperfusion of the posterior inferior frontal gyrus but not the superior temporal gyrus. Wernicke's aphasia was associated with hypoperfusion of the superior temporal gyrus and not the posterior inferior frontal gyrus. Of additional interest, when blood flow was able to be restored within hypoperfused cortical regions, associated aphasia resolved despite an absence of change to the subcortical lesion itself. These results suggest that variations in language profiles seen following subcortical lesions, at least in the case of non-thalamic infarcts, may be attributed to differences in areas of cortical hypoperfusion as a consequence of large-vessel (principally the middle cerebral artery) stenosis or occlusion, independent of the subcortical lesions themselves.

In all, the validity of the aforementioned operative models of subcortical participation in language remains unattested, largely attributed to a previous incapacity to strictly define vascular neuropathology. A further encumbrance to empirical ratification rests with the inadequacy of animal models in providing an appropriate linguistic platform for investigation (Crosson, 1992). The value of model-driven and theoretically founded studies of cognition cannot be overestimated in quests to extricate the subcortico-cortical mechanisms underpinning language (Cappa and Sterzi, 1990). The utilization of existing frameworks, however, in the context of advancing scientific techniques is considered critical to their ultimate interpretation (Crosson *et al.*, 1997b). In line with this proposal, a recent resurgence in functional neurosurgery to treat Parkinson's disease, involving the generation of discrete surgically induced lesions of the subcortical nuclei (Speelman and Bosch, 1998), currently provides an unprecedented opportunity to empirically test contemporary theories of subcortical participation in language.

Directions for future research: Parkinson's disease as a platform for ratifying subcortical language theories

As previously defined in Chapter 2, Parkinson's disease results from nigrostriatal dopaminergic cell degeneration. Reduced dopamine levels have been documented to detrimentally influence the flow of activity through basal ganglia circuits (Kopell *et al.*, 2006). In summary, deficient nigrostriatal dopamine levels observed in Parkinson's disease result in an activity imbalance within dopamine-regulated pathways of the basal ganglia, namely a net increase in indirect pathway activity and a decrease in direct pathway activity (DeLong, 1990) (see Figure 10.2). This change in activity subsequently results in disinhibition or hyperactivity of inhibitory GPi-SNr outputs, causing excessive inhibition or 'braking' of thalamocortical and brain-stem neurones (Kopell *et al.*, 2006). Clinically, these changes in circuitry activity typically manifest as motor symptoms including resting tremor, akinesia, rigidity and postural instability (Lang and Lozano, 1998b; Starr *et al.*, 1998). However, non-motor phenomena have also been reported and include executive dysfunction, apathy and personality changes (Wichmann and DeLong, 1998), as well as high-level language dysfunction (Lewis *et al.*, 1998).

Over the course of the last 17 years, primate research has served to catalyse the development of theoretical frameworks which define the pathophysiology underlying Parkinson's disease (Obeso *et al.*, 2000). An enhanced conceptualization of basal ganglia function has been subsequently accompanied by a revision of available treatment options for people with Parkinson's disease, including neurosurgical procedures (Speelman and Bosch, 1998). The revival of functional stereotactic neurosurgical techniques has been hailed as the most significant therapeutic development in the treatment of Parkinson's disease since the introduction of levodopa (Quinn, 1999). In addition to their potent therapeutic value, these procedures also offer a platform for the empirical validation of subcortical language theories.

Neurosurgical interventions utilized in the treatment of Parkinson's disease

Prior to the clinical inception of levodopa in 1961 (Benabid *et al.*, 1998), functional neurosurgical techniques constituted the primary therapeutic armamentarium against Parkinson's disease for nearly 50 years (Speelman and Bosch, 1998). As summarized by Periera and Aziz (2006), it was Parkinson himself who initially discovered that neurological disruption (i.e. stroke) in Parkinson's disease patients could ameliorate associated motor symptoms (Parkinson, 1817). The basal ganglia were not specifically implicated in Parkinson's disease until 1868 by Hughlings Jackson (Jackson, 1868), and then again by Hunt (1917), who suggested that basal ganglia lesions could cause Parkinsonism, among other movement disorders. Such experimental evidence provided the catalyst to utilize surgical lesions as a potential means of treating Parkinson's disease throughout the first half of the twentieth century (Pereira and Aziz, 2006). In addition to the spine and motor cortex, the majority of early surgical approaches targeted the basal ganglia, with minimal clinical benefit reported, however, clarified which components of the neural axis were influential or in fact not implicated in Parkinson's disease (Pereira and Aziz, 2006).

A turning point in the surgical treatment of Parkinson's disease occurred in 1952 (Espay *et al.*, 2006), whereby the accidental ligation of the anterior choroidal artery in a Parkinson's disease patient resulted in infarction of the globus pallidus and the subsequent resolution of motor symptoms (Cooper, 1953). This finding then lead to the practice of injecting alcohol into the globus pallidus as a means of relieving Parkinsonian symptoms. Then, in 1947, the first stereotactic head frame which permitted the precise localization of brain targets, as opposed to utilizing skull landmarks, heralded a new era in the accuracy of ablative surgery (Spiegel *et al.*, 1947). Indeed, utilizing the stereotactic head frame, Leksell in 1949 successfully relieved bradykinesia and rigidity in excess of 200 Parkinson's patients by lesioning the posteroventral portion of the globus pallidus internus via a thermocoagulation technique (Leksell, 1949; Svennilson *et al.*, 1960; Laitinen, 2000). This was followed by the introduction of thalamic lesioning in the 1950s demonstrated to relieve tremor and rigidity with more reliable results than pallidotomy (Hassler and Riechert, 1954). Consequently, thalamotomy became the most popular surgical technique for treating Parkinson's disease until the 1970s, when levodopa was established as the mainstay of Parkinsonian therapy (Pereira and Aziz, 2006).

Levodopa is a pharmacological precursor to dopamine (Pfann *et al.*, 1997) administered to patients as a drug therapy. Despite its recognized potency with respect to relieving motor deficits associated with Parkinson's disease, the effectiveness of levodopa deteriorates over time and chronic use has been linked to a number of disabling side effects (Brin, 1998). Long-term contraindications include the development of motor fluctuations (i.e. erratic on/off states) and peak-dose dyskinesias. A resurgence of interest in neurosurgical interventions for the treatment of Parkinson's disease during the mid-1970s (Gildenberg, 1984) was prompted by the recognized limitations of dopaminergic pharmacotherapy, as well as technological advancements in surgical and neuroimaging capabilities which proffered enhanced mechanical accuracy and brain resolution (Obeso *et al.*, 1997), relative to formative techniques. The alleviation of neurological deficits represents the principle objective of functional neurosurgical procedures, which typically involve the generation of circumscribed lesions or active stimulation of the brain or spinal cord (Bosch, 1986).

Initially, the most commonly applied functional neurosurgical techniques in the treatment of Parkinsonian symptoms involved the generation of ablative lesions within the thalamus and globus pallidus (to be discussed in Chapter 5) (Lang *et al.*, 1997; Lozano and Lang, 1998; Moro *et al.*, 1999; Kleiner-Fisman *et al.*, 2003; Vitek *et al.*, 2003). Although seemingly counter-intuitive (Pereira and Aziz, 2006), lesioning of overactive subcortical nuclei was hypothesized to re-establish normal activity within relevant neural circuits (Moro and Lang, 2006). Despite evident benefits of these procedures in relieving symptoms of Parkinson's disease, they were also associated with a number of side effects: increased risk when performed bilaterally, absent post-operative decrease in dopaminergic medications and a loss in long-term surgical benefit (Moro and Lang, 2006). In the 1990s, a procedure involving high-frequency electrical stimulation of brain targets (deep-brain stimulation) was documented to produce the same effects as those of ablative lesions (Benabid and Pollak, 1991), with the added advantage of being reversible. This technique now provides an alternative to ablative lesions that has become the surgical norm as opposed to the exception, and will be discussed in detail in Chapter 6. In light of the evident limitations associated with vascular infarct populations in testing contemporary theories of subcortical participation in language, the effects of surgically induced circumscribed lesions of the thalamus and basal ganglia in Parkinsonian patients will be examined in detail in the ensuing chapters (see Chapters 5 and 6).

Summary

Although the concept of subcortical aphasia remains controversial, recent years have seen a growing acceptance of a role for subcortical structures in language. Although the precise nature of that role remains elusive, attempts to explain the clinical manifestations of subcortical aphasia have culminated in the formulation of several theories of subcortical participation in language. These theories, largely developed on the basis of language data collected from subjects who have sustained cerebrovascular accidents involving the thalamus or striatocapsular region, have been expressed as neuroanatomically based models. The most influential of these models include the Subcortical White Matter Pathways model, the RRSF model, the LDM model and the Selective Engagement model. Although each of these models have a number of limitations, they do serve as frameworks for generating experimental hypotheses which can be tested to advance our understanding of subcortical brain mechanisms in language.

References

Afifi, A.K. and Bergman, R.A. (2005). *Functional Neuroanatomy: Text and Atlas*. New York: Lange Medical Books/McGraw-Hill.

Alexander, G.E. and LoVerme, S.R. (1980). Aphasia after left hemisphere intracerebral haemorrhage. *Neurology* 30, 1193–1202.

Alexander, G.E. and DeLong, M.R. (1985a). Microstimulation of the primate neostriatum. I. Physiological properties of striatal microexcitable zones. *Journal of Neurophysiology* 53, 1417–32.

Alexander, G.E. and DeLong, M.R. (1985b). Microstimulation of the primate neostriatum. II. Somatotopic organisation of striatal microexcitable zones and their relation to neuronal response properties. *Journal of Neurophysiology* 53, 1433–46.

Alexander, G.E., DeLong, M.R. and Strick, P.L. (1986). Parallel organisation of functionally segregated circuits linking basal ganglia and cortex. *Annual Review of Neuroscience* 9, 357–81.

Alexander, G.E., Naeser, M.A. and Palumbo, C.L. (1987). Correlations of subcortical CT lesion sites and aphasia profiles. *Brain* 110, 961–91.

Alexander, G.E., Crutcher, M.D. and DeLong, M.R. (1990). Basal ganglia-thalamocortical circuits: parallel substrates for motor, oculomotor, "prefrontal" and "limbic" functions. *Progress in Brain Research* 85, 119–46.

Asanuma, C., Anderson, R.A. and Cowan, W.M. (1985). The thalamic relations of the caudal inferior parietal lobule and the lateral prefrontal cortex in monkeys: divergent cortical projections from cell clusters in the medial pulvinar nucleus. *Journal of Comparative Neurology* 241, 357–81.

Astrup, J., Siesjo, B.K. and Symon, L. (1981). Thresholds in cerebral ischemia-The Ischemic Penumbra. *Stroke* 12, 723–5.

Benabid, A. and Pollak, P. (1991). Long-term suppression of tremor by chronic stimulation of the ventral internediate thalamic nucleus. *Lancet* 337, 403–6.

Benabid, A., Caparros-Lefebvre, D. and Pollak, P. (1998). History of surgery for movement disorders. In I. Germano (ed.), *Neurosurgical Treatment of Movement Disorders* (pp. 19–35). Park Ridge, IL: Thieme.

Bogousslavsky, J., Regli, F. and Uske, A. (1988). Thalamic infarcts: clinical syndromes, aetiology and prognosis. *Neurology* 38, 837–48.

Boivin, M.J., Giordani, B., Berent, S., Amato, D.A., Lehtinen, S. *et al.* (1992). Verbal fluency and positron emission tomographic mapping of regional cerebral glucose metabolism. *Cortex* 28, 231–9.

Bosch, D.A. (1986). *Stereotactic Techniques in Clinical Neurosurgery*. New York: Springer-Verlag.

Brin, M.F. (1998). Pharmacological treatment of movement disorders. In I. Germano (ed.), *Neurosurgical Treatment of Movement Disorders* (pp. 83–104). Park Ridge, IL: Thieme.

Brunner, R.J., Kornhuber, H.H., Seemuller, E., Suger, G. and Wallesch, C.-W. (1982). Basal ganglia participation in language pathology. *Brain and Language* 16, 281–99.

Buckingham, H.W. (1987). Phonemic paraphasias and psycholinguistic production models for neologistic jargon. *Aphasiology* 1, 381–400.

Campos-Ortega, J.A. and Cluver, P.F. (1969). The cortico-thalamic projections from the sensorimotor cortex of galago crassicaudatus. *Journal of Comparative Neurology* 136, 397–418.

Cappa, S.F. and Vignolo, L.A. (1979). Transcortical features of aphasia following left thalamic haemorrhage. *Cortex* 15, 121–30.

Cappa, S.F. and Sterzi, R. (1990). Infarction in the territory of the anterior choroidal artery: a cause of transcortical motor aphasia. *Aphasiology* 4, 213–17.

Cappa, S.F. and Vallar, G. (1992). Neuropsychological disorders after subcortical lesions: implications for neural models of language and spatial attention. In G. Vallar, S. Cappa, F. and C.-W. Wallesch (eds), *Neuropsychological Disorders Associated with Subcortical Lesions* (pp. 7–41). Oxford: Oxford University Press.

Cappa, S.F. and Wallesch, C.-W. (1994). Subcortical lesions and cognitive deficits. In A. Kertesz (ed.), *Localisation and Neuroimaging in Neuropsychology* (pp. 545–66). San Diego: Academic Press.

Cohen, J.A., Gelfer, C.E. and Sweet, R.P. (1980). Thalamic infarction producing aphasia. *Mt Sinai Journal of Medicine* 47, 398–404.

Cooper, I.S. (1953). Ligation of the anterior choroidal artery for involuntary movements: Parkinsonism. *Psychiatric Quarterly* 27, 317–19.

Crosson, B. (1984). Role of the dominant thalamus in language: a review. *Psychological Bulletin* 96, 491–517.

Crosson, B. (1985). Subcortical functions in language: a working model. *Brain and Language* 25, 257–92.

Crosson, B. (1992). *Subcortical Functions in Language and Memory*. New York: The Guilford Press.

Crosson, B. (1999). Subcortical mechanisms in language: lexical-semantic mechanisms and the thalamus. *Brain and Cognition* 40, 414–39.

Crosson, B. and Early, T.A. (1990). *A Theory of Subcortical Functions in Language: Review and Critique*. Unpublished manuscript.

Crosson, B. and Nadeau, S.E. (1998). The role of subcortical structures in linguistic processes: recent developments. In B. Stemmer and H.A. Whitaker (eds), Handbook of neurolinguistics (pp. 431–45). San Diego: Academic Press.

Crosson, B., Moberg, P.J., Boone, J.R., Rothi, L.J.G. and Raymer, A.M. (1997a). Category-specific naming deficit for medical terms after dominant thalamic/capsular haemorrhage. *Brain and Language* 29, 301–14.

Crosson, B., Zawacki, T., Brinson, G., Lu, L. and Sadek, J.R. (1997b). Models of subcortical functions in language: current status. *Journal of Neurolinguistics* 10(4), 277–300.

Crosson, B., Rao, S.M., Woodley, S.J., Rosen, A.C., Bobholz, J.A. *et al.* (1999). Mapping of semantic, phonological and orthographic verbal working memory in normal adults with funtional magnetic resonance imaging. *Neuropsychology* 13, 171–87.

Cummings, J.L. (1993). Frontal-subcortical circuits and human behaviour. *Archives of Neurology* 50, 873–80.

Damasio, A.R., Damasio, H., Rizzo, M., Varney, N. and Gersh, F. (1982). Aphasia with non-hemorrhagic lesions in the basal ganglia and internal capsule. *Archives of Neurology* 29, 15–20.

DeLong, M.R. (1990). Primate models of movement disorders of basal ganglia origin. *Trends in Neuroscience* 13, 281–5.

DeLong, M.R. and Georgopoulos, A.P. (1981). Motor functions of the basal ganglia. In J.M. Brookhart, V.B. Mountcastle and V.B. Brooks (eds), *Handbook of Physiology*, vol. 2 (pp. 1017–61). Betheseda: American Physiology Society.

Demonet, J.-F., Celsis, P., Puel, M., Cardebat, D., Marc-Vergnes, J.P. *et al.* (1992). Thalamic and non-thalamic subcortical aphasia: a neurolinguistic and SPECT approach. In G. Vallar, S.F. Cappa and C.-W.

Wallesch (eds), *Neuropsychological Disorders Associated with Subcortical Lesions* (pp. 397–411). New York: Oxford University Press.

DeMyer, W. (1998). *Neuroanatomy*, 2nd edn. Baltimore: Williams and Wilkins.

DeWitt, L.D., Grek, A.J., Buonanno, F.S., Levine, D.N. and Kistler, J.P. (1985). MRI and the study of aphasia. *Neurology* 35, 861–5.

Divac, I., Oberg, G.E. and Rosenkilde, C.E. (1987). Patterned neural activity: implications for neurology and neuropharmacology. In J.S. Schneider and T.I. Lidsky (eds), *Basal Ganglia and Behaviour: Sensory Aspects of Motor Functioning* (pp. 61–7). New York: Hans Huber.

Eccles, J.C. (1977). *The Self and its Brain*. New York: Springer.

Espay, A.J., Mandybur, G.T. and Revilla, F.J. (2006). Surgical treatment of movement disorders. *Clinics in Geriatric Medicine* 22, 813–25.

Fox, M.W., Ahlskog, J.E. and Kelly, P.J. (1991). Stereotaxic ventrolateralis thalamotomy for medically refractory tremor in post-levodopa era Parkinson's disease patients. *Journal of Neurosurgery* 75, 723–30.

Gentilini, M., De Renzi, E. and Crisi, G. (1987). Bilateral paramedian thalamic artery infarcts: report of eight cases. *Journal of Neurology Neurosurgery and Psychiatry* 50, 900–9.

Gildenberg, P.L. (1984). The present role of stereotactic surgery in the management of Parkinson's disease. In R.G. Hassler and J.F. Christ (eds), *Advances in Neurology*, vol. 40 (pp. 447–52). New York: Raven Press.

Goldenberg, G., Wimmer, A. and Maly, J. (1983). Amnesic syndrome with a unilateral thalamic lesions: a case report. *Journal of Neurology* 229, 79–86.

Goldman-Rakic, P.S. and Selemon, L.D. (1986). Topography of corticostriatal projections in non-human primates and implications for functional parcellation of the neostriatum. In E.G. Jones and A. Peters (eds), *Cerebral Cortex: Sensory-Motor Areas and Aspects of Cortical Connectivity*, vol. 5 (pp. 447–66). New York: Plenum Press.

Goldman-Rakic, P.S. and Selemon, L.D. (1990). New frontiers in basal ganglia research. *Trends in Neuroscience* 13, 241–4.

Goodglass, H. (1993). *Understanding Aphasia*. San Diego: Academic Press.

Graff-Radford, N.R., Eslinger, P.J., Damasio, A.R. and Yamada, T. (1984). Nonhaemorrhagic infarction of the thalamus: behaviour, anatomic and physiological correlates. *Neurology* 34, 14–23.

Groves, P.M. (1983). A theory of the functional organisation of the neostriatum and neostriatal control of voluntary movement. *Brain Research Review* 5, 109–32.

Hassler, R. and Riechert, T. (1954). Indikationen und lokalisations methode der gezielten hirnoperationene. *Nervenarzt* 25, 441.

Hillis, A., Kane, A., Tuffiash, A., Ulatowski, J.A., Barker, P. *et al.* (2002). Reperfusion of specific brain regions by raising blood pressure restores selective language functions in subacute stroke. *Brain and Language* 79, 495–510.

Hillis, A., Baker, P.B., Wityk, R.J., Aldrich, E.M., Restrepo, L. *et al.* (2004). Variability in subcortical aphasia is due to variable sites of cortical hypoperfursion. *Brain and Language* 89, 524–30.

Hunt, R. (1917). Progressive atrophy of the globus pallidus: a contribution to the functions of the corpus striatum. *Brain* 40, 58–148.

Jackson, J.H. (1868). Observations on the physiology and pathology of hemichorea. *Edinburgh Medical Journal* 14, 294–303.

Jackson, J.H. (1932). *Selected Writing*. London: Hodder and Stoughton.

Jonas, S. (1982). The thalamus and aphasia including transcortical aphasia: a review. *Journal of Communication Disorders* 15, 31–41.

Jones, E. (1985). The thalamus. New York: Plenum Press.

Kennedy, M. and Murdoch, B. (1989). Speech and language disorders subsequent to subcortical vascular lesions. *Aphasiology* 3, 221–47.

Kirshner, H.S. (1991). Language disorders. In W.G. Bradley, R.B. Daroff, G.M. Fenichel and D.C. Marsden (eds), *Neurology in Clinical Practice: Principles of Diagnosis and Management*, vol. 1 (pp. 101–15). Boston: Butterworth-Heineman.

Kleiner-Fisman, G., Fisman, D.N. and Sime, E. (2003). Long-term follow up of bilateral deep brain stimulation of the subthalamic nucleus in patients with advanced Parkinson's disease. *Journal of Neurosurgery* 99, 489–95.

Kocsis, J.D., Sugimori, M. and Kitai, S.T. (1977). Convergence of excitatory synaptic inputs to caudate spiny neurons. *Brain Research* 124, 403–13.

Kopell, B.H., Rezai, A., Chang, J.-W. and Vitek, J.L. (2006). Anatomy and physiology of the basal ganglia: implications for deep brain stimulation for Parkinson's disease. *Movement Disorders* 21 (suppl. 14), 238–46.

Kushner, M., Reivich, M., Fieschi, C., Silver, F., Chawluk, J. *et al.* (1987). Metabolic and clinical correlations of acute ischaemic infarction. *Neurology* 37, 1103–10.

Laitinen, L.V. (2000). Leksell's unpublished pallidotomies of 1958–1962. *Stereotactic and Functional Neurosurgery* 74, 1–10.

Lang, A.E. and Lozano, A.M. (1998a). Medical progress: Parkinson's disease (Part II of II). *New England Journal of Medicine* 339, 1130–43.

Lang, A.E. and Lozano, A.M. (1998b). Parkinson's disease (Part I of II). *New England Journal of Medicine* 339, 1044–53.

Lang, A.E., Lozano, A.M., Montgomery, E., Duff, J., Tasker, R. *et al.* (1997). Posteroventral medial pallidotomy in advanced Parkinson's disease. *New England Journal of Medicine* 337, 1036–42.

Lassen, N.A., Olsen, T., Hojgaard, K. and Skriver, E. (1983). Incomplete infarction: a CT negative irreversible ischaemic brain lesion. *Journal of Cerebral Blood Flow and Metabolism* 3 (suppl. 1), 602–3.

Lecours, A.R., Tainturier, M.-J. and Boeglin, J. (1988). Classification of aphasia. In F.C. Rose, R. Whurr and M.A. Wyke (eds), *Aphasia* (pp. 3–22). London: Whurr Publishers Ltd.

Leksell, L. (1949). A stereotaxic apparatus for intracerebral surgery. *Acta Chirurgica Scandanivica* 99, 229–33.

Lewis, F.M., LaPointe, L.L., Murdoch, B.E. and Chenery, H.J. (1998). Language impairment in Parkinson's disease. *Aphasiology* 12(3), 193–206.

Lhermitte, F. (1984). Language disorders and their relationship to thalamic lesions. *Advances in Neurology* 42, 99–113.

Lichtheim, L. (1885). On aphasia. *Brain* 7, 433–84.

Lim, J.S., Ryu, Y.H. and Lee, J.D. (1998). Crossed cerebellar diaschisis due to intracranial hematoma in basal ganglia or thalamus. *Journal of Nuclear Medicine* 39, 2044–7.

Livingstone, M.S. and Hubel, D.H. (1981). Effects of sleep and arousal on the processing of visual information in the cat. *Nature* 291, 554–61.

Lozano, A.M. and Lang, A.E. (1998). Pallidotomy for Parkinson's disease. *Neurosurgical Clinics of North America* 9, 325–36.

Lucchelli, F. and De Renzi, E. (1992). Proper name anomia. *Cortex* 28, 221–30.

Malamut, B.L., Graff-Radford, N.R., Chawluk, J., Grossman, R.I. and Gur, R.C. (1992). Memory in a case of bilateral thalamic infarction. *Neurology* 42, 163–9.

Malapani, C., Pillon, B., Dubois, B. and Agid, Y. (1994). Impaired simultaneous cognitive task performance in Parkinson's disease: a dopamine-related dysfunction. *Neurology* 44, 319–26.

Martin, W.R.W. and Raichle, M.E. (1983). Cerebellar blood flow and metabolism in cerebral hemispheric infarction. *Annals of Neurology* 14, 168–76.

Matzke, H.A. and Foltz, F.M. (1983). *Synopsis of Neuroanatomy*, 4th edn. Oxford: Oxford University Press.

McClelland, J.L., Rummelhart, D.E. and Group, P.R. (1986). *Parallel Distributed Processing*. Cambridge, MA: MIT Press.

McCormick, D.A. and Feeser, H.R. (1990). Functional impications of burst firing and single spike activity in lateral geniculate relay neurons. *Neuroscience* 39, 103–13.

McFarling, D., Rothi, L.J.G. and Heilman, K.M. (1982). Transcortical aphasia from ischaemic infarcts of the thalamus: a report of two cases. *Journal of Neurology Neurosurgery and Psychiatry* 45, 107–12.

Mega, M.S. and Alexander, M.P. (1994). Subcortical aphasia: the core profile of capsulostriatal infarction. *Neurology* 44, 1824–9.

Mega, M.S. and Cummings, J.L. (1994). Frontal-subcortical circuits and neuropsychiatric disorders. *Journal of Neuropsychiatry and Clinical Neurosciences* 6, 358–70.

Metter, E.J. (1987). Neuroanatomy and physiology of aphasia: evidence from positron emission tomography. *Aphasiology* 1, 3–33.

Metter, E.J., Riege, W.H., Hanson, W.R., Kuhl, D.E., Phelps, M.E. *et al.* (1983). Comparisons of metabolic rates, language and memory in subcortical aphasia. *Brain and Language* 19, 33–47.

Mohr, J.P., Watters, W.C. and Duncan, G.W. (1975). Thalamic haemorrhage and aphasia. *Brain and Language* 2, 3–17.

Moro, E. and Lang, A.E. (2006). Criteria for deep brain stimulation in Parkinson's disease: review and analysis. *Expert Review of Neurotherapeutics* 6(11), 1695–1705.

Moro, E., Scerrati, M., Romito, L.M.A., Roselli, R., Tonali, P. *et al.* (1999). Chronic subthalamic nucleus stimulation reduces medication requirements in Parkinson's disease. *Neurology* 53, 85–90.

Murdoch, B. (1987). Aphasia following right thalamic haemorrhage in a dextral. *Journal of Communication Disorders* 20, 459–68.

Murdoch, B. (1990). Subcortical aphasia syndromes. In *Acquired Speech and Language Disorders: a Neuroanatomical and Functional Neurological Approach* (pp. 97–119). London: Chapman and Hall.

Murdoch, B. (1996). The role of subcortical structures in language: clinico-neuroradiological studies of brain-damaged subjects. In B. Dodd, R. Campbell and L. Worrall (eds), *Evaluating Theories of Language: Evidence from Disordered Communication* (pp. 137–60). London: Whurr Publishers.

Murdoch, B., Thompson, D., Fraser, S. and Harrison, L. (1986). Aphasia following non-haemorrhagic lesions in the left striato-capsular region. *Australian Journal of Human Communciation Disorders* 14(2), 5–21.

Murdoch, B., Kennedy, M., McCallum, W. and Siddle, K.J. (1991). Persistent aphasia following a purely subcortical lesion. *Aphasiology* 5, 183–97.

Nadeau, S.E. and Crosson, B. (1997a). Subcortical aphasia. *Brain and Language* 58, 355–402.

Nadeau, S.E. and Crosson, B. (1997b). Subcortical aphasia: response to reviews. *Brain and Language* 58, 436–58.

Nadeau, S.E., Jordan, J.E. and Mishra, S.K. (1993). A prospective evaluation of the utility of clinical data in distinguishing acute large vessel from lacunar cerebral infarctions. *Journal of Stroke and Cerebrovascular Disease* 3, 231–9.

Naeser, M.A., Alexander, G.E., Helm-Estabrooks, N., Levine, H.L., Laughlin, S.A. *et al.* (1982). Aphasia with predominantly subcortical lesion sites: description of three capsular/putaminal aphasia syndromes. *Archives of Neurology* 39, 2–14.

Naeser, M.A., Palumbo, C.L., Helm-Estabrooks, N., Stiassny-Eder, D. and Albert, M.L. (1989). Severe non-fluency in aphasia: role of the medical subcallocal fasciculus and other white matter pathways in the recovery of spontaneous speech. *Brain* 112, 1–38.

Nauta, H.J.W. (1979). A proposed conceptual reorganisation of the basal ganglia and telencephalon. *Neuroscience* 4, 1875–81.

Nolte, J. (1993). *The Human Brain: an Introduction to its Functional Anatomy*, 3rd edn. St Louis: Mosby-Year Book.

Obeso, J.A., Guridi, J. and DeLong, M.R. (1997). Surgery for Parkinson's disease. *Journal of Neurology Neurosurgery and Psychiatry* 62(1), 2–8.

Obeso, J.A., Rodriguez-Oroz, M.C., Rodriguez, M., Macias, R., Alvarez, L. *et al.* (2000). Pathophysiologic basis of surgery for Parkinson's disease. *Neurology* 55 (suppl. 6), S7–12.

Ojemann, G. (1976). Subcortical language mechanisms. In H.A. Whitaker and H. Whitaker (eds), *Studies in Neurolinguistics* (pp. 103–38). New York: Academic Press.

Ojemann, G.A. (1983). Brain organisation for language from the perspective of electrical stimulation mapping. *Behavioral and Brain Sciences* 2, 189–230.

Okuda, B., Tanaka, H., Tachibana, H., Kawabata, K. and Sugita, M. (1994). Cerebral blood flow in subcortical global aphasia: perisylvian cortical hypoperfusion as a crucial role. *Stroke* 25, 1495–9.

Parkinson, J. (1817). *An Essay on the Shaking Palsy*. London: Sherwood Neely and Jones.

Perani, D., Vallar, G., Cappa, S.F., Messa, C. and Fazio, F. (1987). Aphasia and neglect after subcortical stroke: a clinical/cerebral perfusion correlation study. *Brain* 110, 1211–29.

Pereira, E.A.C. and Aziz, T. (2006). Surgical insights into Parkinson's disease. *Journal of the Royal Society of Medicine* 99, 238–44.

Pfann, K.D., Shannon, K.M., Penn, R.D. and Corcos, D.M. (1997). Motor consequences of neurosurgical interventions in Parkinson's disease. *Neurology Report* 21(4), 109–16.

Phillips, C.G. and Porter, R. (1977). *Corticospinal Neurones*. London: Academic Press.

Phillips, C.G., Zeki, S. and Barlow, H.B. (1984). Localisation of function in the cerebral cortex. *Brain* 107, 327–62.

Pujol, J., Vendrell, P., Deus, J., Kulisevsky, J., Marti-Vilalta, J.L. *et al.* (1996). Frontal lobe activation during word generation studied by functional MRI. *Acta Neurologica Scandanivica* 93, 403–10.

Pulvermuller, F., Hauk, O., Nikulin, V.V. and Ilmoniemi, R.J. (2005). Functional links between motor and language systems. *European Journal of Neuroscience* 21, 793–7.

Quinn, N. (1999). Progress in functional neurosurgery for parkinson's disease. *Lancet* 354, 1658–9.

Radanovic, M. and Scaff, M. (2003). Speech and language disturbances due to subcortical lesions. *Brain and Language* 84, 337–52.

Raymer, A.M., Moberg, P.J., Crosson, B., Nadeau, S.E. and Rothi, L.J.G. (1997). Lexical-semantic deficits in two cases of thalamic lesion. *Neuropsychologia* 35, 211–19.

Reivich, M., Alavi, A., Gur, R.C. and Greenberg, J. (1985). Determination of local cerebral glucose metabolism in humans: methodology and applications to the study of sensory and cognitive stimuli. *Research Publications: Association for Research in Nervous and Mental Disease* 63, 105–19.

Robin, D.A. and Schienberg, S. (1990). Subcortical lesions and aphasia. *Journal of Speech and Hearing Disorders* 55, 90–100.

Scheibel, M.E. and Scheibel, A.B. (1972). Specialised organisational patterns within the nucleus reticularis thalami of the cat. *Experimental Neurology* 34, 316–22.

Skinner, J.E. and Yingling, C.D. (1977). Central gating mechanisms that regulate event-related potentials and behaviour. In J.E. Desmedt (ed.), *Attention, Voluntary Contraction and Event-Related Cerebral Potentials* (pp. 30–69). Basel: Karger.

Skyhoj Olsen, T., Bruhn, P. and Oberg, G.E. (1986). Cortical hypoperfusion as a possible cause of 'subcortical aphasia'. *Brain* 109, 393–410.

Sokoloff, L. (1977). Relation between physiological function and energy metabolism in the central nervous system. *Journal of Neurochemistry* 29, 13–26.

Speelman, J.D. and Bosch, D.A. (1998). Resurgence of functional neurosurgery for Parkinson's disease: a historical perspective. *Movement Disorders* 13(3), 582–8.

Spencer, H.J. (1976). Antagonism of cortical excitation of striatal neurons by glutamic acid diethyl ester: evidence for glutamic acid as an excitatory transmitter in the rat striatum. *Brain Research* 102, 91–101.

Spiegel, E.A., Wycis, H.T., Marks, M. and Lee, A J. (1947). Stereotaxic apparatus for operations on the human brain. *Science* 106, 349–50.

Starr, P.A., Vitek, J.L. and Bakay, R.A.E. (1998). Ablative surgery and deep brain stimulation for Parkinson's disease. *Neurosurgery* 43(5), 989–1015.

Steriade, M., Jones, E. and Llinas, R.R. (1990). *Thalamic Oscillations and Signaling.* New York: Wiley.

Steriade, M. and Llinas, R.R. (1988). The functional states of the thalamus and associated neuronal interplay. *Physiology Reviews* 68, 649–742.

Steriade, M., Parent, A. and Hada, J. (1984). Thalamic projections of nucleus reticularis thalami of cat: a study using retrograde transport of horseradish perioxidase and flourescent tracers. *Journal of Comparative Neurology* 229, 531–47.

Svennilson, E., Torvik, A., Lowe, R. and Leksell, L. (1960). Treatment of Parkinsonism by stereotactic thermolesions in the pallidal region. *Acta Psychiatrica et Neurologica Scandinavia* 35, 358–77.

Szentagothai, J. (1975). The 'module-concept' in cerebral cortex architecture. *Brain Research* 95, 475–96.

Vallar, G., Perani, D., Cappa, S.F., Messa, C., Lenzi, G.L. *et al.* (1988). Recovery from aphasia and neglect after subcortical stroke: neuropsychological and cerebral perfusion study. *Journal of Neurology Neurosurgery and Psychiatry* 51, 1269–76.

Van Buren, J.M. (1963). Confusion and disturbance of speech from stimulation in the vicinity of the caudate nucleus. *Journal of Neurosurgery* 20, 148–57.

Van Buren, J.M. (1966). Evidence regarding a more precise localisation of the posterior fronto-caudate arrest response in man. *Journal of Neurosurgery* 24, 416–17.

Van Buren, J.M. and Borke, R.C. (1969). Alterations in speech and the pulvinar: a serial section study of cerebrothalamic relationships in cases of acquired speech disorders. *Brain* 92, 255–84.

Van Hoesen, G.W., Yeterian, E.H. and Lavizzo-Mourey, R. (1981). Widespread cortico-striate projections from temporal cortex of the rhesus monkey. *Journal of Comparative Neurology* 199, 205–19.

Vitek, J.L., Bakay, R.A.E. and Freeman, A. (2003). Randomised trial of pallidotomy versus medical therapy for Parkinson's disease. *Annals of Neurology* 53, 558–69.

Von Monakow, C. (1969). Diaschisis. In K.H. Pribram (ed.), *Brain and Behaviour I: Mood States and Mind* (pp. 27–36). Baltimore: Penguin [1914 article translated by G. Harris].

Wallesch, C.-W. (1985). Two syndromes of aphasia occurring with ischaemic lesions involving the left basal ganglia. *Brain and Language* 25, 357–61.

Wallesch, C.-W. (1990). Repetitive verbal behaviour: functional and neurological considerations. *Aphasiology* 4, 133–54.

Wallesch, C.-W. (1997). Symptomatology of subcortical aphasia. *Journal of Neurolinguistics* 10(4), 267–75.

Wallesch, C.-W. and Papagno, C. (1988). Subcortical aphasia. In F.C. Rose, R. Whurr and M.A. Wyke (eds), *Aphasia* (pp. 256–87). London: Whurr Publishers.

Wallesch, C.-W., Kornhuber, H.H., Brunner, R.J., Kunz, T., Hollerbach, B. *et al.* (1983). Lesions of the basal ganglia, thalamus and deep white matter: differential effects on language functions. *Brain and Language* 20, 286–304.

Weiller, C., Ringelstein, E.B., Reiche, W., Thron, A. and Buell, U. (1990). The large striatocapsular infarct. a clinical and pathophysiological entity. *Archives of Neurology* 47, 1085–91.

Wernicke, C. (1874). *Der aphasische symptomenkomplex.* Breslau: Kohn and Weigert.

Wichmann, T. and DeLong, M.R. (1998). Models of basal ganglia function and pathophysiology of movement disorders. *Neurosurgery Clinics of North America* 9(2), 223–36.

Wodarz, R. (1980). Watershed Infarctions and computed tomography: a topographical study in cases with stenosis or occlusion of the carotid artery. *Neuroradiology* 19, 245–8.

4 Language disorders associated with striatocapsular and thalamic lesions

Introduction

The primary avenue for investigating the role of subcortical brain structures in language has involved observation of 'experiments in nature'; namely, the clinico-neuroanatomical study of language function in individuals with vascular lesions involving the subcortical regions of the dominant hemisphere. Cerebrovascular accidents involving the subcortical region may be centred on either the striatocapsular region (head of the caudate nucleus, putamen, anterior limb of the internal capsule) or thalamus, as these two areas have differing blood supplies (see below). Consequently, the majority of studies which have attempted to explore the notion of subcortical participation in language have investigated the impact of vascular thalamic and striatocapsular lesions on linguistic abilities (Murdoch, 1990), giving rise to syndromes of thalamic and striatocapsular aphasia. Despite the fact that the aphasic symptom complex associated with thalamic lesions appears to approximate a more uniform syndrome than its striatocapsular counterpart, heterogeneity within each aphasic category has been documented with respect to language profiles and recovery rates (Murdoch, 1996). This inconsistency has been partly attributed to methodological limitations, including the wide-ranging scope of language assessments utilized and experimental designs employed.

Kennedy and Murdoch (1990) emphasized that general measures of language function typically utilized in the assessment of subcortical aphasia may have lacked the requisite sensitivity to detect more subtle, high-level linguistic deficits within this population. Furthermore, it has been suggested that the complexity of circulatory dynamics and the protean nature of spontaneous vascular lesions may also have contributed to the inherent variability of symptoms observed (Graff-Radford *et al.*, 1984). Therefore, prior to looking in detail at the variety of language disorders reported to occur in association with lesions in the striatocapsular region and thalamus, it is important to briefly revise the blood supply to these two areas.

Blood supply to the striatocapsular region and thalamus

The distribution of the anterior, middle and posterior cerebral arteries and their deep branches to the subcortical region was detailed in Chapter 2 and consequently will only be summarized here (see Figure 4.1). The medial and lateral striate (also called lenticulostriate) and the anterior choroidal arteries provide the blood supply to the internal capsule. The anterior limb is supplied primarily by the lateral striate branches

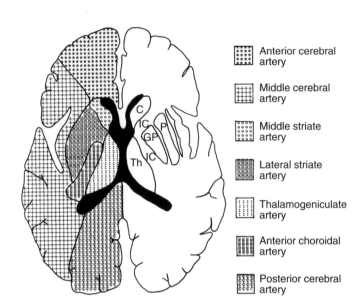

Figure 4.1 Horizontal section of the cerebral hemispheres showing the subcortical distribution of the anterior, middle and posterior cerebral arteries and branches. C, caudate nucleus; GP, globus pallidus; IC, internal capsule; P, putamen; Th, thalamus.

of the middle cerebral artery, the medial striate (also called the recurrent artery of Heubner) from the anterior cerebral artery supplying the rostral-medial tip. Blood supply to the genu comes via some direct branches from the internal carotid or from the lateral striate arteries. The posterior limb of the internal capsule is supplied partly by the anterior choroidal artery (internal carotid) and partly by the lateral striate arteries.

Arterial supply to the corpus striatum is mainly provided by the lateral striate arteries. Part of the head of the caudate nucleus, however, is provided with nourishment by the medial striate artery. Most of the putamen and the body of the caudate are supplied by the lateral striate arteries while the tail of the caudate and posterior portion of the putamen receive blood from the anterior choroidal artery. The majority of the globus pallidus is also supplied by this latter artery.

Whereas the striatocapsular region is supplied by branches of the middle and anterior cerebral arteries, branches of the posterior cerebral artery provide the major blood supply to the thalamus. The medial and anterior regions of the thalamus are supplied by the thalamo-perforating branches while the pulvinar (posterior portion of the thalamus) and lateral aspects of the thalamus are nourished by the thalamo-geniculate branches. The dorsal part of the thalamus is supplied by the posterior choroidal branches of the posterior cerebral artery. Some branches of the anterior choroidal artery are thought to pass to the lateral geniculate body.

Language disorders associated with thalamic lesions

The first clinicopathologic study of thalamic stroke was published by Dejerine and Roussy (1906), who emphasized sensorimotor disturbances. Twenty years later, cognitive deficits after isolated thalamic lesions were described by Hillemand (1925) and

Lhermitte (1936), with 'atypical' aphasia reported in patients with left thalamic lesions. Since that time, evidence to support a role for the thalamus in language function has come from studies of language changes due to surgical destruction and stimulation of thalamic targets as well as from observations of language disturbances following spontaneous thalamic lesions, including neoplastic, infectious and vascular lesions. In most reported cases of thalamic aphasia, the language disorder has been associated with thalamic haemorrhage (Fisher, 1959; Ciemens, 1970; Mohr et al., 1975; Kirshner and Kistler, 1982; Murdoch, 1987). A smaller number of cases has also been reported in association with thalamic tumours (Smyth and Stern, 1938; Cheek and Taveras, 1966), thalamic abscesses (Panchal et al., 1974) and more recently induced thalamic lesions (thalamotomy) for the treatment of Parkinson's disease (Whelan et al., 2002). Because most of these disorders (i.e. thalamic haemorrhage, tumour and abscess) are associated with a considerable mass effect, a number of authors have suggested that the accompanying language deficit may not be directly attributable to the localized damage to the thalamus per se (Mohr et al., 1975). Rather the observed language abnormalities may be the products of the effects of pressure and oedema on other areas of the brain, particularly the left cerebral hemisphere where the known speech and language centres are located. In other words, the aphasia associated with localized thalamic lesions reported in many studies may not be the direct product of thalamic destruction but rather the secondary product of pressure effects on other parts of the brain.

To some extent, the influence of extraneous factors such as pressure effects can be reduced by studying patients with ischaemic infarcts in the thalamus as these are associated with much smaller mass effects. Although rare, several authors have documented such cases of ischaemic infarcts of the thalamus (Gorelick et al., 1984; Graff-Radford et al., 1984) in association with language disorders. These findings lend support to the suggestion that aphasia subsequent to thalamic lesions is the direct result of thalamic damage rather than the product of associated pressure effects. Added to this, left thalamotomy has been reported to impact negatively on high-level linguistic abilities and possibly semantic processing skills (Whelan et al., 2002). Further, thalamic aphasia is more frequently found in lesions of the dominant tuberothalamic (polar) and interpeduncular profunda (paramedian thalamic) arteries, and as these are small vessels there is a low probability that some associated cortical dysfunction may exist (Crosson and Nadeau, 1998).

Language impairment associated with thalamic lesions appears to be much more homogenous than the language profile associated with striatocapsular lesions. Although some variability in the language profile does exist, a number of authors believe that 'thalamic aphasia' has enough defining characteristics to warrant its identification as a 'new' aphasia syndrome. Despite this, thalamic aphasia does not fit neatly into any of the currently accepted cortical aphasias.

Characteristics of thalamic aphasia

Overall, the language disturbance resulting from lesions of the thalamus resembles a transcortical aphasia (Crosson, 1992; Murdoch, 1996), and is characterized by word-finding difficulties, paraphasia (predominantly semantic), neologisms, perseveration, circumlocution, impaired writing abilities and reduced spontaneous speech output in the presence of relatively preserved repetition and variable, but often good, auditory comprehension abilities (Crosson, 1985; Murdoch, 1987). This profile, however, has been reported to vary, including reports of normal language abilities in individuals following thalamic haemorrhage (Cappa *et al.*, 1986).

In particular it is the relative preservation of repetition that indicates similarities between thalamic and transcortical aphasia. The relatively intact repetition abilities of thalamic aphasics in the presence of semantic impairment (semantic paraphasias) suggests that the system for semantic monitoring involves the thalamus, while that involved in the transmission of phonological linguistic information for repetition is separate and does not involve thalamic structures. Crosson (1985) suggested that the arcuate fasciculus is involved in phonological processing. Preservation of repetition further suggests that the aphasia associated with thalamic lesions is not due to compression of adjacent or surrounding brain structures such as the temporal isthmus, as damage to these structures is known to cause aphasia syndromes in which repetition abilities are not preserved (e.g. Wernicke's and conduction aphasia).

Because of the similarities to transcortical aphasia (particularly transcortical sensory), it has been suggested that the language deficits observed in cases of thalamic aphasia may possibly be due to compression of the internal carotid artery intracranially, or its middle and anterior cerebral branches, or both. Such restriction of the internal carotid is known to produce diffuse ischaemic damage in the arterial border zone of the left hemisphere, a condition known to be associated with transcortical aphasias. This theory, however, does not explain why auditory comprehension abilities of thalamic aphasics are often reported to be relatively good whereas in transcortical sensory aphasia comprehension of spoken language is severely defective. Further, as indicated previously, thalamic infarcts are generally caused by occlusion of the posterior cerebral arteries (or their branches), which represent branches of the basilar artery and are therefore supplied by the vertebral artery system rather than the internal carotid system. Although similar, therefore, to transcortical aphasia, thalamic aphasia does show some differences, especially in comprehension abilities. Thalamic aphasics exhibit greater retention of the phonemic level of verbal behaviour than the semantic level, as evidenced by the high number of semantic paraphasic errors present in their speech. The preserved repetition abilities of thalamic aphasics suggest that integrity of the thalamus is not crucial for intentional speech and the phonemic level of verbal behaviour.

Lateralization and thalamic aphasia

The results of studies of patients following surgical intervention in the thalamus are also suggestive of a role for the thalamus in language. These include studies of the effects of surgical ablation of the thalamus (thalamotomy) (Whelan *et al.*, 2002) and thalamic stimulation (Ojemann, 1977; Cappa and Vignolo, 1979). Based on conclusions drawn from these studies, several authors have suggested that thalamic involvement with language is entirely a left thalamic function. For example, the single left thalamotomy case studied by Whelan *et al.* (2002) was reported to exhibit significant post-operative declines in performance on tasks of verbal memory, construction of syntax with contextually constrained boundaries, comprehension of written logical semantic relationships, category-specific generative naming (with an advantage for inanimate concepts) and the temporal processing of words coded for number of meanings and meaning relatedness. In contrast, the right thalamotomy case examined by Whelan *et al.* (2002) demonstrated no significant post-operative changes in language abilities. According to Lhermitte (1984), neither ablation nor stimulation of the right thalamus has been reported to produce effects on language. The lesion has primarily involved the left thalamus rather than the right in most reported cases of acquired thalamic aphasia (Cappa and Vignolo, 1979). Karussis *et al.* (2000) reported that the incidence of aphasia subsequent to left thalamic stroke was 87.5%. Other more traditional researchers advocate a dominant-hemisphere thalamic function. Language disorders have been reported after right thalamic haemorrhage in right-handed (Murdoch, 1987) and left-handed (Kirshner and Kistler, 1982; Chesson, 1983) patients, thereby lending support to the suggestion that thalamic involvement in language is a dominant-hemisphere function.

Role of the thalamus in language

The function of the thalamus in language has been described in terms of an integrative role (Penfield and Roberts, 1959; Schuell *et al.*, 1965), arousal mechanism (Riklan and Cooper, 1975; Luria, 1977; McFarling *et al.*, 1982), modulation and integration of cortical areas to permit language processing (Ojemann, 1983), semantic verification of formulated cortical language segments in verbal production (Cappa and Vignolo, 1979; Wallesch and Papagno, 1988) and managing of verbal memory (Reynolds *et al.*, 1979). More recently, studies have put forward the hypothesis of a thalamic involvement in a mechanism of selective engagement of cortical areas required to perform verbal tasks (Nadeau and Crosson, 1997). This latter concept is close to that of an alerting system activating a mosaic of specific discrete cortical areas appropriate to a particular language-processing mechanism, suggested by Ojemann (1983) on the basis of the findings of electrical stimulation studies of the thalamus. According to this view, the thalamus would not only intervene in activating the cortical area required for a given language task, but also in maintaining other cortical areas in a state of relative disengagement. For further information regarding models of subcortical participation in language, see Chapter 3.

Mechanisms of thalamic aphasia

Despite the above theories, the precise mechanism of thalamic aphasia remains controversial, with several explanations for language impairment occurring subsequent to thalamic lesions having been proposed. As indicated above, thalamic lesions may induce cortical dysfunction by mass effect leading to direct compression of the cortex or via a compromise of the vascular supply to the cortex. Although this explanation may apply in cases of thalamic haemorrhage or tumours, it is unlikely that well-demarcated ischaemic infarcts reported in some cases of thalamic aphasia (e.g. Karussis *et al.*, 2000) could compromise functioning of the cortical language centres by this mechanism. Alternatively, thalamic lesions may lead to metabolic depression of the cerebral cortex by way of diaschisis. This entails a transient functional depression of activity occurring at a distance from a focal lesion. Studies based on techniques such as positron emission tomography (PET) have demonstrated hypoperfusion subsequent to thalamic infarction in the cerebral cortex and subcortical grey matter in addition to the infarcted area of the thalamus (Baron *et al.*, 1986; DeReuck *et al.*, 1995). The severity of aphasia has also been reported to correlate with the severity of cortical hypoperfusion documented by PET scans following left thalamotomy, suggesting that the cortical hypoperfusion is not the outcome of cerebral artery stenosis (Baron *et al.*, 1986, 1992). Rather, it is likely to be due to diaschisis, particularly since the hypoperfusion is observed in the thalamocortical projections from the intralaminar, anterior, medial and lateral nuclei of the thalamus. Recovery of both aphasia and cortical perfusion probably reflects re-establishment of input to cortical areas due to synaptic reorganization (Baron *et al.*, 1986, 1992).

Currently thalamic aphasia is primarily considered to represent a disconnection syndrome between the cortical language areas and the thalamus. Several authors have emphasized the possibility of frontal lobe dysfunction as a prominent disturbance in thalamic stroke (Sandson *et al.*, 1991; Bogousslavsky, 1994). Nagaratnam *et al.* (1999) also proposed that the akinetic mutism and mixed transcortical aphasia observed in their case with left thalamo-mesencephalic infarction was the result of an interruption to frontal-subcortical circuitry.

Prognosis for language disorders associated with thalamic lesions

The reported prognosis for thalamic aphasia varies, some authors reporting a good prognosis for some of their patients and a poor prognosis for others. Riklan and Levita (1970) found that speech disorders associated with left unilateral thalamotomy for Parkinson's disease tended to recover well. Benson (1979) suggested that the language findings following thalamic haemorrhage are transient, with 'recovery often beginning within days or weeks and except in cases complicated by widespread damage, the course is usually one of consistent improvement over a few weeks or months' (p. 96). Although several cases of aphasia following left thalamic haemorrhage have been reported to recover completely, or have been left with only mild deficits, some reports suggest that persistent language deficits, particularly naming problems, may occur (Chesson, 1983; Murdoch, 1987).

Language disorders associated with striatocapsular lesions

The striatocapsular region occupies the deep, central portion of each cerebral hemisphere and is comprised of the basal ganglia (the caudate nucleus, putamen, globus pallidus) and the anterior limb of the internal capsule. With regard to the current state of understanding of the relationship between structures of the striatocapsular region and language function, Kinnier Wilson's (1925) original characterization of the basal ganglia as the dark basements of the brain still rings true today. Various possible functional attributes of these structures have been illuminated through studies of individuals with subcortical vascular lesions, surgical lesions and electrical stimulation during neurosurgical procedures and more recently through functional neuroimaging studies. Despite these findings, the question of whether the structures comprising the striatocapsular region play any role in language functions remains a point of controversy.

The occurrence of language disturbances subsequent to lesions in the striatocapsular region is well documented (Alexander and Lo Verme, 1980; Crosson, 1985; Murdoch *et al.*, 1986; Kennedy and Murdoch, 1993; Nadeau and Crosson, 1997). Although these *in vivo* correlation studies have documented beyond reasonable doubt that language impairments may occur in association with lesions confined to the striatocapsular region of the dominant hemisphere, manifestations of language pathology subsequent to lesions of the basal ganglia and internal capsule have failed to establish a homogeneous symptom complex with no unitary striatocapsular aphasia identified

(Crosson, 1985; Kennedy and Murdoch, 1993; Nadeau and Crosson, 1997). Furthermore, the effects of striatocapsular lesions on language abilities appear, in general, to be more enduring than the impact associated with thalamic lesions (Wallesch *et al.*, 1983). Indeed, reported language profiles extend from normal to severe impairments on the parameters of auditory and reading comprehension, spontaneous speech, repetition, naming and writing (Alexander and Lo Verme, 1980; Damasio *et al.*, 1982; Vallar *et al.*, 1988).

Characteristics of striatocapsular aphasia

The classification of language deficits subsequent to striatocapsular lesions in terms of existing classical aphasia syndromes has been reported to be of limited value. For example, Weiller *et al.* (1993) reported that of 15 aphasic patients with striatocapsular infarcts, four had a Broca's-type aphasia, three exhibited a Wernicke's aphasia, four were anomic, two appeared global and two were unclassifiable. Basso *et al.* (1987) and Cappa *et al.* (1983) also reported cases with striatocapsular lesions fitting all of the classical aphasia syndromes. The considerable number of striatocapsular cases which have presented with an atypical constellation of language deficits (Alexander and Lo Verme, 1980; Damasio *et al.*, 1982; Cappa *et al.*, 1983; Wallesch, 1985) also suggests that an insistence on describing language deficits associated with striatocapsular lesions in terms of classical aphasia syndromes may be of limited benefit.

Despite the documented variability of language disturbances associated with striatocapsular aphasia, some researchers have identified a distinct pattern of impairment which conforms to the anterior-non-fluent/posterior-fluent cortical dichotomy (Cappa *et al.*, 1983). In one of the first systematic studies of this nature, Naeser *et al.* (1982) noted that patients with capsular-putaminal lesions extending into the anterior-superior white matter typically had good comprehension and slow but agrammatical speech. In contrast, those with capsular-putaminal lesions including posterior white matter extension showed poor comprehension and fluent Wernicke's-type speech, while those with both anterior-superior and posterior white matter involvement were globally aphasic. Similarly D'Esposito and Alexander (1995) found that patients with striatocapsular lesions extending anteriorly into the deep frontal white matter were non-fluent, while patients with lesions extending posteriorly into the temporal white matter showed comprehension deficits.

Cappa *et al.* (1983) provided further support for this anterior/posterior distinction by describing an atypical non-fluent aphasia associated with anterior capsular-putaminal lesions (putamen and anterior limb of the internal capsule) and a mild fluent aphasia sometimes associated with posterior striatocapsular involvement (putamen and posterior limb of the internal capsule). Similarly, Murdoch *et al.* (1986) found that patients with striatocapsular lesions involving the anterior limb of the internal capsule exhibited a non-fluent aphasia with semantic paraphasias, while lesions involving the posterior limb of the internal capsule and the posterior putamen resulted in a mild fluent Wernicke's-type aphasia. Damasio *et al.* (1982) also reported that patients with lesions involving the head of the caudate nucleus, the anterior limb of the internal capsule and putamen commonly exhibited semantic paraphasias, but noted that subjects were varied in terms of fluency, comprehension, repetition and the presence of phonemic paraphasias.

Despite this apparent consensus, several other studies have questioned the accuracy and utility of the anterior/posterior dichotomy by describing a number of cases in which the patterns of language impairment could not be accounted for in terms of this anatomical distinction (Wallesch, 1985; Kennedy and Murdoch, 1993). For example, Wallesch (1985) reported that patients with anterior striatocapsular lesions exhibited a Wernicke's-type aphasia with semantic and phonemic paraphasias and later suggested that anterior striatocapsular lesions may be associated with fluent or non-fluent paraphasic output, impaired comprehension and intact repetition (Wallesch, 1997). Puel *et al.* (1984) demonstrated the variability in this area by describing fluent aphasia with semantic paraphasia in patients with anterior putaminocapsular haemorrhage and a non-fluent aphasia with phonemic and semantic paraphasia subsequent to a haemorrhage involving the head of the caudate nucleus and anterior limb of the internal capsule.

Nadeau and Crosson (1997) comprehensively reviewed findings of anterior striatocapsular infarction (involving the head of the caudate nucleus, the putamen and the anterior limb of the internal capsule) and revealed a diverse range and pattern of language deficits in subjects. Findings included fluent paraphasic patients with impaired comprehension, repetition and naming in a syndrome which is more typically associated with posterior cortical lesions, as well as non-fluent cases with or without comprehension deficits.

Accounts also exist of patients with posterior striatocapsular lesions whose language function differs from the symptoms previously noted following lesions of this area (Naeser *et al.*, 1982; Cappa *et al.*, 1983; Murdoch *et al.*, 1986). For example, Weiller *et al.* (1993) cited 12 cases with posterior striatocapsular lesions presenting with no aphasia. Further, Nadeau and Crosson (1997) observed that infarcts of the head of the caudate nucleus, the putamen and the anterior limb of the internal capsule which extend posteriorly to involve the temporal stem result in more significant impairments in comprehension, repetition and naming than in patients without this extension.

Consequently, despite numerous attempts at delineating specific patterns of language impairment subsequent to circumscribed striatocapsular lesions, this area still defies any clear clinico-anatomical picture. As a case in point, Weiller *et al.* (1993) concluded that aphasic syndromes did not differ accordingly to the involvement of particular striatocapsular structures in a study of 57 cases, again bringing into question the validity of any anterior/posterior distinction.

Levels of language processing compromised in striatocapsular aphasia

The different levels of language processing compromised following striatocapsular lesions is somewhat difficult to interpret given that the majority of studies in this area have reported language function only in broad terms of fluency, comprehension, repetition, naming and the presence of paraphasias. Although, as indicated above, the performance of patients with striatocapsular lesions reportedly varies widely on these parameters, some trends are evident. Following striatocapsular lesions, the phonological system – as assessed minimally by repetition and the presence of phonemic paraphasias – may be impaired (Damasio *et al.*, 1982; Naeser *et al.*, 1982; Cappa *et al.*, 1983) but is often spared (Alexander and Lo Verme, 1980; Wallesch, 1985; Murdoch *et al.*, 1986). Repetition of phrases of increasing length and complexity may be compromised (Naeser *et al.*, 1982; Kennedy and Murdoch, 1989). In a more detailed test of phonological discrimination and phonologically based short-term storage, patients with lesions centred on the striatocapsular region performed within normal limits (Valler *et al.*, 1988). Minimal phonemic errors have also been reported in naming tasks (Vallar *et al.*, 1988; Kennedy and Murdoch, 1990).

Auditory comprehension may be impaired to varying degrees (Damasio *et al.*, 1982; D'Esposito and Alexander, 1985) but also is reported to remain intact in other patients (Naeser *et al.*, 1982; Mega and Alexander, 1994). Alexander (1992) reported that subjects in the post-acute phase had no major problems with basic auditory comprehension tasks such as word discrimination, sentence-length requests or two element commands, whereas difficulties were revealed on more complex comprehension tasks. Vallar *et al.* (1988) described mild impairment in sentence comprehension and concluded that this performance might relate to a syntactic or lexical-semantic deficit. Other studies have reported deficits where subjects were required to follow complex sequential commands and comprehend complex instructions (Kennedy and Murdoch, 1993; Mega and Alexander, 1994).

Fluency varies greatly among patients with dominant striatocapsular lesions and Alexander (1992) makes an important distinction between non-fluent speech and non-fluent language production in this population. Non-fluent speech is characterized by impaired articulatory agility, disturbed melodic line, and hypophonia, while non-fluent language is indicated by decreased phrase length and agrammatism. Applying these criteria to 13 subjects with non-thalamic subcortical lesions, Alexander (1992) found that 12 subjects exhibited fluent language using complex grammatical forms and a phrase length greater than seven words, although responses were frequently truncated. In contrast, these subjects exhibited characteristically non-fluent speech. This disassociation between intact language fluency and impaired speech fluency is supported by common findings of grammatical language following striatocapsular lesions (Naeser *et al.*, 1982; Kirk and Kertesz, 1994), although agrammatism has been reported in several instances (Kennedy and Murdoch, 1989; Fabbro *et al.*, 1996).

Evidence suggests that while other aspects of language vary greatly among patients with striatocapsular lesions, lexical-semantic processing is commonly affected (Vallar *et al.*, 1988; Wallesch and Papagno, 1988). There have been numerous reports of confrontation naming deficits, semantic paraphasias and word-finding difficulties subsequent to striatocapsular lesions (Cappa *et al.*, 1983; Wallesch, 1985; Kennedy and Murdoch, 1990, 1993; Mega and Alexander, 1994). Impaired performance on word-fluency and picture-description tasks (Vallar *et al.*, 1988; Kennedy and Murdoch, 1989, 1990; Mega and Alexander, 1994) may also indicate a lexical-semantic deficit, although extra linguistic factors may be involved in the case of word-list generation (Kennedy and Murdoch, 1989).

In summary, a large degree of variability still appears to exist in the reported language profiles of patients with striatocapsular lesions. However, some core features may be present, with Mega and Alexander (1994) proposing the existence of a profile of striatocapsular aphasia comprising impaired generative language accompanied by a naming deficit of varying severity. It is possible that the severity of this profile may vary depending on the extent of damage caused by the lesion and the time post-onset of the lesion.

Cortical dysfunction associated with striatocapsular pathology

Although, as outlined above, language disorders are common subsequent to dominant-hemisphere striatocapsular lesions, it has been suggested that the more overt language symptoms in such cases may be related to concomitant cortical dysfunction via various pathophysiological mechanisms (Nadeau and Crosson, 1997). Nadeau and Crosson (1997) described five potential mechanisms of aphasia associated with subcortical strokes. These included (1) a direct effect of the subcortical lesions indicating that the basal ganglia and other subcortical structures are essential components of the brain networks involved in language function (Damasio *et al.*, 1982), (2) disconnection of cortical structures by white matter lesions that are essential for language (Alexander *et al.*, 1987), (3) impaired 'release' of language segments formulated in the cortex into output (Crosson, 1985, 1992), (4) diaschisis, in which the subcortical lesion 'cuts off' neural input to a remote area of the brain, causing dysfunction of the remote area, as first proposed by Von Monakow (1914) (Metter *et al.*, 1983; Perani *et al.*, 1987) and (5) stenosis or occlusion of the large cerebral vessels that independently cause the subcortical stroke and hypoperfusion of the cortex. Several studies utilizing techniques such as PET and single-photon emission computed tomography (SPECT) have demonstrated cortical hypoperfusion in patients with aphasia associated with striatocapsular lesions (Skyhøj-Olsen, 1986; Vallar *et al.*, 1988; Radanovic and Scoff, 2003). However, it is not clear in these cases if the cortical hypoperfusion is due to the subcortical infarct (through diaschisis as proposed by Metter *et al.* 1983) or an independent phenomenon caused by large-vessel stenosis or occlusion.

Nadeau and Crosson (1997) argued strongly that a direct or indirect effect of the striatocapsular lesion itself should result in a consistent aphasia syndrome. They therefore suggested that the variable aphasias reported in association with striatocapsular lesions (as outlined above) were most probably due to stenosis or occlusion of the large vessels supplying the language cortex, which causes hypoperfusion of a variety of cortical regions, and also causes the striatocapsular infarct by occluding a lenticulostriate artery or the recurrent artery of Heubner. This suggestion is consistent with the wide range of cortical regions that have been shown to be hypoperfused on SPECT after subcortical stroke (Radanovic and Scaff, 2003). Further evidence to support the proposal of Nadeau and Crosson (1997) comes from the findings of Hillis *et al.* (2002). Based on a study of a consecutive series of patients with acute strokes limited to subcortical tissue using magnetic resonance perfusion-weighted imaging as well as diffusion-weighted imaging, the latter authors reported cortical hypoperfusion in all 28 of their aphasic patients and none of their 12 non-aphasic patients. Further they reported that, in those cases in which blood flow could be restored to the cortex within a few days from onset, reperfusion was associated with immediate resolution of aphasia. In a further study, Hillis *et al.* (2004) reported that in their patients with acute left caudate stroke, the variation of speech and language deficits observed could be accounted for by variation in the region of cortical hypoperfusion as demonstrated by magnetic resonance perfusion imaging conducted the same day as language testing. Further, not only did the presence and type of aphasia reflect the regions of hypometabolism, they generally followed predictions based on chronic lesion studies regarding anatomical lesions associated with classic aphasia types.

Although the notion that overlying cortical dysfunction via hypoperfusion is the critical determinant of language impairments associated with striatocapsular lesions has been argued forcefully (Nadeau and Crosson, 1997; Hillis *et al.*, 2004;), there are other views counter to this position (Wallesch and Papagno, 1988; Mega and Alexander, 1994; D'Esposito and Alexander, 1995). Han *et al.* (2003) recently proposed that aphasia associated with subcortical stroke is due to small infarcts in the cerebral cortex that are not visible on computed tomographic or conventional magnetic resonance imaging (MRI) scans, but are seen on diffusion-weighted or delayed conventional

MRI. While this explanation of aphasia would account for the variety of aphasia types observed in patients with so-called subcortical strokes, it does not account for patients with acute aphasia and no cortical infarct on diffusion-weighted imaging.

It remains that the relationship between the structured site and aetiology of the subcortical lesions, time post-onset, the extent of cortical hypometabolism and hypoperfusion and associated language function remains to be fully elucidated. Further, the question of whether language deficits associated with striatocapsular lesions are the sequelae of cortical or subcortical dysfunction should not be considered as necessarily mutually exclusive. Concomitant cortical dysfunction may result in overlying language deficits that mask more subtle changes in language function relating directly to basal ganglia dysfunction. Indeed Metter et al. (1988) provided evidence that striatocapsular structural damage may have direct and indirect (through hypometabolism) effects on certain aspects of language function.

Prognosis of language disorders associated with striatocapsular lesions

Reports in the literature vary as to the prognosis of aphasic disturbances resulting from striatocapsular lesions. Performance on standard aphasia batteries indicates that striatocapsular lesions may result in a transient aphasia or resolve to a mild aphasia (Basso et al., 1987; Vallar et al., 1988; Mega and Alexander, 1994). Other studies have identified long-lasting deficits resulting from left striatocapsular lesions. These latter deficits include the presence of semantic paraphasias and word-finding difficulties in spontaneous speech (Damasio et al., 1982; Murdoch et al., 1986; Kennedy and Murdoch, 1989). Further, although basic auditory comprehension may be intact (Damasio et al., 1982), more subtle long-term deficits have been documented in understanding instructions (Murdoch et al., 1986; Vallar et al., 1988; Kennedy and Murdoch, 1993). Likewise, repetition may be either intact (Damasio et al., 1982; Mega and Alexander, 1994) or impaired in the long term only for low-probability items or sentences (Murdoch et al., 1986; Kennedy and Murdoch, 1989). Confrontation naming may be either normal or chronically impaired (Damasio et al., 1982; Kennedy and Murdoch, 1989; Mega and Alexander, 1994).

Summary

The occurrence of language deficits subsequent to both thalamic and striatocapsular lesions has been widely documented in numerous clinico-anatomical correlation studies published over the past three decades. Commonly, language disturbances resulting from lesions of the thalamus resemble a transcortical aphasia characterized by word-finding difficulties, paraphasias, neologistic output, perseveration and reduced spontaneous speech in the presence of relatively preserved repetition and comprehension abilities. In contrast, manifestations of language pathology subsequent to lesions of the basal ganglia and internal capsule have failed to establish a homogenous symptom complex. Furthermore, the effects of striatocapsular lesions on language abilities appear, in general, to be more enduring than the impact associated with thalamic lesions. Indeed, reported language profiles extend from normal to severe impairments on the parameters of auditory and reading comprehension, spontaneous speech, repetition, naming and writing. Despite the documented variability of language disturbances associated with striatocapsular aphasia, some researchers have identified a distinct pattern of impairment which conforms to the anterior-non-fluent/posterior-fluent cortical dichotomy.

Although the precise mechanism of language dysfunction subsequent to lesions in the thalamus and striatocapsular region remains unknown, it is possible that aspects of the impairments are the outcome of a direct effect of subcortical lesion or represent the secondary effects of the lesion on the cortical language centres via mechanisms such as compression, diaschisis, hypometabolism or hypoperfusion. Consequently, the role of subcortical structures (particularly those in the striatocapsular region) in language remains controversial.

References

Alexander, M.P. (1992). Speech and language deficits after subcortical lesions of the left hemisphere: a clinical CT and PET study. In G. Vellar, S.F. Cappa and C-W. Wallesch (eds), *Neuropsychological Disorders Associated with Subcortical Lesions* (pp. 455–77). Oxford: Oxford University Press.

Alexander, M.P. and Lo Verme, S.R. (1980). Aphasia after left hemisphere intracerebral hemorrhage. *Neurology* 30, 1193–1202.

Alexander, M.P., Naeser, M.A. and Palumbo, C.L. (1987). Correlations of subcortical CT sites and aphasia profiles. *Brain* 110, 961–91.

Baron, J.C., D'Antona, R., Pantano, P., Serdaru, M., Samson, Y. *et al.* (1986). Effects of thalamic stroke on energy metabolism in the cerebral cortex. *Brain* 109, 1243–59.

Baron, J.C., Levasseur, M., Mazoyer, B., Legault-Demare, F., Mauguiere, R. *et al.* (1992). Thalamo-cortical diaschisis: PET study in humans. *Journal of Neurology Neurosurgery and Psychiatry* 55, 935–42.

Basso, A., Della Sala, S. and Farabola, M. (1987). Aphasia arising from purely deep lesions. *Cortex* 23, 29–44.

Benson, D.F. (1979). Neurologic correlates of anomia. In H. Whitaker and H.A. Whitaker (eds), *Studies in Neurolinguistics* (pp. 293–328). New York: Academic Press.

Bogousslavsky, J. (1994). Frontal stroke syndromes. *European Neurology* 34, 306–15.

Cappa, S.F. and Vignolo, L.A. (1979). Transcortical features of aphasia following left thalamic hemorrhage. *Cortex* 15, 121–30.

Cappa, S.F., Cavallotti, G., Guidotti, M., Papagno, C. and Vignolo, L.A. (1983). Subcortical aphasia: two clinical-CT scan correlation studies. *Cortex* 19, 227–41.

Cappa, S.F., Papagno, C., Vallar, G. and Vignolo, L.A. (1986). Aphasia does not always follow left thalamic hemorrhage: a study of five negative cases. *Cortex* 22, 639–47.

Cheek, W.R. and Taveras, J. (1966). Thalamic tumours. *Journal of Neurosurgery* 24, 505–13.

Chesson, A.L. (1983). Aphasia following right thalamic hemorrhage. *Brain and Language* 19, 306–16.

Ciemens, V.A. (1970). Localized thalamic hemorrhage: a cause of aphasia. *Neurology* 20, 776–82.

Crosson, B. (1985). Subcortical functions in language: a working model. *Brain and Language* 25, 257–92.

Crosson, B. (1992). *Subcortical Functions in Language and Memory*. New York: Guildford Press.

Crosson, B. and Nadeau, S.E. (1998). The role of subcortical structures in linguistic processes: recent developments. In B. Stemmer and H.A. Whitaker (eds), *Handbook of Neurolinguistics* (pp. 431–45). San Diego: Academic Press.

Damasio, A.R., Damasio, H., Rizzo, M., Varney, N. and Gersh, F. (1982). Aphasia with non-hemorrhagic lesions in the basal ganglia and internal capsule. *Archives of Neurology* 29, 15–20.

D'Esposito, M. and Alexander, M.P. (1995). Subcortical aphasia: distinct profiles following left putaminal hemorrhage. *Neurology* 45, 38–41.

Dejerine, J. and Roussy, G. (1906). Le syndrome thalamique. *Revue Neurologique* 14, 521–32.

DeReuck, J., Decoo, D., Lemanhieu, I., Strijekmans, K., Goethals, P. *et al.* (1995). Ipsilateral thalamic diaschisis after middle cerebral artery infarction. *Journal of Neurological Science* 134, 130–5.

Fabbro, F., Clarici, A. and Bava, A. (1996). Effects of left basal ganglia lesions on language production. *Perceptual and Motor Skills* 82, 1291–8.

Fisher, C.M. (1959). The pathologic and clinical aspects of thalamic hemorrhage. *Trans American Neurological Association* 33, 56–9.

Gorelick, P.B., Hier, D.B., Benevento, L., Levitt, S. and Tan, W. (1984). Aphasia after left thalamic infarction. *Archives of Neurology* 41, 1296–8.

Graff-Radford, N.R., Eslinger, P.J., Damasio, A.R. and Yamada, T. (1984). Nonhemorrhagic infarction of the thalamus: behaviour, anatomic and physiological correlates. *Neurology* 34, 14–23.

Han, M., Kang, D., Bae, H., Oh, G., Jeong, S. *et al.* (2003). Aphasia in striatocapsular infarction may be explained by concomitant small cortical infarctions of cortical language zones. *Stroke* 34, 259.

Hillemand, P. (1925). *Contribution à l'étude des syndromes thalamiques*. Paris: Thèse.

Hillis, A.E., Kane, A., Tuffiash, E., Ulatowski, J., Barker, P. *et al.* (2002). Reperfusion of specific brain regions by raising blood pressure restores selective language function in subacute stroke. *Brain and Language* 79, 495–510.

Hillis, A.E., Barker, P.B., Wityk, R.J., Aldrich, E.M., Restrepo, L. *et al.* (2004). Variability in subcortical aphasia is due to variable sites of cortical hypoperfusion. *Brain and Language* 89, 524–30.

Karussis, D., Leker, R.R. and Abramsky, O. (2000). Cognitive function following thalamic stroke: a study of 16 cases and review of the literature. *Journal of the Neurological Sciences* 172, 25–9.

Kennedy, M. and Murdoch, B.E. (1989). Speech and language disorders subsequent to subcortical vascular lesions. *Aphasiology* 3, 221–47.

Kennedy, M. and Murdoch, B.E. (1990). Persistent word fluency deficit in patients with dominant hemisphere striatocapsular lesions: further evidence for a subcortical role in language? *Australian Journal of Human Communication Disorders* 18, 3–20.

Kennedy, M. and Murdoch, B.E. (1993). Chronic aphasia subsequent to striatocapsular and thalamic lesions in the left hemisphere. *Brain and Language* 44, 284–95.

Kirk, A. and Kertesz, A. (1994). Cortical and subcortical aphasias compared. *Aphasiology* 8, 65–82.

Kirshner, H.S. and Kistler, K.H. (1982). Aphasia after right thalamic hemorrhage. *Archives of Neurology* 39, 667–9.

Lhermitte, J. (1936). Symptomatologie de l'hémorragie du thalamus. *Revue Neurologique* 65, 89–93.

Lhermitte, J. (1984). Language disorders and their relationship to thalamic lesions. *Advances in Neurology* 42, 99–113.

Luria, A.R. (1977). On quasi-aphasic speech disturbances in lesions of the deep structures of the brain. *Brain and Language* 4, 432–59.

McFarling, D., Rothi, L.J. and Heilman, K. (1982). Transcortical aphasia from ischaemic infarcts of the thalamus: a report of two cases. *Journal of Neurology Neurosurgery and Psychiatry* 45, 107–12.

Mega, M.S. and Alexander, M.P. (1994). Subcortical aphasia: the core profile of capsulostriatal infarction. *Neurology* 44, 1824–9.

Metter, E.J., Riege, W.H., Hanson, W.R., Kuhl, D.E., Phelps, M.E. *et al.* (1983). Comparison of metabolic rates, language and memory in subcortical aphasias. *Brain and Language* 19, 33–47.

Metter, E.J., Riege, W.H., Hanson, W.R., Jackson, C.A., Kempler, D. *et al.* (1988). Subcortical structures in aphasia: an analysis on (F-18)-Fluorodeoxyglucose, positron emission tomography and computed tomography. *Archives of Neurology* 45, 1229–34.

Mohr, J.P., Watters, W.C. and Duncan, G.W. (1975). Thalamic hemorrhage and aphasia. *Brain and Language* 2, 3–17.

Murdoch, B.E. (1987). Aphasia following right thalamic hemorrhage in a dextral. *Journal of Communication Disorders* 20, 459–68.

Murdoch, B.E. (1990). *Acquired Speech and Language Disorders: a Neuroanatomical and Functional Neurological Approach*. London: Chapman and Hall.

Murdoch, B.E. (1996). The role of subcortical structures in language: clinico-neuroradiological studies of brain damaged subjects. In B. Dodd, R. Campbell and L. Worrall (eds), *Evaluating Theories of Language: Evidence from Disordered Communication* (pp. 137–60). London: Whurr Publishers.

Murdoch, B.E., Thompson, D., Fraser, S. and Harrison, L. (1986). Aphasia following non-haemorrhagic lesions in the left striatocapsular region. *Australian Journal of Human Communication Disorders* 14, 5–21.

Nadeau, S.E. and Crosson, B. (1997). Subcortical aphasia. *Brain and Language* 58, 355–402.

Naeser, M.A., Alexander, M.P., Helm-Estabrooks, N., Levine, H.L., Laughlin, S.A. *et al.* (1982). Aphasia with predominantly subcortical lesion sites: description of three capsular/putaminal aphasia syndromes. *Archives of Neurology* 39, 2–14.

Nagaratnam, N., McNeil, C. and Gilhotra, J.S. (1999). Akinetic mutism and mixed transcortical aphasia following left thalamo-mesencephalic infarction. *Journal of Neurological Sciences* 163, 70–3.

Ojemann, G.A. (1977). Asymmetric function of the thalamus in man. *Annals of the New York Academy of Science* 299, 380–96.

Ojemann, G.A. (1983). Brain organization for language from the perspective of electrical stimulation mapping. *Behavioural and Brain Sciences* 2, 189–230.

Panchal, V.G., Parikh, V.R. and Karapurkar, A.P. (1974). Thalamic abscesses. *Neurology (India)* 22, 106–10.

Penfield, W. and Roberts, L. (1959). *Speech and Brain Mechanisms*. Princeton: Princeton University Press.

Perani, D., Vallar, G., Cappa, S.F., Messa, C. and Fazio, F. (1987). Aphasia and neglect after subcortical stroke: a clinical/cerebral perfusion correlation study. *Brain* 110, 1211–29.

Puel, M., Demonet, J.F., Cardebat, D., Bonafe, A., Gazounaud, Y. *et al.* (1984). Aphasies sous-corticales: etude neurolinguistique avec scanner X de 25 cas. *Revue Neurologique* 140, 695–710.

Radanovic, M. and Scaff, M. (2003). Speech and language disturbances due to subcortical lesions. *Brain and Language* 84, 337–52.

Reynolds, A.F., Turner, P.T., Harris, A.B., Ojemann, G.A. and Davis, L.E. (1979). Left thalamic hemorrhage with dysphasia: a report of five cases. *Brain and Language* 7, 62–73.

Riklan, M. and Cooper, I.S. (1975). Psychometric studies of verbal functions following thalamic lesions in humans. *Brain and Language* 2, 45–64.

Riklan, M. and Levita, E. (1970). Psychological studies of thalamic lesions in humans. *Journal of Nervous and Mental Disorders* 150, 251–65.

Sandson, T.A., Daffner, K.R., Carvalho, P.A. and Meslman, M.M. (1991). Frontal lobe dysfunction following infarction of the left-sided medial thalamus. *Archives of Neurology* 8, 1300–3.

Schuell, H., Jenkins, J.J. and Jimenez-Pabon, E. (1965). *Aphasia in Adults*. New York: Harper Row.

Skyhøj-Olsen, T., Bruhn, P. and Öberg, R.G. (1986). Cortical hypoperfusion as a possible cause of subcortical aphasia. *Brain* 106, 393–410.

Smyth, G.E. and Stern, K. (1938). Tumours of the thalamus: a clinicopathological study. *Brain* 61, 339–60.

Vallar, G., Papagno, C. and Cappa, S.F. (1988). Latent dysphasia after left hemispheric lesions: a lexical-semantic and verbal memory deficit. *Aphasiology* 2, 463–78.

Von Monakow, C. (1914). *Die lokalisation im grosshirn und der abbau der funktionen durch corticale herde*. Wiesbaden: Bergmann.

Wallesch, C.-W. (1985). Two syndromes of aphasia occurring with ischemic lesions involving the left basal ganglia. *Brain and Language* 25, 357–61.

Wallesch, C.-W. (1997). Symptomatology of subcortical aphasia. *Journal of Neurolinguistics* 10, 267–75.

Wallesch, C.-W. and Papagno, C. (1988). Subcortical aphasia. In F.C. Rose, R. Whurr and M.A. Wyke (eds), *Aphasia* (pp. 256–287). London: Whurr Publishers.

Wallesch, C.-W., Kornhuber, H.H., Brunner, R.J., Kunz, T., Hollerbach, B. *et al.* (1983). Lesions of the basal ganglia, thalamus and deep white matter: differential effects on language functions. *Brain and Language* 20, 286–304.

Weiller, C., Willmes, K., Reiche, W., Thron, A., Isensee, C. *et al.* (1993). The case of aphasia or neglect after striatocapsular infarction. *Brain* 116, 1509–25.

Whelan, B.-M., Murdoch, B.E., Theodoros, D.G., Silburn, P. and Hall, B. (2002). A role for the dominant thalamus in language? The linguistic comparison of two cases subsequent to unilateral thalamotomy procedures in dominant and non-dominant hemispheres. *Aphasiology* 16, 1213–26.

Wilson, S.A.K. (1925). Disorders of motility and muscle tone with special reference to the striatum. *Lancet* 2, 1–10.

5 Pallidal and thalamic involvement in language: evidence from stereotactic surgical studies

Introduction

As outlined in Chapter 3, neurosurgical procedures are now commonly applied techniques in the management of Parkinson's disease, involving circumscribed lesioning or high-frequency stimulation of specific subcortical nuclei. The mid-1970s and 1980s heralded a resurgence of interest in neurosurgical interventions for the treatment of Parkinson's disease, largely instigated by observed long-term limitations of drug therapy and a better understanding of pathophysiological models of Parkinson's disease (i.e. the rationale for intervention at specific targets), as well as improvements in stereotactic techniques (e.g. brain imaging) and equipment (e.g. intraoperative recording techniques) (Gildenberg, 1984; Lang and Lees, 2002; Speelman and Bosch, 2002). The current chapter focuses on the effects of ablative lesions of specific nuclei within basal ganglia–thalamocortical circuitry on language function.

Ablative techniques

Ablative techniques were originally the most commonly applied procedures during the neurosurgical renaissance of the 1970s and 1980s, typically involving the generation of permanent lesions in the thalamus (i.e. thalamotomy) or globus pallidus (i.e. pallidotomy) (Kleiner-Fisman *et al.*, 2003; Vitek *et al.*, 2003) by way of radiofrequency-mediated electrocoagulation, which aims to permanently disrupt or inactivate the relevant target (Benabid *et al.*, 1998). In re-referencing models of Parkinson's disease, a loss of dopaminergic neurones within the substantia nigra pars compacta results in hyperactivity of the indirect pathway and reduced activity in the direct pathway, causing disinhibition of globus pallidus internus (GPi)-substantia nigra pars reticulata (SNr) inhibitory outputs to the thalamus and brain stem (Lang and Lozano, 1998) (see Figure 10.2, p. 224). This alteration in neurophysiology leads to the manifestation of cardinal Parkinsonian symptoms including akinesia, bradykinesia, rigidity and tremor. Ablative lesions within motor components of this circuit aim to reduce excessive inhibitory outflow from the GPi-SNr complex (Obeso *et al.*, 1997a) via the inactivation of target nuclei (Lang and Lees, 2002). In relation to target specificity, neurosurgical procedures pinpoint three primary structures which may be functionally overactive as a result of the Parkinson's disease process; namely the thalamus, globus pallidus or subthalamic nucleus (STN) (Lang and Lees, 2002). The ventral intermedius (Vim) thalamus, posteroventral portion of the GPi and dorsolateral STN constitute sensorimotor subdivisions of these structures and hence optimal neurosurgical targets.

Variability may exist between patients with Parkinson's disease in relation to primary symptom presentation, perhaps as a consequence of individual pathophysiological mechanisms or the same mechanisms influencing distinct motor subcircuits (Wichmann and DeLong, 1998). As a result, different surgical targets may be selected between patients. Lesioning the Vim thalamus (i.e. Vim thalamotomy) has been shown to be effective in relieving tremor-dominant symptoms; lesioning of posteroventral portion of the GPi (i.e. posteroventral pallidotomy, PVP) and high-frequency stimulation or lesioning of the dorsolateral STN have been reported to ameliorate the symptoms of akinesia, rigidity, drug-induced dyskinesias, gait and postural disturbances (Lang and Lees, 2002). The effects of Vim thalamotomy and PVP on language will be discussed in the current chapter. The influence of STN stimulation and lesioning on language processes will be discussed in Chapter 6.

Surgical methodology relative to ablative lesions

In preparation for surgery patients are withdrawn from anti-Parkinson medication and a magnetic resonance imaging (MRI) scan of the head is obtained to identify critical anatomical reference points: the anterior and posterior commissures (Starr *et al.*, 1998). The thalamus or globus pallidus are then indirectly identified by measuring established distances from the intercommisural line (Obeso *et al.*, 1997b). The ablative surgical technique summarised in this chapter was largely adopted from the methodology established by the resident Movement Disorders Group at the Radcliffe Infirmary, Oxford, United Kingdom (Scott *et al.*, 1998). Subsequent to pre-operative MRI, general anaesthetic is administered and a Cosman-Roberts-Wells stereotactic head frame fixed to the patient's skull, in a parallel position to the anterior-commissure–posterior-commissure line. A computed tomography image of the brain with the stereotactic head frame in place is then acquired. Radionics Image Fusion™ software is utilized to fuse and spatially correct the pre-operative MRI to the stereotactic computed tomography scan. The fused image is then loaded into a Stereoplan™ workstation where the target lesion site is localized and a surgical trajectory determined. The coordinates of the surgical trajectory are then transferred to the stereotactic head frame. Utilizing the stereotactic head frame as a guide, a twist-drill craniotomy is then performed and a Radionics™ lesioning electrode passed to the target site. Macrostimulation of the calculated target is then undertaken, by way of passing a current through the lesioning electrode, providing a physiological guidance mechanism for target accuracy (Starr *et al.*, 1998). During the course of macrostimulation, neurological signs and impedance values are monitored. When optimal symptom relief is achieved, a temporary lesion within the localized target is made and the patient evaluated for adverse side effects. If the patient responds favourably, multiple overlapping lesions are then generated incrementally (via electrocoagulation) within the functional target. Following surgery, a post-operative MRI is acquired to compare the actual lesion site with pre-operative target coordinates.

Proposed roles for the basal ganglia and thalamus in language

As mentioned in Chapter 3, a number of models of subcortical participation in language postulate roles for the basal ganglia and/or thalamus in the mediation of language processes (Crosson, 1985; Wallesch and Papagno, 1988; Nadeau and Crosson,

1997). These models collectively propose roles for the striatum, globus pallidus, thalamus (specifically the ventral anterior (VA) and ventral lateral (VL) nuclei, pulvinar, centrum medianum and nucleus reticularis) and cerebral cortex in language processing, executed via the presence of these structures within a hypothesized basal ganglia–thalamocortical language circuit.

The focus of this chapter will be the impact of ablative pallidal and thalamic lesions – otherwise known as pallidotomy and thalamotomy, respectively – on language function. As mentioned previously, the motor and/or sensory subdivisions of subcortical nuclei are typically targeted in neurosurgical procedures used in treating the motor anomalies associated with Parkinson's disease. In relation to the globus pallidus, the internal segment of this structure (GPi) represents the motor subdivision. GPi outputs primarily project to the motor nuclei of the thalamus (i.e. VA and VL nuclei) (Sohn and Hallett, 2005), which in turn project to the supplementary motor, anterior cingulate and premotor areas of the cerebral cortex (Schell and Strick, 1984; Jones, 1985). The Vim portion of the thalamus has been reported to constitute components of the ventral lateral posterior as well as ventral posterolateral nuclei, which demonstrate sensory as well as motor connectivity (Lenz et al., 1993, 1995). As a general rule of thumb, lesions in the posteroventral portion of the GPi have been demonstrated to be effective in relieving akinesia, rigidity and drug-induced dyskinesias, and lesions of the Vim have been shown to be effective in alleviating tremor. Here we will attempt to empirically validate roles for the GPi and Vim in the mediation of language processes by reporting the findings of studies that have documented the behavioural profiles of cohorts with surgically induced circumscribed lesions of these structures.

Hypothesized contribution of the internal segment of the globus pallidus to language function

The GPi represents the anatomical linchpin of proposed closed corticostriatal circuits mediating motor and cognitive functions, in that it provides the primary output channel of the basal ganglia (Middleton and Strick, 1994). Amplified GPi activity has been identified in individuals with Parkinson's disease as a consequence of hypothetical dopamine-dependent alterations to direct and indirect basal ganglia pathway dynamics (Alexander et al., 1990; Lang and Lozano, 1998). Ablative lesions of the GPi (i.e. pallidotomy) reportedly serve to temper immoderate thalamocortical inhibition in Parkinson's disease (Stebbins et al., 2000). PVP has been specifically hypothesized to eradicate abnormal Parkinsonian GPi signals or 'noise' in basal ganglia–thalamocortical motor circuits by destroying the primary outflow path for that signal, resulting in enhanced motor performance (Stebbins et al., 2000).

Research pertaining to the functional organization of the basal ganglia, in particular the globus pallidus, has focused primarily on motor circuitry (Lacritz et al., 2000). Topographically organized output from the basal ganglia includes the projection of 'motor-related' neurones within specific portions of the GPi and SNr to motor regions of the cerebral cortex (Hoover and Strick, 1999). In relation to motor behaviour, the basal ganglia have been implicated in the regulation of sequential, manual motor tasks (Lieberman, 2000), and basal ganglia dysfunction associated with the manifestation of motor sequencing abnormalities, such as those observed in Parkinson's disease (Harrington and Haaland, 1991).

Two distinct motor control functions have been assigned to the human basal ganglia: (1) the execution of automatic action via the facilitation of cortically driven motor activity and the suppression of superfluous muscular activation, and (2) the modification of ongoing action in novel contexts, including the re-organization of cortically driven motor behaviour (Marsden and Obeso, 1994). Recent evidence, however, suggests that the basal ganglia may also contribute to cognitive functions, as shown by evidence for the manifestation of progressive neuropsychological deficits in tandem with motor impairments in individuals with Parkinson's disease (Owen *et al.*, 1998). If thought is perceived as mental action without motion, the basal ganglia may serve to regulate routine thought and to orchestrate alterations in the sequencing of thought processes in response to novel contexts, in a parallel fashion to the mediation of motor behaviour (Marsden and Obeso, 1994). In this way, basal ganglia dysfunction has been hypothesized to result in cognitive as well as motor inflexibility (Marsden and Obeso, 1994), and may indeed include language deficits.

Neuropsychological investigations pertaining to the impact of PVP on cognition have largely focused on unilateral lesions (Turner *et al.*, 2002). Furthermore, this corpus of research presents a range of methodological shortcomings and, consequently, highly variable outcomes (York *et al.*, 1999). A functional dissociation relative to post-PVP motor and cognitive abilities, however, represents a well-documented finding (Stebbins *et al.*, 2000), common to both unilateral and bilateral PVP cohorts, with improvements in motor function and declines in cognitive function being a typical profile.

In relation to bilateral PVP, reports of enhanced motor outcomes concomitant with declines in certain aspects of cognition dominate the scant compendium of literature (Scott *et al.*, 1998, 2002; Ghika *et al.*, 1999; Lang *et al.*, 1999; Turner *et al.*, 2002). These findings suggest not only that surgically induced lesions targeting motor portions of the GPi impact upon cognitive functions, but that this procedure evokes differential effects within hypothetically segregated yet parallel motor and cognitive circuits. The infiltration of proximal cognitive circuits which encompass prefrontal and inferotemporal areas of the cerebral cortex (Middleton and Strick, 2000), as a consequence of large, surgically induced lesions of motor portions of the GPi, may represent the most plausible mechanism responsible for manifestations of the aforementioned symptom complex (Middleton and Strick, 2000). Alternatively, these results may support the notions of circuitry 'convergence' (Percheron and Filion, 1991) or 'integration' (Joel and Weiner, 1994) challenging currently accepted models of functional organization of the basal ganglia.

In Parkinson's disease, cognitive impairments have been hypothesized to occur as a result of anomalous basal ganglia outflow (Owen *et al.*, 1998). This conclusion was drawn subsequent to the observation of highly significant inverse correlations between Parkinsonian and normal cohorts with respect to regional cerebral blood flow rates in the right GPi during high-level cognitive tasks involving planning and spatial working memory (Owen *et al.*, 1998). Increased blood flow was observed consistently in control subjects during such tasks, in contrast to reduced regional cerebral blood flow and cognitive performance in the Parkinson's disease cohort.

Task-oriented alterations in GPi activity have been postulated to reflect frontostriatally mediated indirect/direct pathway alterations to basal ganglia outflow, which ultimately aim to enhance performance (Mink and Thach, 1991). For example, indirect-pathway-governed excitation of GPi neurones results in the hypothetical inhibition of cortical regions considered superfluous to task demands. In contrast, direct-pathway-mediated reductions in GPi inhibition result in thalamocortical disinhibition, facilitating a 'focusing' of function in utilitarian cortical regions. In Parkinson's disease, task-related reductions in GPi activity may reflect disturbed indirect/direct pathway dynamics as a consequence of dopamine depletion (Owen *et al.*, 1998). Disturbed basal ganglia outflow consequently impacts upon the nature of information transfer through frontostriatal circuits and hence frontal lobe functions, resulting in impaired cognitive performance. Similarly, functional inhibition of the GPi subsequent to pallidotomy may also evoke excessive disinhibition of thalamo-cortical outputs and a consequent inability to temper superfluous cortical activity, resulting in cognitive deficits (Stebbins *et al.*, 2000).

Of note, post-operative improvements in performance on a number of cognitive variables have also been reported subsequent to bilateral PVP, particularly when individual profiles as opposed to group-wise comparisons are considered (Scott *et al.*, 1998, 2002). It has been hypothesized that idiosyncratic performance profiles with respect to directions of post-operative change relating to cognitive parameters may represent variations in functional basal ganglia output channels subsequent to the lesion, and consequently to ensuing neural activity within innervated cortical regions (Middleton and Strick, 2000).

With regard to language, two theoretical frameworks promote a role for the GPi in the mediation of linguistic processes (Crosson, 1985; Wallesch and Papagno, 1988). The Response-Release Semantic Feedback model (Crosson, 1985) (see Chapter 3) postulates the GPi to participate in the tonic arousal of the cerebral cortex as well as regulating the release of semantically verified language segments for verbal output, in tandem with the caudate nucleus. Lesions of the GPi are hypothesized to result in fluent language pathology, including the generation of extraneous verbal output such as semantic paraphasias, as a consequence of thalamic disinhibition and overexcitation of the anterior language cortex (Crosson, 1992). The Lexical Decision Making model (Wallesch and Papagno, 1988) (see Chapter 3) incorporates the GPi within a frontal lobe system, capable of manipulating multiple degrees of freedom with respect to the temporal isochronization of cortically generated lexical and contextual modules (Wallesch, 1990). On the basis of this model, GPi lesions are predicted to result in a range of potential language impairments including inappropriate lexical output and speech-initiation difficulties, as well as an increased dependency upon contextual constraints.

Hypothesized contribution of the thalamus to language function

Situated downstream from the globus pallidus in basal ganglia–thalamocortical circuits, the thalamus dualistically constitutes the principal recipient of basal ganglia outflow dispensed by the GPi and SNr, as well as a subcortical–cortical nexus, which ultimately governs the regulation of cortical activity. In relation to operative theories of subcortical participation in language, the thalamus has been characteristically established as a critical co-operative nucleus, given its direct affiliation with the cerebral cortex (Wallesch and Papagno, 1988). Indeed, the VA and VL and non-specific thalamic nuclei (i.e. nucleus reticularis, centrum medianum and parafascicular nucleus) have each been hypothesized to play a role in linking and perhaps procuring language-dedicated cortical regions, by way of facilitating the transmission and even modulation of linguistic information, travelling via cortico-subcortico-cortical circuits (Crosson, 1985; Wallesch and Papagno, 1988; Nadeau and Crosson, 1997). Within these circuits the thalamus has been specifically postulated to support a number of possible functions, including (1) the facilitation of pre-verbal semantic monitoring and the release of semantically verified language segments for verbal production (Crosson,

1985), (2) the synchronization and gating of cortically generated lexical information (Wallesch and Papagno, 1988; Wallesch, 1997) and (3) the selective engagement of cortical nets involved in semantically driven lexical retrieval and declarative memory processes (Nadeau and Crosson, 1997). On the basis of these postulates, therefore, the thalamus has been generally perceived to represent a linguistic fulcrum relative to lexical-semantic processes.

In relation to the abovementioned theoretical frameworks of subcortical participation in language, a specific function for the Vim nucleus of the thalamus has not been proposed. Rather, only specific roles for the VA, VL and non-specific thalamic nuclei (i.e. nucleus reticularis, centrum medianum and parafascicular nucleus) have been offered. On this basis, predictions pertaining to the impact of Vim lesions on language processes are difficult to make, yet some assumptions may be drawn, particularly in light of paradoxical clinico-anatomical findings relative to functional thalamic organization. For example, comparable aphasic profiles have been reported in cases presenting lesions both within and external to thalamic systems, hypothetically implicated in the mediation of linguistic processes (Crosson, 1984), suggesting a potential inter-relationship between anterior and posterior thalamic nuclei relative to language mechanisms (Crosson, 1999). Given the small size of the thalamus as a neural structure and the close proximity of individual nuclei to each other, circumscribed Vim lesions may influence language function in a similar manner to lesions within the general ventral region of the thalamus (e.g. VA and VL), or lesions incorporating the nucleus reticularis, connected to and responsible for manipulating the firing mode of almost all thalamic output nuclei. In this case, in terms of the Lexical Decision Making, Response-Release Semantic Feedback and Selective Engagement models, Vim lesions may result in (1) inappropriate lexical content (e.g. semantic paraphasias) as a consequence of disturbed thalamic gating mechanisms (Wallesch and Papagno, 1988; Crosson, 1992), (2) reduced spontaneous speech and paraphasic verbal output as a consequence of disturbed VA-mediated semantic release mechanisms and/or impaired cortical arousal systems mediated by intralaminar nuclei innervated by the reticular formation (Crosson, 1985, 1992) or (3) deficits in semantically driven lexical retrieval and access to declarative memory as a consequence of disturbed thalamic engagement of language production and comprehension mechanisms (Nadeau and Crosson, 1997).

The impact of contemporary pallidotomy and thalamotomy on language function: clinical evidence

As mentioned in Chapter 3, the post-levodopa era resurgence in the use of functional neurosurgery to treat Parkinson's disease has provided a novel platform from which theories of subcortical participation in language may be tested. Typically, contemporary studies pertaining to the impact of pallidotomy and thalamotomy on cognitive functions, including language, have been neuropsychologically based. The main aim of baseline neuropsychological evaluations within Parkinsonian populations has been to identify whether cognitive and behavioural profiles are consistent with the diagnosis of Parkinson's disease, and an absence of co-existing dementia and/or neurological and psychiatric comorbidity (Saint-Cyr and Trepanier, 2000). It has been documented that patients with Parkinson's disease characteristically demonstrate difficulty on cognitive tasks that involve the functioning of striato-frontal circuitry (Dubois and Pillon, 1991). Consequently, anticipated cognitive deficits encompass the following skills: complex visuospatial functions, free recall memory, working memory, effort-demanding tasks (e.g. rapid processing and complex problem solving), set-formation and set-shifting entailing the internal control of attention, sequencing, temporal order and recency discrimination, as well as executive function (Saint-Cyr and Trepanier, 2000). Neuropsychological test batteries, therefore, typically include the following psychometric domains: brief cognitive screens (e.g. Mini-mental status evaluation, Mattis dementia rating scale), estimates of pre-morbid and current intelligence quotients (e.g. New adult reading test, Weschler Adult Intelligence Scale, Kaufman-brief intelligence test), attention/working memory/psychomotor processing speed (e.g. digit span, trail-making test (A and B), frontal executive functioning (e.g. odd man out, Wisconsin card-sorting test, Stroop test, Tower of London test, Raven's progressive matrices), language (e.g. Boston naming test, phonemic and semantic fluency, alternating fluency), verbal learning/memory (e.g. California verbal learning test, Rey auditory verbal learning test, Hopkins verbal learning test), visuospatial learning/memory (e.g. Rey–Osterrieth complex figure test), mood and frontal personality/behavioural symptoms (e.g. Beck depression inventory, Geriatric depression scale, Beck anxiety inventory, Frontal lobe personality scale) (Saint-Cyr and Trepanier, 2000).

Literature relating to the effects of ablative neurosurgical procedures on neuropsychological performance can be broadly divided into three groups: (1) bilateral PVP (BPVP), (2) unilateral PVP (UPVP) and (3) unilateral Vim thalamotomy. A general summary of post-operative cognitive findings is provided below.

Unilateral and bilateral pallidotomy: neuropsychological findings and implications for language

In relation to pallidotomy, conflicting results between studies have been reported in reference to the effects of this procedure on cognitive functioning. The main corpus of neuropsychological literature has focused primarily on the effects of unilateral lesions (Turner *et al.*, 2002). The comparatively smaller number of published BPVP studies may reflect the finding of a higher incidence of cognitive decline and speech dysfunction following BPVP (Lang *et al.*, 1999). Indeed, BPVP has been described as a more psychologically toxic procedure when compared to the effects of UPVP (Trepanier *et al.*, 2000), with unacceptably high rates of adverse effects limiting its general application (Alkhani and Lozano, 2001; Parkin *et al.*, 2002). Bilateral lesions have drawn special attention, given that data report more frequent declines in cognitive performance as a consequence of left-sided lesions (Obwegeser *et al.*, 2000). Consequently, bilateral lesions may be associated with greater risks to general levels of cognitive functioning. Within the scant BPVP cognitive literature, however, the following post-operative findings have been reported across studies: reduced verbal fluency scores (Scott *et al.*, 1998; Ghika *et al.*, 1999); absence of decline in verbal fluency, but presence of deficits in planning (Turner *et al.*, 2002); confrontation naming abilities, attention, verbal memory, visuospatial abilities and executive functioning (Ghika *et al.*, 1999).

In reference to UPVP, inconsistent cognitive outcomes have also been reported across studies, with some investigations revealing declines in neuropsychological functioning as a consequence of the procedure (Rilling *et al.*, 1996; Manning *et al.*, 1997; Uitti *et al.*, 1997, 2000; Crowe *et al.*, 1998; Masterman *et al.*, 1998; Scott *et al.*, 1998; Trepanier *et al.*, 1998, 2000; Troster *et al.*, 1998, 2002, 2003; Junque *et al.*, 1999; Yokoyama *et al.*, 1999; Alegret *et al.*, 2000, 2003; Kubu *et al.*, 2000; Lacritz *et al.*, 2000; Lombardi *et al.*, 2000; Obwegeser *et al.*, 2000; Rettig *et al.*, 2000; Schmand *et al.*, 2000; Stebbins *et al.*, 2000; de Bie *et al.*, 2001; Demakis *et al.*, 2002, 2003; Green *et al.*, 2002; Carr *et al.*, 2003; York *et al.*, 2003; Olzak *et al.*, 2006), others failing to identify any post-operative changes in cognitive functioning (Baron *et al.*, 1996; Cullum *et al.*, 1997; Soukup *et al.*, 1997; Cahn *et al.*, 1998; Fukuda *et al.*, 2000; Kuzis *et al.*, 2001; Gironell *et al.*, 2003), and still others reporting improvements in a range of cognitive skills (Junque *et al.*, 1999; Lacritz *et al.*, 2000; Obwegeser *et al.*, 2000; Rettig *et al.*, 2000; Trepanier *et al.*, 2000; Alegret *et al.*, 2003). In general, declines in verbal fluency have been reported as most common following UPVP, followed by declines in working memory as well as verbal learning and memory (Carr *et al.*, 2003). Less common changes and mixed post-operative results have been reported for executive functioning, visual memory, psychomotor speed, visuospatial abilities and naming (Carr *et al.*, 2003).

Despite the above inconsistencies, definitive hemispheric effects have been identified following UPVP (Rettig *et al.*, 2000). Of specific interest to the speech-language pathologist is the finding of significant declines in verbal fluency scores as a consequence of UPVP, in greater than 70% of studies which assess this variable (Troster *et al.*, 2003). Furthermore, out of 20 studies which have documented declines in semantic and/or phonemic fluency following pallidotomy, left-sided lesions were responsible for 65% (13/20) of these decrements (Troster *et al.*, 2003). In contrast, right-sided lesions have been more commonly associated with changes in visuospatial functions and visual memory (Carr *et al.*, 2003; Olzak *et al.*, 2006). Consequently, it has been postulated that the right and left basal ganglia, respectively, differentially mediate visuospatial and verbal abilities (Green and Barnhart, 2000), akin to the cerebral cortex.

Verbal fluency has been described as a complex task involving the engagement of numerous cognitive modules typically described as semantic or executive in nature (e.g. conceiving and application of retrieval strategy, shifting between sub-categories, accessing vocabulary and semantic processing) (De Gaspari *et al.*, 2006). The identification, via functional neuroimaging studies, of a frontotemporal network mediating verbal fluency tasks give credence to the above explanation, in that the inferior frontal gyrus incorporating Broca's area (Brodmann areas 44 and 45), the anterior cingulate cortex and superior temporal regions (Schlosser *et al.*, 1998; Gourovitch *et al.*, 2000) have been observed as the neural substrates underpinning semantic and executive functions (De Gaspari *et al.*, 2006). The reliable finding of impaired verbal fluency as a consequence of pallidotomy suggests that language systems, specifically those involving complex word-retrieval mechanisms which demand frontal lobe participation, may be seriously implicated as a consequence of basal ganglia lesions.

An inherent limitation of previous studies is that they have failed to routinely assess both semantic and phonemic fluency within the same test battery (Troster *et al.*, 2003). Of 18 studies which have simultaneously assessed phonemic and semantic fluency in UPVP patients, 33% (6/18) reported an exclusive decline in phonemic fluency, and only one study (6%) showed an exclusive decline in semantic fluency (Gironell *et al.*, 2003; Troster *et al.*, 2003). Troster *et al.* (2003) extrapolated these results further by demonstrating that patients undergoing left-sided UPVP ($N = 16$) presented greater declines in phonemic fluency performance than those undergoing right-sided UPVP ($N = 11$), with no similar observable interaction for semantic fluency. These findings suggest that phonemic fluency may be more susceptible to the effects of UPVP in the left hemisphere.

Indeed, measures of frontal lobe function have been reported as more sensitive to the effects of left UPVP lesions (Green and Barnhart, 2000). Evident verbal fluency deficits as a consequence of pallidal lesions have been attributed to disruptions in the functioning of frontal-basal ganglionic circuits involved in word-search and -retrieval processes, rather than as a result of more typical language disturbances associated with aphasia (Troster *et al.*, 2003). In support of this proposal, phonemic fluency has been conceptualized to involve executive processes and therefore to be more reliant on the frontal lobes as opposed to semantic fluency, which is dependent upon semantic networks within the temporal lobes (Troyer *et al.*, 1998).

Furthermore, qualitative analyses of verbal fluency performance post-UPVP have also revealed interesting findings which further support suggestions of frontal lobe dysfunction as a consequence of this procedure. For example, the integrity of two dissociable component processes, known as clustering and switching, determines performance success relative to verbal fluency tasks (Troyer *et al.*, 1997). Clustering refers to the ability to generate words within subcategories or clusters, and switching refers to the ability to change between clusters. Relative to UPVP populations, a significantly reduced number of switches, but not clusters, has been identified on both phonemic and semantic fluency tasks (York *et al.*, 1999, 2003; Troster *et al.*, 2002; Demakis *et al.*, 2003), and patients with left UPVP have been observed to present significantly greater declines in number of switches post-operatively, when compared to those with right UPVP (York *et al.*, 2003). Importantly, cluster size has been reported as dependent upon temporal lobe integrity and access to semantic stores (Troyer *et al.*, 1998), and switching, upon frontal-subcortical circuit integrity mediating cognitive flexibility and mental set-shifting (Troyer *et al.*, 1997).

Thalamotomy: neuropsychological findings and implications for language

In comparison to the vast body of literature detailing the affects of pallidotomy on cognitive function, the impact of thalamotomy has been modestly represented. Perhaps this is a consequence of negative early thalamotomy reports, with estimates of over 30% of unilateral lesions and 60% of bilateral lesions associated with language and memory dysfunction (Burchiel, 1995). Analogous to pallidotomy research, however, studies investigating the effects of thalamotomy on cognitive status have been for the most part neuropsychologically based, overtly lacking in-depth language analyses (Welman, 1971; Jurko and Andy, 1973; Van Buren *et al.*, 1973; Vilkki, 1978; Petrovici, 1980; Rossitch *et al.*, 1988; Hugdahl *et al.*, 1990; Lund-Johansen *et al.*, 1996; Wester and Hugdahl, 1997; Fukuda *et al.*, 2000; Hugdahl and Wester, 2000; Johnson and Ojemann, 2000). Similar again to pallidotomy findings, general reports of impairments in cognitive function (Almgren *et al.*, 1972; Van Buren *et al.*, 1973; Modesti and Blumetti, 1980) and no change in cognitive status (Levita *et al.*, 1967; Fukuda *et al.*, 2000) may be found, as well as improvements in cognitive functioning (Lund-Johansen *et al.*, 1996; Hugdahl and Wester, 2000). It must be stated, however, that such inconsistencies between reports may be largely due to the fact that the majority of early thalamotomy studies targeted different thalamic nuclei (i.e. ventrolateral) to contemporary studies (i.e. ventralintermediate) (Troster *et al.*, 1998), making the generalization of results difficult.

Nonetheless, laterality effects have also been investigated in relation to thalamotomy and cognition, with interesting implications for language/verbal functioning. It has been reported that left thalamotomy lesions incur greater deficits in verbal fluency

(Riklan *et al.*, 1969; Riklan and Levita, 1970; Vilkki and Laitinen, 1974, 1976; Petrovici, 1980; Schuurman *et al.*, 2002), executive functioning (Almgren *et al.*, 1969, 1972; Schuurman *et al.*, 2002), receptive and expressive verbal 'performance' (Vilkki and Laitinen, 1976; Modesti and Blumetti, 1980), attention (Modesti and Blumetti, 1980), dichotic listening (Wester and Hugdahl, 1997) and remembering word pairs (Almgren *et al.*, 1969). In addition, a greater incidence of language deficits of a high-level nature have been reported following left-sided as well as bilateral thalamotomy lesions (Darley *et al.*, 1975). A paucity of bilateral thalamotomy outcomes may be related to the belief that bilateral thalamic lesions present a greater risk of neurobehavioural anomalies than unilateral lesions (Troster, 2000), and as such are not discussed more fully in this chapter.

Pallidotomy and thalamotomy: application of comprehensive language assessments

As demonstrated by the above discussion, the majority of studies to date investigating the effects of pallidotomy and thalamotomy on cognition and, consequently, language operations have been largely neuropsychologically based. Assessment batteries have typically included cognitive measures of intelligence, attention, memory, executive functioning, language and visuospatial abilities. Regarding language, the effects of pallidotomy and thalamotomy on confrontation naming, verbal learning and of course verbal fluency have been given some consideration; however, the impact of these procedures on a wider range of linguistic processes which incorporate complex comprehension and sentential-level production tasks has, until recently, remained unknown.

A series of recently conducted investigations have attempted to better assess the impact of pallidotomy and thalamotomy procedures on language functions (Murdoch *et al.*, 2003, 2004; Whelan *et al.*, 2002, 2004, 2005). These studies represent the most comprehensive of their type published to date, utilizing measures of both general and high-level linguistic functioning (which incorporated single-word and sentential-level comprehension and production tasks), not routinely included within neuropsychological test batteries, as well as measures of on-line semantic processing (see Box 5.1).

The following discussion represents a summary of the aforementioned studies. The reader is referred to the full papers for a more detailed account of the findings. The specific aims of the aforementioned research were to (1) evaluate the effects of bilateral pallidotomy and unilateral thalamotomy on language function utilizing a comprehensive language test battery and (2) to discuss post-operative language profiles within the context of working theories of subcortical participation in language. As mentioned previously, ablative lesions within basal ganglia–thalamocortical circuitry components aim to reduce excessive inhibitory outflow from the GPi-SNr complex (Obeso *et al.*, 1997a) via the inactivation of target nuclei (Lang and Lees, 2002). Functionally, pallidotomy results in inhibition/inactivation of the GPi, resulting in reduced inhibition of thalamus-mediated cortical excitation. With respect to language, this alteration in circuitry dynamics results in thalamic disinhibition, which was hypothesized to result in the following: (1) extraneous verbal output as a result of disturbed preverbal semantic monitoring mechanisms and heightened anterior language cortex activity (Crosson, 1985) or (2) lexical selection deficits and speech-initiation difficulties resulting from disturbed thalamic gating mechanisms and the random excitation of inhibitory cortical interneurones (Wallesch and Papagno, 1988). In contrast,

Box 5.1 Language-assessment battery utilized to assess the impact of pallidotomy and thalamotomy on language.

Battery 1 General language

■ Neurosensory Centre Comprehensive Examination of Aphasia (NCCEA) (Spreen and Benton, 1977)
■ Boston Naming Test (BNT) (Kaplan *et al.*, 1983)

Battery 2 High-level linguistics

■ Test of Language Competence-Expanded edition (TLC-E) (Wiig and Secord, 1989)
Subtests:
 1 **Ambiguous sentences** (e.g. providing two essential meanings for ambiguous sentences (e.g. *Right then and there the man drew a gun*))
 2 **Listening comprehension: making inferences** (e.g. utilizing causal relationships or chains in short paragraphs to make logical inferences)
 3 **Oral expression: recreating sentences** (e.g. formulating grammatically complete sentences utilizing key semantic elements within defined contexts (e.g. defined context = *At the ice-cream store*; key semantic elements = *some, and, get*)
 4 **Figurative language** (e.g. interpreting metaphorical expressions (e.g. *There is rough sailing ahead for us*) and correlating structurally related metaphors (e.g. *We will be facing a hard road*) according to shared meanings)
 5 **Remembering word pairs** (e.g. recalling paired word associates)
■ The Word Test-Revised (TWT-R) (Huisingh *et al.*, 1990)
 1 **Associations** (e.g. identifying semantically unrelated words within a group of four spoken words (e.g. knee, shoulder, *bracelet*, ankle) and providing an explanation for the selected word in relation to the category of semantically related words (e.g. *The rest are parts of the body*))
 2 **Synonym generation** (e.g. generation of synonyms for verbally presented stimuli (e.g. *afraid = scared*))
 3 **Semantic absurdities** (e.g. identifying and repairing semantic incongruities (e.g. My grandfather is the youngest person in my family = My grandfather is the oldest person in my family)
 4 **Antonym generation** (e.g. generating antonyms for verbally presented stimuli (e.g. *alive = dead*))
 5 **Formulating definitions** (e.g. identify and describe critical semantic features of specified words (e.g. *house = person + lives*))
 6 **Multiple definitions** (e.g. provision of two distinct meanings for series of spoken homophonic words (e.g. *down = position/feathers/feeling*)
■ **Conjunctions and transitions subtest** of the Test of Word Knowledge (TOWK) (Wiig and Secord, 1992) (e.g. evaluation of logical relationships between clauses and sentences (e.g. *It is too cold to play outside now. We will play outside* (until/when/where/while) *it gets warmer*)
■ Wiig–Semel Test of Linguistic Concepts (WSTLC) (Wiig and Semel, 1974) (e.g. comprehension of complex linguistic structures (e.g. *John was hit by Eric. Was John hit?*))
■ Animal and tool verbal fluency

Battery 3 Semantic processing

■ On-line lexical decision task incorporating written legal non-words (i.e. pronounceable but meaningless letter strings (e.g. *BELF*)) and real word stimuli (e.g. *TRAP*) classified by number of meanings and meaning relatedness (Azuma and Van Orden, 1997) thalamotomy results in functional inhibition/inactivation of the thalamus, associated with a reduction in thalamus-mediated excitation of the cerebral cortex. With respect to language, this alteration in circuitry dynamics results in thalamic inhibition, which was hypothesized to result in the following: (1) inappropriate lexical content (e.g. semantic paraphasias) as a consequence of disturbed thalamic gating mechanisms (Wallesch and Papagno, 1988; Crosson, 1992), (2) reduced spontaneous speech and paraphasic verbal output as a consequence of disturbed VA-mediated semantic release mechanisms and/or impaired cortical arousal systems mediated by intralaminar nuclei (Crosson, 1985, 1992) or (3) any combination of language comprehension and production deficits as a result of indiscriminate or inappropriate thalamic engagement of cortical regions subserving linguistic processes (Nadeau and Crosson, 1997). These hypotheses were tested via the compilation of language profiles obtained subsequent to pallidotomy and thalamotomy procedures.

A number of interesting findings were generated from this research. Similar to neuropsychologically based studies, it was revealed that pallidotomy and thalamotomy may effect variable changes in language performance, including both improvements and declines in functioning.

Study 1: group-wise study of six patients with BPVP

Study 1 investigated the effects of BPVP (i.e. 3 months following surgery) on language function within a group of six surgical subjects, utilizing the comprehensive general and high-level language-assessment batteries summarized in Box 5.1 (Whelan *et al.*, 2004). A non-surgical Parkinson's disease (NSPD) and normative control group were also recruited for comparative purposes. When results were analysed in a group-wise fashion, no significant differences in language performance were demonstrated between groups. A case-by-case analysis of subject profiles, however, revealed a greater proportion of reliable declines in performance by the BPVP group on the Boston Naming Test and tool fluency task, as compared to the NSPD group.

The results of this research suggested that BPVP has the capacity to affect language-processing mechanisms. In particular, the above findings imply that GPi lesions may specifically impact upon semantically driven lexical retrieval mechanisms, such as the semantic gating of appropriate lexical competitors for verbal production (Wallesch and Papagno, 1988), or preverbal semantic monitoring mechanisms (Crosson, 1985).

Study 2: exploring the notion of akinetic and dyskinetic linguistic homologues in two BPVP cases over time

The next series of studies investigated the notion of akinetic and dyskinetic language homologues in two patients with Parkinson's disease over a 12 month period following BPVP (Murdoch *et al.*, 2003; Whelan *et al.*, 2005). Two patients with Parkinson's disease with opposing symptom complexes (i.e. akinetic versus dystonic/dyskinetic) served as experimental subjects in this research. When language profiles relative to general and high-level language measures (as per Box 5.1) at baseline, 3 months and 12 months following surgery were compared to a normative control group, a number of interesting findings were revealed. For instance, reliable changes in performance (including both improvements and declines) were largely restricted to higher-level language operations across subjects. Furthermore, dyskinetic symptoms were associated with an initial overall improvement in high-level language function which diminished over time. Hypokinetic symptoms, however, were associated with a more stable longitudinal linguistic profile, albeit defined by higher proportions of reliable decline versus improvement in post-operative assessment scores over time.

One subject (subject 1; akinetic) failed to demonstrate overall reliable median changes in general or high-level language abilities at 3 or 12 months following BPVP. A median trend towards reliable decline, however, was observed in relation to high-level language performance at 12 months post-BPVP. Furthermore, when case-by-case reliable change indices achieved were examined across subtests and test phases, both reliable improvements and declines in performance were identified on a number of assessment variables. At the 3 month post-operative assessment phase, subject 1 demonstrated reliable changes in performance on a total of 13 subtests collapsed across assessment batteries. Thirty-one (4/13) per cent were classified as reliable improvements and 69% (9/13) were classified as declines in performance. At the 12 month post-operative assessment phase a similar profile was revealed. Subject 1 demonstrated reliable changes on a total of 19 variables collapsed across test batteries; 32% (6/19) constituted reliable improvements and 68% (13/19) constituted reliable declines in performance. Across testing phases, reliable changes were typically observed on more complex language tasks involving lexical-semantic operations relative to elaborate linguistic relationships, the repetition and manipulation of lengthy verbal material and the production of divergent, novel language at both single-word and sentential levels.

Similarly, in relation to the other subject (subject 2; dyskinetic), a failure to demonstrate a trend towards reliable post-operative improvement or decline was observed relative to general and high-level language abilities. Again, when individual reliable change indices achieved were examined across subtests and test phases, both reliable improvements and declines in performance were identified on a number of assessment variables. At the 3 month post-operative test phase, subject 2 demonstrated reliable changes in performance on a total of 19 subtests collapsed across assessment batteries. Sixty-three (12/19) per cent were classified as reliable improvements and 37% (7/19) as reliable declines in performance. At 12 months following surgery, subject 2 demonstrated reliable changes in performance on a total of 15 subtests collapsed across assessment batteries, 47% (7/15) constituting reliable improvements in performance and 53% (8/15) constituting reliable declines. Similarly to subject 1, reliable changes in post-operative performance were typically observed on more complex linguistic measures involving lexical-semantic operations relative to elaborate linguistic relationships, the repetition and manipulation of lengthy verbal material and the production of divergent, novel language at both single-word and sentential levels.

The findings of this research lent support to the hypothesis of hyper- and hypokinetic linguistic correlates, paralleling Parkinsonian motor behaviour. Within the two cases presented, variations in performance stability over time were observed between subjects, as were subtle differences in individual language variables affected. Akinetic motor symptoms were associated with a relatively stable long-term performance profile, albeit defined by predominant proportions of reliable decline in language abilities across testing phases. Dyskinetic motor symptoms, however, were associated with a more volatile performance profile, with possible evidence of a decrescendo effect relative to surgical beneficence over time. Intersubject variability with respect to magnitudes and directions of reliable post-operative change over time was also evident. Discernable changes (i.e. both improvements and decrements) were, however, typically restricted to tasks demanding complex linguistic operations across subjects, endorsing a role for the GPi in cognitive 'focusing' and 'scaling' (Brown and Marsden, 1998) mechanisms, which potentially underpin frontal lobe-mediated lexical-semantic manipulation and selection, and possibly cognitive-linguistic resource allocation. In relation to theories of subcortical participation in language, behaviours observed lent most support to models which included the GPi as part of a frontal lobe system mediating language functions; in particular, a role in manipulating multiple competing lexical elements in both the context of verbal expression (Wallesch and Papagno, 1988) and comprehension (Nadeau and Crosson, 1997).

Studies 3 and 4: investigating a subcortical chain of command in the regulation of language processes: cerebellum versus GPi; cerebellum versus thalamus

Study 3 examined differences in language profiles between a group ($N = 5$) of patients with left primary cerebellar lesion (i.e. of vascular origin) and a group ($N = 5$) of patients with BPVP, in reference to 16 non-neurologically impaired controls (Murdoch *et al.*, 2004). Significant between-group differences were identified on a number of subtests. Post-hoc analyses revealed more pronounced decreases in high-level language skills as a consequence of cerebellar ($P \leq 0.01$) versus GPi ($P \leq 0.05$) lesions. In addition, the scope of significantly reduced scores was broader in the cerebellar group (i.e. 13 as opposed to seven variables).

The results of this study demonstrated that although GPi and cerebellar lesions implicate similar linguistic abilities, the magnitude and scope of deficits was more pronounced for the cerebellar group. These findings suggest the presence of a potential ascending neuroregulatory hierarchy corresponding to the neural axis, whereby the cerebellum influences the overall efficiency with which other brain regions (perhaps including the GPi) mediate complex lexico-semantic operations.

Study 4 examined differences in language profiles between two cases with spontaneous vascular infarcts of the left cerebellar hemisphere and two cases with Parkinson's disease and surgically induced lesions of the left Vim thalamus, in reference to 16 non-neurologically impaired controls (Whelan and Murdoch, 2005). Evident deficits were largely restricted to complex language functions, irrespective of lesion type; however, certain trends in performance were observed between groups. When compared to cerebellar lesions, thalamic lesions were associated with a higher overall proportion (i.e. 30% for thalamotomy (18/60 language variables) versus 12% for cerebellar lesions (7/60 language variables)) of below-normal test scores as well as greater magnitudes of decline from normal (average z score for reduced variables for thalamotomy was 6.01 compared with 3.04 for cerebellar lesions).

These findings support hypotheses of subcortical participation in language, and also suggest that the thalamus may play a superordinate role to the cerebellum in the regulation of higher-level lexical-semantic processes.

Study 5: examining thalamic language dominance in two cases

Study 5 investigated the role of the dominant thalamus in language (Whelan *et al.*, 2002). Experimental subjects in this research consisted of two right-handed males with tremor-dominant Parkinson's disease and unilateral lesions of the left and right Vim thalamus, respectively. The results indicated a role for the dominant thalamus in language, specifically in relation to performance on tasks of high-level language processing and the temporal processing of semantic information.

Each subject underwent a comprehensive language assessment of general and high-level language abilities as well as on-line semantic processing skills (as per Box 5.1). The surgical subjects were assessed up to 1 month prior to and 3 months following surgically induced lesions of the left or right Vim thalamus. Pre- and post thalamotomy scores were compared to the mean performance scores of a normal control and NSPD group. Post-operative changes in performance were essentially restricted to measures of high-level language functioning and, potentially, semantic processing following left thalamotomy (i.e. subject 1). Significant post-operative declines on the Test of Language Competence-Expanded edition (TLC-E) were attributed to reductions in performance on subtests of recreating sentences and remembering word pairs. Subject 2 (i.e. right thalamotomy recipient) demonstrated no significant changes in post-operative language performance.

The findings of this study support the hypothesis of a cortico-subcortico-cortical circuit subserving language function, which incorporates the dominant thalamus (Crosson, 1985; Nadeau and Crosson, 1997; Wallesch and Papagno, 1988). Lesioning of the left Vim thalamus impacted negatively on high-level language abilities and possibly the speed of lexical retrieval. Despite the fact that a specific role for the Vim nucleus of the thalamus has not been previously proposed in models of subcortical participation in language, it is postulated that post-thalamotomy neurophysiological changes in nuclei which lie in close proximity to the Vim target, including those previously implicated in language (e.g. VA, VL, pulvinar and nucleus reticularis), may account for the results observed.

An example of the high-level language errors produced by subject 1 (i.e. left Vim thalamotomy) and their possible interpretation in relation to models of subcortical participation in language have been provided below. Subject 1 demonstrated significant post-operative declines on a number of high-level linguistic measures including the recreating sentences and remembering word pairs subtests of the TLC-E (see Box 5.1), when compared to both the normal control and NSPD groups. When asked to recreate a sentence combining the lexical units *difficult*, *nonetheless* and *now* within the context of *moving house*, subject 1 responded 'Now the movers were . . . moving the difficult . . . (uhm . . .) . . . no wait . . . furniture . . . nonetheless'. Such a response demonstrated an inability to consistently and efficiently combine specified linguistic units within semantically, syntactically and pragmatically appropriate sentences. When consulting theories of subcortical participation in language, this result suggests that left Vim thalamotomy may disrupt the efficient organization, integration and production of specified lexical content (Wallesch and Papagno, 1988) within appropriate syntactic structures, or alternatively, thalamocortical disconnection may result in concept-generation deficits which include vague conceptual markers and a lack of detail in verbal expression (Nadeau and Crosson, 1997). In addition, subject 1's reduced performance in the ability to recall word pairs was consistent with the findings of Almgren *et al.* (1972) who suggested that Vim thalamotomy may impair the processing of verbal language and the subsequent ability to retrieve words from short-term memory. This hypothesis was consistent with the models of (1) Crosson (1985) based on the work of Ojemann (1975, 1976), that the thalamus acts to influence attentional mechanisms that gate the storage and retrieval of items held in short-term memory, and (2) Nadeau and Crosson (1997), that left thalamotomy may prohibit the selective engagement of cortical nets dedicated to the storage and generation of verbal language.

In relation to performance on the semantic processing/lexical decision making task, subject 1 demonstrated prolonged reaction times for all word types, with a possible reaction-time advantage for words with few meanings. In terms of spreading activation theory (Rubenstein *et al.*, 1970), it was hypothesized that left Vim thalamotomy may have served to alter word processing mechanisms, or rather, implicate the efficiency of information transfer via nodal networks. This explanation fits well with Nadeau and Crosson's (1997) selective engagement theory, whereby thalamic lesions are postulated to interfere with thalamus-mediated engagement of lexical-semantic cortical nodes. For example, after left thalamotomy word recognition may become dependent on the number of nodes shared, with an efficiency advantage for minimal nodal distribution, as per an active competition hypothesis (McClelland and Rumelhart, 1981). As such, reduced processing demands (i.e. number of meanings) result in faster recognition and/or responses for words with fewer meanings. This explanation must be considered with a degree of caution, however, in light of the lack of available data with which to compare subject 1's results (i.e. data on pre- and post-right Vim thalamotomy lexical decision making are unavailable).

Summary and caveats

On the basis of the above findings, it is apparent that a range of language alterations may result as a consequence of functionally inhibiting the GPi or Vim thalamus. The current BPVP and unilateral Vim thalamotomy language research revealed: (1) both post-operative improvements and/or decrements in language functioning, (2) greater vulnerability of higher-level language processes compared to general language processes with each procedure, (3) support for akinetic and dyskinetic language homologues, (4) possible evidence of a subcortical hierarchy whereby the cerebellum influences the overall efficiency with which other subcortical brain regions, excluding the thalamus, mediate complex lexico-semantic operations and (5) evidence of a laterality effect in relation to a thalamic contribution to language processing.

Of particular relevance to both the researcher and clinician is the evident variability in post-operative language profiles produced by pallidotomy and thalamotomy procedures across subjects. Divergent profiles were evident across subjects in relation to affected subtests, as well as magnitudes and directions of change across variables. Such variability warrants statistical and clinical caution, suggesting that pallidotomy and thalamotomy patients may be best considered on a case-by-case basis. A case-study example is provided below.

Previous researchers have eluded to the fact that potential performance heterogeneity in Parkinsonian populations may conceal significant individual differences within group comparisons (Fields et al., 1997; Trepanier et al., 1998). This finding has lead to the exploration of alternative methods of data analysis for such experimental cohorts, including the calculation of reliable change indices (RCIs) (McCarter et al., 2000). The RCI represents a standardized difference score (McCarter et al., 2000) which defines clinically significant change in individual patients, relative to a control population. As a final note, it must also be mentioned that the small sample sizes utilized in the previously summarized language research limit the generalization potential of results reported, yet provide valuable direction for future studies of the role of the GPi and Vim thalamus in mediating language processes.

Individual case study: bilateral pallidotomy

The following vignette is a brief summary of a case previously published by the authors (Whelan et al., 2000). The reader is referred to this publication for a more detailed examination of the effects of BPVP on language function.

Case history

LM was a 73 year-old, right-handed, English-speaking female with idiopathic Parkinson's disease and 10 years of formal education. Age at disease onset was 62 years and primary symptom presentation at the time of assessment was bilateral dyskinesia, dystonia and unpredictable 'on' and 'off' states. No previous history of head injury, cerebrovascular accident, cerebral tumour or abscess, coexisting neurological disease, substance abuse, psychiatric disorder, developmental language disorder or speech and/or language disturbance prior to the onset of Parkinson's disease was reported. Pre-operative neuropsychological assessment revealed executive functioning to be largely intact, with no evidence of comorbid dementing illness or indicators of anxiety or depression. Pre-operative MRI revealed nil focal brain abnormalities. LM was deemed by a neurologist an appropriate candidate for BPVP. Pre-operative daily medication regimen included: Parlodel (5 mg), Sinemet 100/25 mg, Sinemet 250/25 mg, Sinemet CR 200/50 mg, Inderal 40 mg and thyroxine 100 mg. Post-operative medication regimen included: Solprin 300 mg, Inderal 40 mg, Pravochol 40 mg, Probanthine 15 mg, Parlodel 2.5 mg, Sinemet 250/25 mg, Sinemet CR 200/50 mg and Madopar 200/50 mg. See Figure 5.1 for a post-operative MRI of bilateral lesion placement.

Language profile
LM was administered a general and high-level language-assessment battery 1 month prior to and 3 months following BPVP, within perceived 'on' periods, as well as a semantic processing/lexical decision task post-operatively (see Box 5.1). LM's general language skills remained relatively intact subsequent to BPVP; however, declines on a number of high-level language skills were evident, such as scores achieved on verbal fluency (i.e. reduced number of items produced on the phonemic fluency task) and definition-formulation tasks (e.g. when asked to define the word *scribble*, requiring the essential semantic elements of *write/colour/draw* + *without order/meaning*, LM responded 'used to take notes'; when asked to provide multiple definitions for the word *park*, LM responded 'parking a car' and 'to park yourself'). Although the phonemic fluency task was incorporated within the general language battery, it is actually considered higher level in nature and was therefore considered as a higher-level task. Some high-level language improvements in performance were also observed post-operatively, including scores achieved on the figurative language and remembering

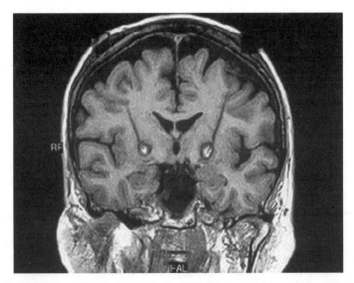

Figure 5.1 Post-operative MRI data demonstrating LM's bilateral posteroventral pallidotomy lesions.

word pairs subtests of the TLC-E, as well as some scores on the complex comprehension subtests of the Wiig-Semel Test of Linguistic Concepts. Pre-operative semantic processing/lexical decision scores were unable to be obtained for LM, therefore, post-operative performance was not discussed further within this summary (again the reader is referred to the published article (Whelan *et al.*, 2000) for a detailed discussion of post-operative semantic processing performance).

Interpretation

From the above profile it was interpreted that BPVP may impact upon language performance, with evidence of both declines and improvements in skills which were predominantly higher level in nature. In relation to reduced performance, it was hypothesized that GPi lesions resulted in semantically inadequate definitions in terms of critical attributes (e.g. circumlocutory responses or extraneous verbal output) as a consequence of thalamic disinhibition and hyperactivation of the anterior language area, consistent with predictions made on the basis of Crosson's model (Crosson, 1985). Furthermore, stimulus-bound responses on the multiple definitions task were consistent with predictions made on the basis of Wallesch and Papagno's (1988) model, in that GPi lesions resulted in a reduced capacity to accurately select or gate multiple competing definitions for expression. As a result, the same definition reference was selected more than once for production. Lesions of the GPi may disrupt thalamic gating mechanisms, resulting in disinhibited thalamic excitation of inhibitory cortical interneurones, preventing the processing of competing alternatives. Indeed, it has been previously observed that lesions of the basal ganglia system typically impair performance on tasks where degrees of freedom, in relation to possible responses, are large (Wallesch and Papagno, 1988). A similar explanation may be utilized in interpreting reduced post-operative performance on the phonemic fluency task.

Improvements in performance on some tasks, however, also suggested that BPVP may serve to equilibrate the functioning of basal ganglia–thalamocortical circuits involved in language. An explanation as to why performance on similar tasks (e.g. all divergent expressive language tasks such phonemic fluency, definition formulation, figurative language interpretation, ambiguity interpretation, synonym and antonym generation, etc.) was not affected in the same way (i.e. uniform improvement) within the same subject, remains difficult to explain. The post-operative inconsistencies (i.e. decrements and improvements in performance on comparable linguistic tasks) observed in the current case may be more accurately interpreted as the result of disruption to, or the disorganization of, the regulation of language processes along reciprocal cortico-subcortical loops (Crosson, 1985; Wallesch and Papagno, 1988). The capacity for lexical alternatives to also be gated via thalamo-frontal and fronto-thalamic circuits which bypass the basal ganglia, in addition to the assumption of functional plasticity within a disordered neural network (Wallesch and Papagno, 1988), may explain in part some of the post-operative inconsistencies in performance observed in a subject with long-standing basal ganglia pathology.

Summary

Contemporary theories of subcortical participation in language have been largely based on clinico-neuroradiological correlation studies of patients with subcortical vascular lesions involving the thalamus or striatocapsular region. Unfortunately vascular lesions are rarely confined to single subcortical nuclei (e.g. caudate nucleus, globus pallidus, etc.), often extending to involve surrounding subcortical white matter pathways. The recent renaissance of surgical interventions for the treatment of Parkinson's disease, such as pallidotomy and thalamotomy, provide an opportunity to study the effects of circumscribed lesions in the globus pallidus and thalamus on language function. The findings of several studies of the language abilities of patients who have undergone pallidotomy or thalamotomy have demonstrated both improvements and decrements in language function subsequent to these techniques but typically restricted to tasks demanding complex linguistic operations. In general, the findings of these studies suggest that subcortical structures underpin a frontal-lobe-mediated language system involved in the regulation of higher-level lexical semantic processes.

References

Alegret, M., Vendrell, P., Junque, C., Valldeoriola, F., Nobbe, F.A. *et al.* (2000). Effects of unilateral posteroventral pallidotomy on 'on-off' cognitive fluctuations in Parkinson's disease. *Neuropsychologia* 38, 628–33.

Alegret, M., Valldeoriola, F., Tolosa, E., Vendrell, P., Junque, C. *et al.* (2003). Cognitive effects of unilateral posteroventral pallidotomy: a four years follow-up study. *Movement Disorders* 18(3), 323–8.

Alexander, G.E., Crutcher, M.D. and DeLong, M.R. (1990). Basal ganglia-thalamocortical circuits: parallel substrates for motor, oculomotor, 'prefrontal' and 'limbic' functions. *Progress in Brain Research* 85, 119–46.

Alkhani, A. and Lozano, A.M. (2001). Pallidotomy for Parkinson's disease: a review of contemporary literature. *Journal of Neurosurgery* 94(1), 43–9.

Almgren, P.E., Andersson, A.L. and Kullberg, G. (1969). Differences in verbally expressed cognition following left and right ventrolateral thalamotomy. *Scandinavian Journal of Psychology* 10(4), 243–9.

Almgren, P.E., Andersson, A.L. and Kullberg, G. (1972). Long-term effects on verbally expressed cognition following left and right ventrolateral thalamotomy. *Confina Neurologica* 34, 162–8.

Azuma, T. and Van Orden, G.C. (1997). Why SAFE is better than FAST: the relatedness of a word's meaning affects lexical decision times. *Journal of Memory and Language* 36, 484–504.

Baron, M.S., Bakay, R.A.E., Green, J., Kaneoke, Y., Hashimoto, T. *et al.* (1996). Treatment of advanced Parkinson's disease by posterior gpi pallidotomy: one-year results of a pilot study. *Annals of Neurology* 40, 335–66.

Benabid, A.L., Caparros-Lefebvre, D. and Pollak, P. (1998). History of surgery for movement disorders. In I. Germano (ed.), *Neurosurgical Treatment of Movement Disorders* (pp. 19–35). Park Ridge, IL: Thieme.

Brown, P. and Marsden, C.D. (1998). What do the basal ganglia do? *Lancet* 351, 1801–4.

Burchiel, K.J. (1995). Thalamotomy for movement disorders. *Neurosurgery Clinics of North America* 6, 55–71.

Cahn, D.A., Sullivan, E.V., Shear, P.K., Heit, G., Lim, K.O. *et al.* (1998). Neuropsychological and motor functioning after unilateral anatomically guided posterior ventral pallidotomy. *Neuropsychiatry, Neuropsychology, and Behavioural Neurology* 11(3), 136–45.

Carr, J.A.R., Honey, C.R., Marci Sinden, P., Phillips, A.G. and Martzke, J.S. (2003). A waitlist control-group study of cognitive, mood, and quality of life outcome after posteroventral pallidotomy in Parkinson disease. *Journal of Neurosurgery* 99, 78–88.

Crosson, B. (1984). Role of the dominant thalamus in language: a review. *Psychological Bulletin* 96, 491–517.

Crosson, B. (1985). Subcortical functions in language: a working model. *Brain and Language* 25, 257–92.

Crosson, B. (1992). *Subcortical Functions in Language and Memory*. New York: The Guilford Press.

Crosson, B. (1999). Subcortical mechanisms in language: lexical-semantic mechanisms and the thalamus. *Brain and Cognition* 40, 414–39.

Crowe, S.F., O'Sullivan, J.D., Peppard, R F., McNeill, P.M., Bardenhagen, F. *et al.* (1998). Left posteroventral pallidotomy results in a deficit in verbal memory. *Behavioural Neurology* 11, 79–84.

Cullum, C.M., Lacritz, L., Frol, A.B., Brewer, K., Ciller, C. *et al.* (1997). Effects of pallidotomy on cognitive function in Parkinson's disease. *Journal of the International Neuropsychological Society* 3, 61.

Darley, F., Brown, J. and Swenson, M. (1975). Language changes after neurosurgery for Parkinsonism. *Brain and Language* 2, 65–70.

de Bie, R.M.A., Schuurman, P.R., Bosch, D.A., de Haan, R.J., Schmand, B. *et al.* (2001). Outcome of unilateral pallidotomy in advanced Parkinson's disease: cohort study of 32 patients. *Journal of Neurology, Neurosurgery and Psychiatry* 71, 375–82.

De Gaspari, D., Siri, C., Di Gioia, M., Antonini, A., Isella, V. *et al.* (2006). Clinical correlates and cognitive underpinnings of verbal fluency impairment after chronic subthalamic stimulation in Parkinson's disease. *Parkinsonism and Related Disorders* 12, 289–95.

Demakis, G.J., Mercury, M.G., Sweet, J.J., Rezak, M., Eller, T. *et al.* (2002). Motor and cognitive sequelae of unilateral pallidotomy in intractable Parkinson's disease: electronic measurement of motor steadiness is a useful outcome measure. *Journal of Clinical and Experimental Neuropsychology* 24(5), 655–63.

Demakis, G.J., Mercury, M.G., Sweet, J.J., Rezak, M., Eller, T. *et al.* (2003). Qualitative analysis of verbal fluency before and after unilateral pallidotomy. *The Clinical Neuropsychologist* 17(3), 322–30.

Dubois, B. and Pillon, B. (1991). Cognitive deficits in Parkinson's disease. *Journal of Neurology* 244, 2–8.

Fields, J.A., Troster, A.I., Wilkinson, S.B. and Koller, W.C. (1997). Preliminary observations of effects on cognitive function following unilateral stimulating electrode implantation in Globus Pallidus Interna (GPI) for treatment of refractory Parkinson's disease. *Journal of the International Neuropsychological Society* 3, 67.

Fukuda, M., Kameyama, S., Yoshino, M., Tanaka, R. and Narabayashi, H. (2000). Neuropsychological outcome following pallidotomy and thalamotomy for Parkinson's disease. *Stereotactic and Functional Neurosurgery* 74, 11–20.

Ghika, J., Ghika-Schmid, F., Fankhauser, H., Assal, G., Vingerhoets, F. *et al.* (1999). Bilateral contemporaneous posteroventral pallidotomy for the treatment of Parkinson's disease: neuropsychological and neurological side effects. *Journal of Neurosurgery* 91, 313–21.

Gildenberg, P.L. (1984). The present role of stereotactic surgery in the management of parkinson's disease. In R.G. Hassler and J.F. Christ (eds), *Advances in Neurology*, vol. 40 (pp. 447–52). New York: Raven Press.

Gironell, A., Kulisevsky, J., Rami, L., Fortuny, N., Garcia-Sanchez, C. *et al.* (2003). Effects of pallidotomy and bilateral subthalamic stimualtion on cognitive function in Parkinson disease: a controlled comparative study. *Journal of Neurology* 250, 917–23.

Gourovitch, M.L., Kirkby, B.S., Goldberg, T.E., Weinberger, D.R., Gold, J.M. *et al.* (2000). A comparison of rCBF patterns during letter and semantic fluency. *Neuropsychology* 14, 353–60.

Green, J. and Barnhart, H. (2000). The impact of lesion laterality on neuropsychological change following posterior pallidotomy: a review of current findings. *Brain and Cognition* 42, 379–98.

Green, J., McDonald, W.M., Vitek, J.L., Haber, M., Barnhart, H. *et al.* (2002). Neuropsychological and psychiatric sequelae of pallidotomy for PD: clinical trial findings. *Neurology* 58, 858–65.

Harrington, D.L. and Haaland, K.Y. (1991). Sequencing in Parkinson's disease: abnormalities in programming and controlling movement. *Brain* 114, 99–115.

Hoover, J.E. and Strick, P.L. (1999). The organisation of cerebello- and pallido-thalamic projections to primary motor cortex: an investigation employing retrograde transneuronal transport of herpes simplex virus type I. *Journal of Neuroscience* 19, 1446–63.

Hugdahl, K. and Wester, K. (2000). Neurocognitive correlates of stereotactic thalamotomy and thalamic stimulation in parkinson's patients. *Brain and Cognition* 42, 231–52.

Hugdahl, K., Wester, K. and Asbjornsen, A. (1990). The role of the left and right thalamus in language asymmetry: dichotic listening in Parkinson's patients undergoing stereotactic thalamotomy. *Brain and Language* 39, 1–13.

Huisingh, R., Barrett, M., Zachman, L., Blagden, C. and Orman, J. (1990). *The Word Test-Revised: a Test of Expressive Vocabulary and Semantics*. East Moline, IL: Linguisystems.

Joel, D. and Weiner, I. (1994). The organisation of the basal ganglia-thalamocortical circuits: open inter-connected rather than closed segregated. *Neuroscience* 63, 363–79.

Johnson, M. and Ojemann, G. (2000). The role of the human thalamus in language and memory: evidence from electrophysiological studies. *Brain and Cognition* 42, 218–30.

Jones, E. (1985). *The Thalamus*. New York: Plenum Press.

Junque, C., Alegret, M., Nobbe, F.A., Valldeoriola, F., Pueyo, R. *et al.* (1999). Cognitive and behavioural changes after unilateral posteroventral pallidotomy: relationship with lesional data from MRI. *Movement Disorders* 14(5), 780–9.

Jurko, M.F. and Andy, O.J. (1973). Psychological changes correlated with thalamotomy site. *Journal of Neurology, Neurosurgery and Psychiatry* 36(5), 846–52.

Kaplan, E., Goodglass, H. and Weintraub, S. (1983). *Boston Naming Test*. Philadelphia, PA: Lippincott Williams and Wilkins.

Kleiner-Fisman, G., Fisman, D.N. and Sime, E. (2003). Long-term follow up of bilateral deep brain stimulation of the subthalamic nucleus in patients with advanced Parkinson's disease. *Journal of Neurosurgery* 99, 489–95.

Kubu, C.S., Grace, G.M. and Parrent, A.G. (2000). Cognitive outcome following pallidotomy: the influence of side of surgery and age of patient at disease onset. *Journal of Neurosurgery* 92, 384–9.

Kuzis, G., Sabe, L., Tiberti, C., Dorrego, F., Starkstein, S. *et al.* (2001). Neuropsychological effects of pallidotomy in patients with Parkinson's disease. *Journal of Neurology, Neurosurgery and Psychiatry* 71, 563–4.

Lacritz, L.H., Munro Cullum, C., Frol, A.B., Dewey, R.B. and Giller, C.A. (2000). Neuropsychological outcome following unilateral stereotactic pallidotomy in intractable Parkinson's disease. *Brain and Cognition* 42, 364–78.

Lang, A.E. and Lozano, A.M. (1998). Medical progress: Parkinson's disease (Part II of II). *New England Journal of Medicine* 339(15), 1130–43.

Lang, A.E. and Lees, A. (2002). Management of Parkinson's disease: an evidence-based review. *Movement Disorders* 17 (suppl. 4), S128–47.

Lang, A.E., Duff, J., Saint-Cyr, J.A., Trepanier, L.L., Gross, R.E. *et al.* (1999). Posteroventral medial pallidotomy in Parkinson's disease. *Journal of Neurology* 246(II), 28–41.

Lenz, F.A., Vitek, J.L. and DeLong, M.R. (1993). Role of the thalamus in Parkinsonian tremor: evidence from studies in patients and primate models. *Stereotactic and Functional Neurosurgery* 60, 94–103.

Lenz, F.A., Normand, S. and Kwan, H.C. (1995). Statistical prediction of the optimal site for thalamotomy in Parkinsonian tremor. *Movement Disorders* 10, 318–28.

Levita, E., Riklan, M. and Cooper, D.B. (1967). Psychological comparison of unilateral and bilateral thalamic surgery. *Journal of Abnormal Psychology* 72(3), 251–4.

Lieberman, P. (2000). *Human Language and our Reptilian Brain: the Subcortical Bases of Speech, Syntax, and Thought*. Cambridge, MA: Harvard University Press.

Lombardi, W.J., Gross, R.E., Trepanier, L.L., Lang, A.E., Lozano, A.M. *et al.* (2000). Relationship of lesion location to cognitive outcome following microelectrode-guided pallidotomy for Parkinson's disease: support for the existence of cognitive circuits in the human pallidum. *Brain* 123, 746–58.

Lund-Johansen, M., Hugdahl, K. and Wester, K. (1996). Cognitive function in patients with Parkinson's disease undergoing stereotaxic thalamotomy. *Journal of Neurology, Neurosurgery and Psychiatry* 60, 564–71.

Manning, C.A., Bennett, J.P., Wilkniss, S.M., Jones, M.G. and Laws, E.R. (1997). Comprehensive neuropsychological assessment of cognitive functioning pre- and post-unilateral posteroventral pallidotomy. *Neurology* 48, A252.

Marsden, C.D. and Obeso, J.A. (1994). The functions of the basal ganglia and the paradox of stereotaxic surgery in Parkinson's disease. *Brain* 117, 877–97.

Masterman, D., DeSalles, A., Baloh, R.W., Frysinger, R., Foti, D. *et al.* (1998). Motor, cognitive and behavioural performance following unilateral ventroposterior pallidotomy for Parkinson's disease. *Archives of Neurology* 55, 1201–8.

McCarter, R.J., Walton, N.H., Rowan, A.F., Gill, S.S. and Palomo, M. (2000). Cognitive functioning after subthalamic nucleotomy for refractory Parkinson's disease. *Journal of Neurology, Neurosurgery and Psychiatry* 69, 60–6.

McClelland, J.L. and Rumelhart, D.E. (1981). An interactive activation model of context effects in letter perception: Part 1. An account of the basic findings. *Psychological Review* 88, 375–407.

Middleton, F.A. and Strick, P.L. (1994). Anatomical evidence for cerebellar and basal ganglia involvement in higher cognitive function. *Science* 266, 458–61.

Middleton, F.A. and Strick, P.L. (2000). Basal ganglia output and cognition: evidence from anatomical, behavioural, and clinical studies. *Brain and Cognition* 42, 183–200.

Mink, J.W. and Thach, W.T. (1991). Basal ganglia motor control. I. Nonexclusive relation of pallidal discharge to five movement modes. *Journal of Neurophysiology* 65, 273–300.

Modesti, L.M. and Blumetti, A.E. (1980). Long term effects of stereotaxic thalamotomy on parameters of cognitive functioning. *Acta Neurochirurgica: Supplementum* 30, 401–3.

Murdoch, B.E., Whelan, B.-M., Theodoros, D.G., Hall, B. and Silburn, P. (2003). Correlating motor and cognitive behaviour: exploring the notion of akinetic and dyskinetic linguistic homologues. *Brain and Language* 87, 192.

Murdoch, B.E., Whelan, B.-M., Theodoros, D.G. and Cahill, L. (2004). A subcortical chain of command involved in the regulation of linguistic processes? *Brain and Language* 91, 175–6.

Nadeau, S.E. and Crosson, B. (1997). Subcortical aphasia. *Brain and Language* 58, 355–402.

Obeso, J.A., Rodriguez, M.C., Gorospe, A., Guridi, J., Alvarez, L. *et al.* (1997a). Surgical treatment of Parkinson's disease. *Bailliere's Clinical Neurology* 6(1), 125–45.

Obeso, J.A., Guridi, J. and DeLong, M.R. (1997b). Surgery for Parkinson's disease. *Journal of Neurology, Neurosurgery and Psychiatry* 62(1), 2–8.

Obwegeser, A.A., Uitti, R., Lucas, J.A., Witte, R.J., Turk, M.F. *et al.* (2000). Predictors of neuropsychological outcome in patients following microelectrode-guided pallidotomy for Parkinson's disease. *Journal of Neurosurgery* 93, 410–20.

Ojemann, G. (1975). Improved performance in some dysnomic states after human ventrolateral thalamic stimulation. *Journal of Neurology, Neurosurgery and Psychiatry* 38, 408.

Ojemann, G. (1976). Subcortical language mechanisms. In H.A. Whitaker and H. Whitaker (eds), *Studies in Neurolinguistics* (pp. 103–38). New York: Academic Press.

Olzak, M., Laskowska, I., Jelonek, J., Michalak, M., Szolna, A. *et al.* (2006). Psychomotor and executive functioning after unilateral posteroventral pallidotomy in patients with Parkinson's disease. *Journal of the Neurological Sciences* 248, 97–103.

Owen, A.M., Doyon, J., Dagher, A., Sadikot, A. and Evans, A.C. (1998). Abnormal basal ganglia outflow in Parkinson's disease identified with PET: implications for higher cortical functions. *Brain* 121, 949–65.

Parkin, S.G., Gregory, R.P., Scott, R., Bain, P., Silburn, P. *et al.* (2002). Unilateral and bilateral pallidotomy for idiopathic Parkinson's disease: a case series of 115 patients. *Movement Disorders* 17(4), 682–92.

Percheron, G. and Filion, M. (1991). Parallel processing in the basal ganglia: up to a point. *Trends in Neuroscience* 14, 55–9.

Petrovici, J.N. (1980). Speech disturbances following stereotaxic surgery in ventrolateral thalamus. *Neurosurgical Review* 3(3), 189–95.

Rettig, G.M., York, M.K., Lai, E.C., Jankovic, J., Krauss, J.K. *et al.* (2000). Neuropsychological outcome after unilateral pallidotomy for the treatment of Parkinson's disease. *Journal of Neurology, Neurosurgery and Psychiatry* 69, 326–36.

Riklan, M. and Levita, E. (1970). Psychological studies of thalamic lesions in humans. *Journal of Nervous and Mental Disease* 150, 251–65.

Riklan, M., Levita, E., Zimmerman, J. and Cooper, I.S. (1969). Thalamic correlates of language and speech. *Journal of the Neurological Sciences* 8, 307–28.

Rilling, L.M., Filoteo, J.V., Roberts, J.W. and Heilbrun, M.P. (1996). Neuropsychological functioning in patients with Parkinson's disease pre- and post-pallidotomy. *Archives of Clinical Neurophysiology* 11, 60.

Rossitch, E., Zeidman, S., Nashold, B., Horner, J., Walker, J. *et al.* (1988). Evaluation of memory and language function pre- amd post-thalamotomy with an attempt to define those patients at risk for postoperative dysfunction. *Surgical Neurology* 29, 11–16.

Rubenstein, H., Garfield, L. and Millikan, J. (1970). Homographic enteries in the internal lexicon. *Verbal Learning and Verbal Behaviour* 9, 484–94.

Saint-Cyr, J.A. and Trepanier, L.L. (2000). Neuropsychologic assessment of patients for movement disorder surgery. *Movement Disorders* 15(5), 771–83.

Schell, G.R. and Strick, P.L. (1984). The origin of thalamic inputs to the arcuate premotor and supplementary motor areas. *Journal of Neuroscience* 4, 539–60.

Schlosser, R., Hutchinson, M., Joseffer, S., Rusinek, H., Saarimaki, A. *et al.* (1998). Functional magnetic resonance imaging of human brain activity in a verbal fluency task. *Journal of Neurology, Neurosurgery and Psychiatry* 64, 492–8.

Schmand, B., de Bie, R.M.A., Koning-haanstra, M., de Smet, J.S., Speelman, J.D. *et al.* (2000). Unilateral pallidotomy in PD: a controlled study of cognitive and behavioural effects. *Neurology* 54, 1058–64.

Schuurman, P.R., Bruins, J., Merkus, M.P., Bosch, D.A. and Speelman, J.D. (2002). A comparison of neuropsychological effects of thalamotomy and thalamic stimulation. *Neurology* 59, 1232–9.

Scott, R.B., Gregory, R., Hines, N., Carroll, C., Hyman, N. *et al.* (1998). Neuropsychological, neurological and functional outcome following pallidotomy for Parkinson's disease: a consecutive series of eight simultaneous bilateral and twelve unilateral procedures. *Brain* 121, 659–75.

Scott, R.B., Harrison, J., Boulton, C., Wilson, J., Gregory, R. *et al.* (2002). Global attentional-executive sequelae following surgical lesions to globus pallidus interna. *Brain* 125, 562–74.

Sohn, Y.H. and Hallett, M. (2005). Basal ganglia, motor control and Parkinsonism. In N. Galvez-Jimenez (ed.), *Scientific Basis for the Treatment of Parkinson's Disease* (pp. 33–51). London: Taylor and Francis.

Soukup, V.M., Ingram, F., Schiess, M.C., Bonnen, J.G., Nauta, H.J.W. *et al.* (1997). Cognitive sequelae of unilateral posteroventral pallidotomy. *Archives of Neurology* 54, 947–50.

Speelman, J.D. and Bosch, D.A. (2002). Neurosurgical treatment modalities in Parkinson's disease. *Movement Disorders* 17 (suppl. 2), S83–5.

Spreen, O. and Benton, A.L. (1977). *Neurosensory Centre Comprehensive Examination for Aphasia*. Victoria: University of Victoria.

Starr, P.A., Vitek, J.L. and Bakay, R.A.E. (1998). Ablative surgery and deep brain stimulation for Parkinson's disease. *Neurosurgery* 43(5), 989–1015.

Stebbins, G.T., Gabrieli, J.D.E., Sannon, K.M., Penn, R.D. and Goetz, C.G. (2000). Impaired frontostriatal cognitive functioning following posteroventral pallidotomy in advanced Parkinson's disease. *Brain and Cognition* 42, 348–63.

Trepanier, L.L., Saint-Cyr, J.A., Lozano, A.M. and Lang, A.E. (1998). Neuropsychological consequences of posteroventral pallidotomy for the treatment of Parkinson's disease. *Neurology* 51, 207–15.

Trepanier, L.L., Kumar, R., Lozano, A.M., Lang, A.E. and Saint-Cyr, J.A. (2000). Neuropsychological outcome of GPi pallidotomy and GPi or STN deep brain stimulation in Parkinson's disease. *Brain and Cognition* 42, 324–47.

Troster, A. (2000). Introduction to neurobehavioural issues in the neurosurgical treatment of movement disorders: basic issues, thalamotomy, and non-ablative treatments. *Brain and Cognition* 42, 173–82.

Troster, A., Wilkinson, S.B., Fields, J., Miyawaki, K. and Koller, W.C. (1998). Chronic electrical stimulation of the left ventrointermediate thalamic nucleus for the treatment of pharmacotherapy-resistant Parkinson's disease: a differential impact on access to semantic and episodic memory? *Brain and Cognition* 38, 125–49.

Troster, A., Woods, S.P., Fields, J., Hanisch, C. and Beatty, W.W. (2002). Declines in switching underlie verbal fluency changes after unilateral pallidal surgery in Parkinson's disease. *Brain and Cognition* 50, 207–17.

Troster, A., Woods, S.P. and Fields, J. (2003). Verbal fluency declines after pallidotomy: an interaction between task and lesion laterality. *Applied Neuropsychology* 10(2), 69–75.

Troyer, A.K., Moscovitch, M. and Winocur, G. (1997). Clustering and switching as two components of phonemic fluency: evidence from younger and older healthy controls. *Neuropsychology* 11, 138–46.

Troyer, A.K., Moscovitch, M., Winocur, G., Alexander, M.P. and Stuss, D. (1998). Clustering and switching on verbal fluency: the effects of focal frontal and temporal-lobe lesions. *Neuropsychologia* 36, 499–504.

Turner, K.R., Reid, W.G., Homewood, J. and Cook, R.J. (2002). Neuropsychological sequelae of bilateral posteroventral pallidotomy. *Journal of Neurology, Neurosurgery and Psychiatry* 73, 444–6.

Uitti, R.J., Wharen, R.E., Turk, M.F., Lucas, J.A., Finton, M.J. *et al.* (1997). Unilateral pallidotomy for Parkinson's disease: comparison of outcome in younger versus elderly patients. *Neurology* 49, 1072–7.

Uitti, R., Wharen, R., Duffy, J.A., Lucas, J.A., Schneider, S.L. *et al.* (2000). Unilateral pallidotomy for Parkinson's disease: speech, motor, and neuropsychological outcome measurements. *Parkinsonism and Related Disorders* 6, 133–43.

Van Buren, J.M., Shapiro, D.Y., Henderson, W.G. and Sadowsky, D.A. (1973). A qualitative and quantitative evaluation of Parkinsonians three to six years following thalamotomy. *Confina Neurologica* 35(4), 202–35.

Vilkki, J. (1978). Effects of thalamic lesions on complex perception and memory. *Neuropsychologia* 16(4), 427–37.

Vilkki, J. and Laitinen, L.V. (1974). Differential effects of left and right ventrolateral thalamotomy on receptive and expressive verbal performances and face matching. *Neuropsychologia* 12, 11–19.

Vilkki, J. and Laitinen, L.V. (1976). Effects of pulvinotomy and ventrolateral thalamotomy on some cognitive functions. *Neuropsychologia* 14, 67–78.

Vitek, J.L., Bakay, R.A.E. and Freeman, A. (2003). Randomised trial of pallidotomy versus medical therapy for Parkinson's disease. *Annals of Neurology* 53, 558–69.

Wallesch, C.-W. (1990). Repetitive verbal behaviour: functional and neurological considerations. *Aphasiology* 4, 133–54.

Wallesch, C.-W. (1997). Symptomatology of subcortical aphasia. *Journal of Neurolinguistics* 10(4), 267–75.

Wallesch, C.-W. and Papagno, C. (1988). Subcortical aphasia. In F.C. Rose, R. Whurr and M.A. Wyke (eds), *Aphasia* (pp. 256–87). London: Whurr Publishers.

Welman, A.J. (1971). Neuropsychological examination of Parkinson's disease patients: before and after thalamotomy. *Schweizer Archiv fuer Neurologie, Neurochirurgie und Psychiatrie* 108(1), 175–88.

Wester, K. and Hugdahl, K. (1997). Thalamotomy and thalamic stimulation: effects on cognition. *Stereotactic and Functional Nuerosurgery* 69, 80–5.

Whelan, B.-M. and Murdoch, B.E. (2005). Unravelling subcortical linguistic substrates: comparison of thalamic versus cerebellar cognitive-linguistic regulation mechanisms. *Aphasiology* 19(12), 1097–1106.

Whelan, B.-M., Murdoch, B.E., Theodoros, D.G., Silburn, P. and Harding-Clark, J.A. (2000). Towards a better understanding of the role of subcortical nuclei participation in language: the study of a case following bilateral pallidotomy. *Asia Pacific Journal of Speech, Language and Hearing* 5, 93–112.

Whelan, B.-M., Murdoch, B.E., Theodoros, D.G., Silburn, P. and Hall, B. (2002). A role for the dominant thalamus in language? A linguistic comparison of two cases subsequent to unilateral thalamotomy procedures in the dominant and non-dominant hemispheres. *Aphasiology* 16(12), 1213–26.

Whelan, B.-M., Murdoch, B., Theodoros, D.G., Silburn, P. and Hall, B. (2004). Redefining functional models of basal ganglia organisation: a role for the posteroventral pallidum in linguistic processing. *Movement Disorders* 19(11), 1267–78.

Whelan, B.-M., Murdoch, B.E., Theodoros, D.G., Silburn, P. and Hall, B. (2005). Borrowing from models of motor control to translate cognitive processes: evidence for hypokinetic-hyperkinetic linguistic homologues? *Journal of Neurolinguistics* 18, 361–81.

Wichmann, T. and DeLong, M.R. (1998). Models of basal ganglia function and pathophysiology of movement disorders. *Neurosurgery Clinics of North America* 9(2), 223–36.

Wiig, E.H. and Semel, E. (1974). Development of comprehension of logical grammatical sentences by grade school children. *Perceptual and Motor Skills* 38, 171–6.

Wiig, E.H. and Secord, W. (1989). *Test of Language Competence-Expanded Edition*. New York: The Psychological Corporation.

Wiig, E.H. and Secord, W. (1992). *Test of Word Knowledge*. New York: The Psychological Corporation.

Yokoyama, T., Imamura, Y., Sugiyama, K., Nishizawa, S., Yokota, N. *et al.* (1999). Prefrontal dysfunction following unilateral posteroventral pallidotomy for Parkinson's disease. *Journal of Neurosurgery* 90, 1005–10.

York, M., Levin, H.S., Grossman, R.G. and Hamilton, W.J. (1999). Neuropsychological outcome following unilateral pallidotomy. *Brain* 122, 2209–20.

York, M., Levin, H.S., Grossman, R.G., Lai, E.C. and Krauss, J.K. (2003). Clustering and switching in phonemic fluency following pallidotomy for the treatment of Parkinson's disease. *Journal of Clinical and Experimental Neuropsychology* 25(1), 110–21.

6 A role for the subthalamic nucleus in language

Introduction

The theoretical models of subcortical participation in language, previously summarized in Chapter 3, failed to consider a role for the subthalamic nucleus (STN), a subcortical structure positioned inferiorly to the thalamus (see Chapter 2). Neglecting the STN was considered a shortcoming by the current authors, given that contemporary studies have revealed evidence of robust STN-mediated excitatory effects upon basal ganglia nuclei (Parent and Hazrati, 1995b; Rodriguez-Oroz *et al.*, 2000) positioned within subcortical language circuits (Crosson, 1985; Wallesch and Papagno, 1988; Nadeau and Crosson, 1997). This discovery prompted a revision of the aforementioned language models, with the aim of incorporating an anatomical and functional role for the STN within existing subcortical language schemas (Whelan *et al.*, 2003a).

The exclusion of the STN from previous subcortical language models may be attributed to the fact that seminal schemas of basal ganglia–thalamocortical circuitry (Nauta, 1979; DeLong and Georgopoulos, 1981; DeLong *et al.*, 1983; Alexander *et al.*, 1986) neglected to establish the STN as an intrinsic regulatory component of the basal ganglia, with the potential to influence motor, and possibly cognitive, functions. Rather, the STN (Nauta and Cole, 1978) was originally considered to represent one of a group of nodal foci within subsidiary circuits, postulated to have the capacity to externally modulate activity within primary cortico-striato-pallido (i.e. globus pallidus internus, GPi)-thalamo-cortical pathways (Alexander *et al.*, 1986). The precise way in which these nodal foci were hypothesized to modulate basal ganglia and hence thalamocortical activity, however, was not afforded salient consideration. Accordingly, theories of subcortical participation in language founded upon formative frameworks of basal ganglia–thalamocortical organization have proffered what we currently recognize as the *direct pathway* (i.e. cortico-striato-GPi-thalamo-cortical) to represent the neural highway underpinning linguistic processes (Crosson, 1985; Wallesch and Papagno, 1988).

The subsequent expansion of functional schemas of basal ganglia organization since the inception of these language models, however, has culminated in the conceptualization of a *direct/indirect* basal ganglia pathway dichotomy, which proposes an *indirect neural pathway* (i.e. cortico-striato-globus pallidus externus (GPe)-STN-GPi-substantia nigra pars reticulata (SNr)-thalamo-cortical) to lie in parallel to the aforementioned *direct pathway* (Albin *et al.*, 1989; Alexander and Crutcher, 1990) (see Figure 2.3, p. 23). The route via which the striatum innervates the GPi-SNr complex provides the basis for the designation of the basal ganglia pathways. More specifically, a monosynaptic striato-GPi-SNr channel represents the direct pathway, and a disynaptic striatal channel incorporating the GPe and STN, constitutes the indirect pathway (Parent and Hazrati, 1995b). As mentioned previously, the respective pathways have been documented to exert oppositional effects upon output nuclei of the basal ganglia, largely by way of differential neurotransmission mechanisms (i.e.excitatory versus inhibitory), yet to each facilitate the transfer of striatally processed cortical inputs to the output nuclei of the basal ganglia (Smith *et al.*, 1998).

Representing a crucial component of the classical indirect pathway, the STN facilitates communication between striatal efferents (i.e. pathways travelling away from the striatum) and principal output nuclei of the basal ganglia (i.e. GPi-SNr) by way of an intermediary GPe-STN projection (Parent and Hazrati, 1995b). Contemporary research has acclaimed the STN as the driving force of basal ganglia outputs, intrinsically involved in the regulation of motor behaviour (Benazzouz and Hallet, 2000). STN dysfunction, defined by an increase in neuronal firing rate (Hutchinson *et al.*, 1998), has even been postulated as the pathophysiological linchpin of Parkinson's disease (Guridi *et al.*, 1996). In Parkinsonian primates, excessive excitatory output from the STN has been reported to result in the tonic inhibition of thalamic motor nuclei as a consequence of heightened GPi-SNr inhibitory output (DeLong, 1990). Thalamic inhibition subsequently results in reduced activity within cortical motor neurones. Of note, in addition to a dorsolateral sensorimotor subdivision, ventromedial associative and medial limbic STN territories have also been identified (Parent and Hazrati, 1995b), suggesting that STN contributions to human behaviour may extend beyond the domain of motor control to cognitive functions, including language.

Furthermore, with respect to prevailing conceptualizations of basal ganglia organization, novel tracing studies have more recently disclosed additional indirect pathways with the potential to influence STN activity (Parent and Hazrati, 1995b; Smith *et al.*, 1998). In addition to sharing a pallido-subthalamic link, the primary constituents of the classical indirect pathway (i.e. GPe and STN), have also been reported to independently demonstrate wide-ranging afferent and efferent subcortical and/or cortical connections, which serve to directly and indirectly influence GPi-SNr activity). These findings subsequently challenge the classical direct/indirect pathway dichotomy mentioned previously which represents the most widely accepted axiomatic schema of functional organization within the basal ganglia (Parent and Hazrati, 1995b). The above evidence, in addition to the fact that established maxima of basal ganglia stratification fail to consistently support predictions of basal ganglia dysfunction (Lang and Lozano, 1998), necessitated the current authors to revise the established models of basal ganglia–thalamocortical organization, specifically those which subserve the mediation of linguistic processes.

Subthalamic nucleus connections and potential implications for proposed basal ganglia–thalamocortical circuits subserving language processes

In relation to operative models of subcortical participation in language, the striatum, GPi and a range of thalamic nuclei (including ventral anterior (VA) and ventral lateral (VL) nuclei, pulvinar, centrum medianum (CM) and nucleus reticularis (NR)) have been hypothesized to facilitate the activation, integration, transfer and/or modulation of cortically generated context-specific and linguistic information by way of cortico-subcortico-cortical circuits (Crosson, 1985; Wallesch and Papagno, 1988; Nadeau and Crosson, 1997). The STN, however, has also been postulated to have the capacity to regulate activity within thalamocortical projection neurones, by way of its robust excitatory influences upon the principal output nuclei of the basal ganglia (Benazzouz et al., 2001), and as such may also play a role in the regulation of language processes.

Notably, recent revisions of basal ganglia anatomy and physiology have indicated that the neural domain of STN influence extends well beyond that of the GPi and SNr (Parent and Hazrati, 1995b). Reportedly, output neurones of the STN also innervate the striatum, cerebral cortex, substantia nigra pars compacta and, perhaps of most note, the GPe (Jackson and Crossman, 1981; Kita and Kitai, 1987). Traditionally, the GPe has been conceptualized as a relay structure, which indirectly links striatal effer- ents and basal ganglia output nuclei, by way of the STN (Albin et al., 1989; Alexander and Crutcher, 1990). In addition to the classical indirect GPe-STN connection, the GPe has now been shown to project outputs to other core components of the basal ganglia (i.e. striatum, GPi-SNr) and related nuclei, including the NR of the thalamus and the pedunculopontine tegmental nucleus (Hazrati et al., 1990; Hazrati and Parent, 1991; Parent et al., 1991). Thus, net STN neuronal activity has been hypothesized to repre- sent the endpoint of complex chemospecific neuronal interactions, which in addition to the systems mentioned above is also influenced by cortical, centromedian/para- fascicular complex (CMPFC) and substantia nigra pars compacta input (Parent and Hazrati, 1995b).

Most recently disclosed indirect circuits with potential influences on STN activity and other subcortical nuclei implicated within language circuits, include (1) glutama- tergic (i.e. excitatory) STN-GPe projections (Nauta and Cole, 1978), (2) glutamatergic cortical-STN projections (Kita, 1994), (3) GABAergic (i.e. inhibitory) GPe projections to GPi-SNr and NR (Smith et al., 1998), (4) glutamatergic CMPFC-STN projections (Parent and Hazrati, 1995b) and (5) GABAergic GPi-CM projections (Parent and Hazrati, 1995a). It has been acknowledged that STN-striatal projections may also serve to influence language, possibly via the augmentation of excitatory cortico- and thalamo-striatal inputs which serve to regulate striatal activity (Parent and Hazrati, 1995b). The relative sparseness of STN-striatal in comparison to pallidal and SNr innervations (Parent and Hazrati, 1995b), however, precluded further detailed discus- sion of the functional significance of this pathway within this chapter. The ensuing summary attempts to extrapolate working models of subcortical participation in lan- guage by way of incorporating the abovementioned indirect basal ganglia pathways in existing theoretical schemas.

Revised theoretical schemas of subcortical participation in language: incorporating a role for the subthalamic nucleus

Together with the striatum, the STN has been documented to receive a diffuse array of cortical outputs (Hazrati and Parent, 1993), with some reports detailing projections from the entire cortical mantle (Rouzaire-Dubois and Scarnati, 1985). This anatomical schema supports a potential role for the STN in the processing of cortical information, which may include input from language-dedicated cortical regions. The integration of cortico-striatal and cortico-subthalamic outputs, however, has been postulated to occur at the level of the globus pallidus, given that striatal and STN axons have been observed to terminate upon homogeneous neurones within the GPi and GPe (Hazrati and Parent, 1992). Thus, the STN may represent an essential component of a language-processing circuit, with the ability to integrate cortical inputs and regulate basal ganglia outputs by way of direct connections with the internal and external segments of the globus pallidus.

Of note, further revisions of STN anatomy and function have revealed that sub-thalamo-pallidal projections violate the inherent segregated pathway principle of basal ganglia organization (Haber *et al.*, 1994). More specifically, primary STN inputs reportedly find their origin in the associative portion of the GPe; however, major outputs of the STN have been documented to project to motor divisions of the GPe and GPi (Weiner, 1997). As a result, the STN has been postulated to have the capacity to facilitate 'cross talk' (Feger *et al.*, 1994) between functionally distinct regions of the basal ganglia. These neural substrates, in addition to the recent identification of pallido-pallido (GPe-GPi-SNr), thalamo-subthalamic (CMPFC-STN) and pallido-thalamic (GPe-NR and GPi-CM) projections, which may potentially influence thalamus-mediated cortical activation, imply unequivocal ramifications for established theories of subcortical participation in language.

Based on the above evidence, the current authors have proposed the integration of indirect basal ganglia pathways within established cortico-striato-GPi-thalamo-corti-cal linguistic circuits to impact upon cortico-subcortical, subcortico-subcortical and subcortico-cortical interactions (Whelan *et al.*, 2003a, 2003b). As stated previously, the striatum and STN simultaneously receive cortical inputs (Hazrati and Parent, 1993), and provide the source of major projections to the GPe and GPi-SNr (Parent and Hazrati, 1995b). By way of apparent similarities in their anatomical configuration, the conceptualization of the striatum and STN as equipotential or symbiotic basal ganglia components subserving language processes was deemed a tenable hypothesis. The precise nature of definitively complex striato- and subthalamo-pallidal interactions, however, is yet to be determined (Parent and Hazrati, 1995b). Current evidence has highlighted that the activation of excitatory or inhibitory neurochemical pathways typically results in complex or subtle alterations in the neuronal firing patterns of target cells, as opposed to a net inhibitory or excitatory effects (Parent and Hazrati, 1995b). The existence of oppositional striato-pallidal and STN-pallidal neurochemical transmission mechanisms (i.e. excitatory versus inhibitory), therefore, suggests a potential counterbalancing function for these nuclei relative to the firing patterns of pallido-thalamic output neurones subserving language functions. The hypothesized impact of pallido-pallidal, thalamo-subthalamic and pallido-thalamic interactions upon linguistic functions will be afforded detailed consideration within the ensuing sections, in relation to operative theories of subcortical participation in language which proffer established roles for the globus pallidus and thalamus.

Lending models of motor dysfunction to predict the nature of language impairments following subthalamic nucleus lesions

Lesions of the STN have been documented to produce the hyperkinetic anomaly known as hemiballism (Hamada and DeLong, 1992b), characterized by violent limb movements (Wichmann and DeLong, 1998). Electrophysiological studies have identi-fied reduced GPe and GPi activity as the mechanism largely responsible for manifesta-tions of hyperkinesia following STN lesions (Hamada and DeLong, 1992a). In relation to theories of motor control, STN lesions hypothetically compromise the integrity of the indirect pathway, and cause the direct pathway to assume control of GPi-SNr outputs (Wichmann and DeLong, 1998). Governing striato-pallidal inhibition of GPi-SNr inhibitory outputs reportedly results in thalamic disinhibition and a subsequent increase in the firing rate of thalamic neurones.

In relation to language, the aforementioned model of motor dysfunction predicts STN lesions to potentially impact upon pallidal and thalamic mechanisms involved in the mediation of linguistic processes, principally by way of altering GPi-SNr-governed thalamic outputs to the cerebral cortex. The precise nature of hypothesized linguistic impairments resulting from an activity imbalance between the direct and indirect basal ganglia pathways will now be discussed in the context of established Response-Release Semantic Feedback (RRSF) (Crosson, 1985; Crosson and Early, 1990), Lexical Decision Making (LDM) (Wallesch and Papagno, 1988) and Selective Engagement (Nadeau and Crosson, 1997) models of subcortical participation in language, which were initially presented in Chapter 3.

Revised Response-Release Semantic Feedback model
In a manner similar to the striatum, the current authors have proposed a potential role for the STN in the processing of cortical information from language- and non-language-dedicated regions, in addition to the regulation of pallidal outflow to thalamic nuclei which ultimately govern linguistic processes (Whelan et al., 2003b). In contrast to GABAergic striato-GPi-SNr and -GPe projections, the STN influences pallidal activity by way of glutamatergic outputs to both the GPi-SNr and GPe. This counterpolarity with respect to striatal and STN neurochemical transmission mechanisms suggests a potential basal ganglia-mediated push–pull system (Alexander, 1994), possibly underpinning the thalamic excitation of language-dedicated cortices, with the striatum and STN in direct competition.

In relation to the established Response-Release Semantic Feedback (RRSF) model (Crosson, 1985; Crosson and Early, 1990), the caudate head was identified as the locus of a response-release mechanism responsible for mediating the cortical release of semantically verified language segments as speech (see Chapter 3). Following the integration of the indirect pathway within the RRSF schema, the STN, in concert with the striatum, is hypothesized to potentially regulate the release of semantically verified language segments, by way of the aforementioned push–pull system. More specifically, discriminatory anterior language centre (ALC) and posterior language centre (PLC) excitation of STN neurones is postulated to alter indirect pathway activity and consequently GPi-SNr output. In turn, GPi-SNr efferents, also under striatal influence, would serve to mediate activation and deactivation of the ALC and subsequently speech production, by way of disinhibiting or inhibiting the thalamus (see Figure 6.1).

Consistent with the original schema, the current revision proposes that the semantic verification of language segments occurs as a consequence of thalamic mechanisms which facilitate the transfer of formulated language from the ALC to the PLC for monitoring and refinement of semantic content (see Chapter 3). In a similar fashion to cortico-striatal interactions, the ALC was postulated to orchestrate a state of hyper-excitability within STN- GPi-SNr neurones while awaiting the semantic verification of a language segment. Heightened excitation of inhibitory GPi-SNr output neurones is predicted to result in thalamocortical inhibition, prohibiting verbal output. Once the language segment has achieved semantic verification, however, the PLC is postulated to potentially overexcite STN-GPe projections, in preference to GPi-SNr efferents, resulting in heightened GPe inhibition of GPi-SNr outputs, disinhibition of the

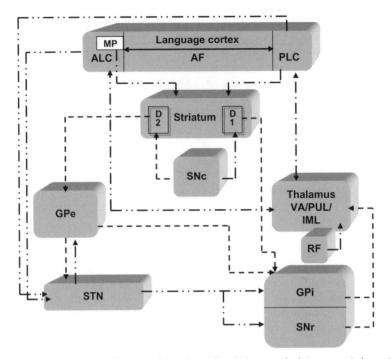

Figure 6.1 Revised schematic diagram of basal ganglia–thalamocortical Response-Release Semantic Feedback model (adapted from Crosson, 1985; 1992; Alexander *et al.*, 1990; Lang and Lozano, 1998) integrating the STN. ALC, anterior language centre; PLC, posterior language centre; MP, motor programming cortex; AF, arcuate fasciculus; D1, striatal output neurone receptor type D1; D2, striatal output neurone receptor type D2; SNc, substantia nigra pars compacta; GPe, globus pallidus externus; GPi, globus pallidus internus; SNr, substantia nigra pars reticulata; RF, reticular formation; VA, ventral anterior thalamic nucleus; IML, internal medullary lamina; PUL, pulvinar; dotted and dashed arrows, excitatory pathway; dashed arrows, inhibitory pathway.

thalamus and consequent activation of the ALC. This model of basal ganglia organization supports the proposal that the GPe may superordinately influence GPi-SNr activity, relative to the striatum and STN (Parent and Hazrati, 1993).

Based on the above schema, lesions of the STN resulting in direct pathway control of pallidal outputs were predicted to disrupt response-release and potentially semantic monitoring mechanisms as a consequence of thalamic disinhibition. Unimpeded thalamic excitation of the ALC was hypothesized to result in manifestations of fluent language pathology, including the production of semantically inappropriate output such as semantic paraphasias.

Revised Lexical Decision Making model

The Lexical Decision Making (LDM) model proffers a frontal lobe system (i.e. the caudate nucleus, GPi, VA and VL thalamic nuclei and ALC) to subserve the synchronization of language and non-language cortical modules processed in parallel, in addition to the regulation of cortical activity within the ALC (Wallesch and Papagno, 1988; Wallesch, 1997). Extending this frontal lobe system to include previously disregarded indirect basal ganglia pathways proposes implications for net pallidal activity, principally by way of STN-GPe and STN-GPi-SNr innervations (see Figure 6.2).

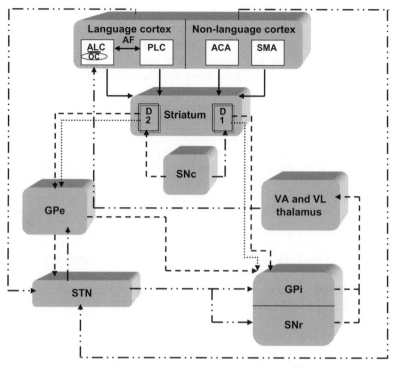

Figure 6.2 Revised schematic diagram of the basal ganglia–thalamocortical Lexical Decision Making model integrating the STN (adapted from Wallesch and Papagno, 1988; Alexander *et al.*, 1990; Crosson, 1992; Lang and Lozano, 1998). OC, output channel; ACA, anterior cingulate area; SMA, supplementary motor area; other abbreviations are as for Figure 6.1; dashed arrows, inhibitory pathway; dotted arrows, disinhibitory pathway; dotted and dashed arrows, excitatory pathway.

Given evidence of GPe and wide-ranging cortical inputs, in addition to a previously proposed ability to 'cross talk' between functionally distinct regions of the basal ganglia, the STN was postulated to represent a subcortical component with the ability to consolidate and perhaps permutate multiplex cortical modules. Within this schema, the striatum would continue to be involved in the communication of cortical modules or 'mini loops', to the GPe and GPi. The STN would receive an identical array of cortical inputs to the striatum (see Figure 6.2), however, and would potentially execute associative-limbic integration of those mini loops, by way of previously defined cross-talk mechanisms. The most appropriate module would be sanctioned for verbal production by way of STN-mediated excitation of homogenous neuronal terminations within the GPe and GPi, relative to the striatum. Communication of a 'central command' or the most appropriate module to the ALC was postulated to occur as a consequence of graded STN-mediated GPi-SNr inhibition of thalamic output neurones. The most appropriate lexical alternative would be associated with subtle or muted thalamic firing rates as a consequence of heightened GPi-SNr inhibition. Subtle thalamic firing rates relative to the activation of inhibitory cortical interneurones would permit cortical processing of the respective module and subsequent production as speech.

Of note, the postulated potential for striatal mechanisms to both inhibit and disinhibit the globus pallidus (Groves, 1983) suggests that within the current schema striato-pallidal projections may have the capacity to manipulate activation thresholds relative to individual cortical modules awaiting STN selection. Prior to associative (i.e. linguistic)-limbic integration within the STN, homogenous pallidal activation thresholds relative to each lexical representation are predicted to preside. The STN determines which representation is the most appropriate for verbal production, via associative-limbic cross-talk mechanisms which consequently overshoot the activation threshold for the relevant representation. A reduction in GPe activity coupled with an increase in GPi-SNr inhibitory output to the thalamus is postulated to represent the net effect of the proposed overshooting mechanism, which subsequently permits cortical processing of the most appropriate module. Consistent with the seminal LDM model, the fittest module among multiple modular contenders achieves terminal cortical processing.

STN lesions were therefore predicted to primarily produce non-fluent language disturbances (e.g. difficulty initiating speech) as a consequence of enforced 'direct' pathway dominance, resulting in thalamic disinhibition and the unmitigated excitation of inhibitory cortical interneurones. In addition, disturbed associative-limbic integration mechanisms as a result of STN lesions may be responsible for the presentation of inappropriate semantic content in verbal output (e.g. semantic paraphasias). Inappropriate striatal activation of subordinate alternatives may offer an explanation for manifestations of this behaviour, in the presence of STN lesions.

Revised Selective Engagement model
Despite the absence of an accepted role for the basal ganglia in original schemas (Nadeau and Crosson, 1997), recently disclosed inhibitory GPe-GPi-SNr, GPe-NR (i.e. NR), GPi-CM and excitatory CMPFC-STN projections propose potential implications for Selective Engagement theory. In the presence of reciprocal GPe connections and abundant GPi-SNr efferents, the STN was postulated to have the capacity to indirectly regulate thalamic engagement of the cerebral cortex, via its robust excitatory influences upon the internal and external segments of the globus pallidus. The GPi and GPe regulate thalamic output directly and indirectly, respectively.

It has been documented, however, that STN influences extend well beyond the domain of the globus pallidus. The entire cortical mantle has been reported to innervate the STN (Rouzaire-Dubois and Scarnati, 1985). In a similar yet reciprocal manner to the STN, intralaminar thalamic nuclei (including the CM) have been reported to project to the majority of the cortex (Jones, 1985). Cortical-STN, STN-GPe, GPe-NR, GPe-GPi-SNr, STN-GPi-SNr, CMPFC-STN, GPi-CM and CM-cortical projections propose a feedback mechanism promoting the STN as the interface of cortico-subcortical interactions (see Figure 6.3), which potentially govern Selective Engagement mechanisms.

Selective Engagement theory proposes a frontal-inferior thalamic peduncle (ITP)-NR-CM system to principally regulate cortical functions by way of the NR and its inherent ability to modulate the firing mode of thalamic output neurones, relative to cortical activation (Nadeau and Crosson, 1997). Excitatory STN influences upon pallidal outputs have the potential to indirectly regulate the thalamic engagement of language cortices. The existence of reciprocal STN-GPe innervations and concomitant inhibitory GPe projections to the NR suggest that this regulatory role may indeed extend to the establishment of the firing mode of thalamic output nuclei hypothesized to underpin language processes, including the pulvinar and CMPFC (see Chapter 3). Furthermore, evidence of STN-GPi-SNr, GPi-CM, CMPFC-STN and diffuse CM-cortical projections supports the notion of a potential STN contribution to the selective

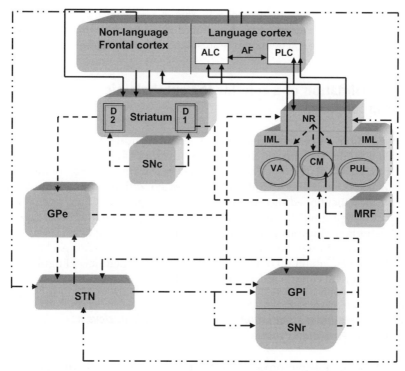

Figure 6.3 Revised schematic diagram of potential basal ganglia–thalamocortical influences (incorporating the STN) upon Selective Engagement mechanisms dedicated to language and non-language cortical regions (adapted from Crosson, 1985; Wallesch and Papagno, 1988; Parent and Hazrati, 1995a, 1995b; Nadeau and Crosson, 1997; Lang and Lozano, 1998). NR, nucleus reticularis; IML, internal medullary lamina; CM, centrum medianum; MRF, midbrain reticular formation; other abbreviations are as for Figure 6.1; dotted and dashed arrows, excitatory pathway; dashed arrows, inhibitory pathway.

engagement of language cortices, by way of regulating frontal-ITP-CM-NR system activity. Observations of language pathology in four cases subsequent to tuberothalamic and paramedian territory infarcts which infiltrated components of a frontal-ITP-NR-CM system provided the clinico-anatomical basis of Selective Engagement theory (Nadeau and Crosson, 1997). Precise roles pertaining to the individual components of and potential contributors to the frontal-ITP-NR-CM system are yet to be determined. Based on theories of motor control, however, lesions of the STN have been postulated to instigate 'direct' pathway control of striato-pallidal interactions, via STN-GPe and STN-GPi-SNr disconnection. Of most note, STN-GPe disconnection was postulated to have the most impact upon Selective Engagement mechanisms, by way of altering GPe-NR interactions. Aberrant or defunct GPe-NR exchanges are hypothesized to result in the production of aberrant firing modes, relevant to thalamic nuclei subserving the engagement of language-dedicated cortical components, namely the pulvinar and CM. In relation to seminal Selective Engagement theory, deficits in semantically driven lexical retrieval and access to declarative memory have been indexed as the most common linguistic impairments associated with damage to frontal-ITP-NR-CM mechanisms. Lesions of the STN may contribute to manifestations of this symptom complex by disrupting basal ganglia mechanisms that regulate the switching of thalamocortical engagement between neural nets (Malapani *et al.*,

1994). Relevant to language, disturbed switching mechanisms may involve disruption to the temporal synchronization of differential firing modes within thalamic nuclei subserving access to lexical-semantic representations and declarative memory.

Empirical validation of a role for the subthalamic nucleus in language

The extrapolations of contemporary models of subcortical participation in language summarized within the current chapter were much needed in order to fit with contemporary schemas of functional basal ganglia organization. By way of incorporating previously neglected indirect basal ganglia pathways within existing linguistic frameworks, the aforementioned theoretical extensions propose an unprecedented role for the STN and the indirect basal ganglia pathway, in the mediation of language processes. Attempts to empirically validate hypotheses pertaining to a STN contribution to language ensue in the current chapter. Investigations of the impact of surgically induced functional inhibition of the STN on general and high-level linguistic abilities within Parkinsonian cohorts are reported in detail.

Non-ablative deep-brain stimulation of the subthalamic nucleus as a treatment for Parkinson's disease

In contrast to the ablative procedures described in Chapter 5 which permanently destroy neural tissue, deep-brain stimulation (DBS) involves minimal destruction of brain tissue (Lozano and Mahant, 2004) via the implantation of electrodes within a range of potential subcortical targets (Wichmann and DeLong, 2006). The implanted electrodes deliver high-frequency electrical signals to the target nuclei by way of attachments to pulse generators, inserted within the chest wall. Targets utilized in the management of Parkinson's disease include the GPi, STN, thalamus and pedunculopontine nucleus; however, the STN (specifically the dorsolateral motor nucleus) is currently recognized as the preferred target, given that stimulation in this region is associated with potent anti-Parkinsonian effects (Wichmann and DeLong, 2006). The DBS procedure has been hailed as the gold standard in surgery for movement disorders, given that its side effects are reversible (i.e. via removal or turning 'off' electrodes) and its parameters adjustable in terms of maximizing clinical benefit (i.e. stimulation parameters may be programmed to different therapeutic levels) (Kopell et al., 2006).

Application of the DBS technique arose from the observation that high-frequency stimulation (i.e. >100 Hz) of estimated surgical targets during ablative procedures resulted in the relief of motor symptoms (Walter and Vitek, 2004). The procedure was pioneered in the 1980s by Benabid who used stimulation of the thalamus to alleviate tremor in patients with essential tremor and Parkinson's disease (Wichmann and DeLong, 2006). In the management of Parkinson's disease, STN-DBS has been shown to eradicate the gamut of associated motor deficits (Starr et al., 1998), as well as to support a significant reduction in levodopa dosages required (Krack et al., 1998; Garcia et al., 2005). In fact, the effects of STN-DBS have been compared to a long-duration response to levodopa (Moro et al., 2002). The manner in which DBS achieves these outcomes, however, is not known particularly in light of the fact that clinical applications of the technique have preceded a sound scientific interpretation of its precise mechanism of action (McIntyre *et al.*, 2004).

As stated previously, within models of Parkinson's disease a dopaminergic deficit causes the manifestation of Parkinsonian symptoms via an imbalance of direct/indirect pathway activity (Lozano and Mahant, 2004). Reduced activity within the indirect pathway causes hyperactivity within STN and consequently GPi neurones, resulting in the inhibition of thalamocortical activity (Kopell *et al.*, 2006). Neuronal hyperactivity within the STN and GPi has been commonly translated as an increase in neuronal firing rates within these structures (Miller and DeLong, 1987). Functionally, such neuronal hyperactivity has been associated with increased metabolic rates within the pallidum (Eidelberg and Edwards, 2000) as well as reduced downstream metabolic rates and blood flow within the motor cortices, both of which are similarly reversed in the presence of dopaminergic therapy (Ceballos-Baumann, 2003) and STN-DBS (Asanuma *et al.*, 2006). Factors such as neuronal firing patterns and spatial coding of information, however, may also need to be considered in Parkinson's disease, and when trying to understand the effects of DBS (Lozano and Mahant, 2004).

In addition to increases in firing rates, consistent alterations in patterns of activity within STN, GPi and thalamic neuronal pools have also been documented in Parkinson's disease, including frequent discharge bursts and more synchronized oscillations between neighbouring neurones in these structures (Wichmann *et al.*, 2000). How DBS modulates these abnormal neuronal activity patterns is yet to be determined. The mechanism of DBS was initially thought to mimic that of ablative lesions involving a functional inactivation of the target, given similarities between lesion and DBS effects (Lozano and Mahant, 2004; Kopell *et al.*, 2006). Current research, however, suggests that the precise mechanism of action may be of a more complex nature (Wichmann and DeLong, 2006), involving the adjustment of pathological activity (Garcia *et al.*, 2005). In fact, recently reported experimental data suggest that DBS mechanisms may involve inhibition and excitation effects, as well as changes to network synchrony (Kopell *et al.*, 2006).

Despite this perplexity, two fundamental mechanisms (i.e. silencing ('less' mechanism) and excitation ('more' mechanism)), perhaps working in combination, have been proposed as the neurophysiological processes mediating the effects of DBS (Garcia *et al.*, 2005). Specifically, DBS acts to dampen ('less' mechanism) disturbed STN activity, and to introduce high-frequency discharge rates ('more' mechanism) within the STN. In this way, DBS removes detrimental neuronal activity and replaces it with a more regular pattern of activity, associated with normal behavioural functioning.

It has been postulated that in untreated Parkinson's disease patients, pathological low-frequency (i.e. 11–30 Hz) oscillations exist within STN and GPi neurones (Levy *et al.*, 2002). Improved function as a consequence of STN-DBS has been hypothesized to result from the reduction of the aforementioned pathological frequency band and the introduction of high-frequency (i.e. >70 Hz) oscillation bands (Montgomery and Baker, 2000; Williams *et al.*, 2002; McIntyre *et al.*, 2004). Regardless of the mechanisms of action, however, evidence is mounting to suggest that the effects of DBS are network-wide (McIntyre *et al.*, 2004). In relation to functional activity within Parkinsonian brains, importantly STN-DBS has been shown to effect the normalization of frontal lobe activity during neuroimaging studies (Grafton *et al.*, 2006), and consequently to affect behaviour.

Surgical methodology relative to deep-brain stimulation

Target localization and intraoperative techniques are identical to those utilized for the previously described ablative procedure (see Chapter 5) and typically involve neuroradiographic identification and neurophysiological confirmation of the proposed lesion site prior to the implantation of permanent stimulating electrodes and pulse generators (Broggi, 1998; Liu *et al.*, 2001). More specifically, once macrostimulation of a clinically effective lesion site has been confirmed, the Radionics™ lesioning electrode is removed and replaced with a permanent tetrapolar stimulating electrode. The electrode is then connected to an extension cable which is tunnelled subcutaneously from the scalp to a subclavicular incision, where a pulse generator is inserted. A post-operative computed tomography (CT) scan is undertaken to confirm the electrode location with the pre-operative target. The pulse generators are then programmed by a neurologist within 48 h of surgery and stimulation parameters calibrated to achieve optimal motor performance and symptom relief. Most favourable clinical results have been reported using the following DBS parameters within the STN: 60–200 μs pulse duration, 1–5 V amplitude, delivered at a frequency of 120–180 Hz (Garcia *et al.*, 2005).

Impact of deep-brain stimulation of the subthalamic nucleus on language function: clinical evidence

The impact of bilateral STN-DBS on motor systems has been well established in comparison to its effects on non-motor functions (Voon *et al.*, 2006). In general, STN-DBS has been described as having relatively benign effects on cognition, yet there is documented evidence of both improvements and decrements in certain domains of cognition in some research reports (Voon *et al.*, 2006), confusing perceptions relating to the genuine impact of this procedure.

STN-DBS: neuropsychological findings and implications for language

Post-operative STN-DBS improvements in mental flexibility (Jahanshahi *et al.*, 2000; Alegret *et al.*, 2001; Witt *et al.*, 2004), working memory (Jahanshahi *et al.*, 2000), visuo-motor sequencing (Ardouin *et al.*, 1999; Jahanshahi *et al.*, 2000; Pillon *et al.*, 2000; Daniele *et al.*, 2003), conceptual reasoning (Jahanshahi *et al.*, 2000; Daniele *et al.*, 2003) and general cognitive functioning (Daniele *et al.*, 2003) have been reported in a number of studies; however, other reports have identified declines in verbal memory (Saint-Cyr *et al.*, 2000; Trepanier *et al.*, 2000; Alegret *et al.*, 2001; Dujardin *et al.*, 2001; Daniele *et al.*, 2003; Morrison *et al.*, 2004; Wojtecki *et al.*, 2006), conditional associative learning (Jahanshahi *et al.*, 2000), visuospatial memory (Saint-Cyr *et al.*, 2000; Trepanier *et al.*, 2000; Alegret *et al.*, 2001), processing speed (Saint-Cyr *et al.*, 2000) and certain indices of executive functioning (Trepanier *et al.*, 2000). Similar to ablative lesions, it is apparent that studies pertaining to the impact of STN-DBS on cognition have been largely neuropsychological. Perhaps of most interest to the speech-language pathologist again is the fact that reduced verbal fluency scores are the most consistently reported neuropsychological sequelae of STN-DBS in patients with Parkinson's disease (Ardouin *et al.*, 1999; Moro *et al.*, 1999; Pillon *et al.*, 2000; Saint-Cyr *et al.*, 2000; Alegret *et al.*, 2001; Berney *et al.*, 2002; Woods et al, 2002; Daniele *et al.*, 2003; Gironell *et al.*, 2003; Moretti *et al.*, 2003; Schroeder *et al.*, 2003; Funkiewiez *et al.*, 2004; Morrison *et al.*, 2004; De Gaspari *et al.*, 2006a, 2006b; Smeding *et al.*, 2006; Wojtecki *et al.*, 2006). The reliable finding of impaired verbal fluency as a consequence of STN-DBS suggests that language systems, specifically those involving complex word-retrieval mechanisms which demand frontal lobe participation, may be seriously implicated as a consequence of STN disruption.

STN-DBS: application of comprehensive language assessments

To date, studies investigating the effects of STN-DBS on language function have utilized a narrow scope of measures (Whelan *et al.*, 2005). As can be seen from the neuropsychological results above, assessment batteries have typically included cognitive measures of attention, memory, concentration visuospatial abilities and executive functioning. Regarding language, the effects of STN-DBS on confrontation naming, verbal learning and – of course – verbal fluency have been given some consideration; however, the impact of this procedure on a wider range of linguistic processes which incorporate complex comprehension and sentential-level production tasks, has until recently, remained unknown.

A series of recently conducted investigations have attempted to better assess the impact of STN-DBS on language functions (Whelan *et al.*, 2003b, 2004, 2005). These studies represent the most comprehensive of their type, utilizing measures of both general and high-level linguistic functioning (see Box 5.1, p. 122) incorporating single-word and sentential-level comprehension and production tasks, not routinely included in neuropsychological test batteries. The following discussion represents a summary of the above studies. The reader is referred to the full papers for a more detailed account of the findings.

The specific aims of the aforementioned research were to (1) evaluate the immediate and long-term effects of bilateral and unilateral STN-DBS on language function utilizing a comprehensive test battery and (2) to discuss post-operative language profiles in the context of working theories of subcortical participation in language. As mentioned previously, STN-DBS has been hypothesized to alter the functioning of basal ganglia circuitry. Essentially, DBS results in functional inhibition of the STN, governing the direct pathway to largely assume control of GPi-SNr outputs (Wichmann and DeLong, 1998). With respect to language, this alteration in circuitry dynamics results in thalamic disinhibition which was hypothesized to result in the following: (1) extraneous verbal output as a result of disturbed preverbal semantic monitoring mechanisms and heightened anterior language cortex activity (Crosson, 1985), (b) lexical selection deficits and speech-initiation difficulties resulting from disturbed thalamic gating mechanisms and the random excitation of inhibitory cortical interneurones (Wallesch and Papagno, 1988) or (c) any combination of language comprehension and production deficits as a result of indiscriminate or inappropriate thalamic engagement of cortical regions subserving linguistic processes (Nadeau and Crosson, 1997). These hypotheses were tested via a comparison of language profiles obtained subsequent to DBS or lesioning of STN.

A number of interesting findings were generated from this research. Similar to neuropsychologically based studies, it was revealed that STN-DBS may affect variable changes in language performance, including both improvements as well as declines in functioning.

Study 1: group-wise study of five patients with bilateral STN-DBS

When the language profiles of a group ($N = 5$) of patients having undergone bilateral STN-DBS were compared to a group ($N = 16$) of non-surgical Parkinson's disease patients matched for age, education and disease duration a limited number of significant language changes were revealed within the STN-DBS group (Whelan *et al.*,

2003b). The only significant statistical results related to post-operative prolongations in reaction times for a range of word types in a semantic processing/lexical decision task. Interestingly, however, when examined on a case-by-case basis, a different profile was revealed. The STN-DBS patients demonstrated a significantly greater proportion of reliable improvement on the The Word Test-Revised (TWT-R) than the non-surgical Parkinson's disease group, attributed to performance on a single subtest (i.e. multiple definition formulation), as well as a greater proportion of reliable decline in the ability to accurately identify real words with many meanings and high degree of relatedness between meanings (MH words).

In reference to higher-level language skills (i.e. TWT-R), these findings suggested that pre-operative STN dysfunction as a result of Parkinson's disease may have moderated the efficiency of direct/indirect pathway push–pull mechanisms subserving higher-level language mechanisms. STN-DBS served to equilibrate basal ganglia activity, including the potential enhancement of synaptic efficiency particularly within neural circuits mediating linguistic flexibility in the production of definitions constrained by semantically distinct criteria. This profile speaks to the LDM model (Wallesch and Papagno, 1988) whereby enhanced basal ganglia circuitry dynamics result in more flexible lexical selection mechanisms which are active during complex or frontally taxing language tasks. Uncertainty remains, however, as to why additional high-level linguistic assessments that also required the formulation of self-generated complex language (e.g. synonym and antonym generation, semantic absurdity explanation, verbal fluency) failed to reveal a similar profile of significant post-operative improvement.

In interpreting semantic processing performance evidenced as a generalized post-operative prolongation of reaction times for all word types and reduced accuracy of decisions relating to MH words, spreading activation theory was consulted. According to this theory, word recognition is dependent upon the coherence of orthographic, phonological and semantic features, made possible by the correlation of activation patterns between lexical (i.e. orthographic/phonological input) and semantic nodes (Van Orden and Goldinger, 1994). Rapid coherence and consequently reaction time are contingent upon strong correlations. DBS has been hypothesized to disrupt neural networks through the production of artificial nerve impulses, a phenomenon defined as neural jamming (Benazzouz and Hallet, 2000). Our findings suggest that STN-DBS may indeed alter the efficiency of neural communication at the lexical-semantic interface, resulting in delayed or contaminated coherence correlations, perhaps as a consequence of neural jamming. In relation to theories of subcortical participation in language, STN-DBS may disturb GPe-NR exchanges resulting in abnormal firing modes within thalamic nuclei subserving the efficient engagement of lexical and semantic nodes (Nadeau and Crosson, 1997). STN-DBS may result in unimpeded thalamocortical activation and, in relation to language, the engagement of multiplex versus definitive lexical-semantic representations. A post-lesional inability to suppress or disengage subordinate lexical-semantic alternatives would hypothetically result in increased reaction times on the lexical decision task.

Words with many meanings have been hypothesized to have a probability advantage for nodal activation, given a high concentration of interrelated nodes (Rubenstein et al., 1970). In the present research, reduced accuracy of lexical decisions pertaining to MH words was interpreted as a reflection of inefficient coherence mechanisms whereby intricate nodal networks underlying MH words are perhaps more susceptible to neural disturbances facilitated by DBS. In relation to Selective Engagement theory (Nadeau and Crosson, 1997), MH words may have failed to reach recognition thresholds with respect to the coherence of orthographic and semantic representations. STN-DBS may have disturbed the assimilation of lexical information within convoluted neural networks resulting in 'incoherence' and the subsequent engagement of subordinate representations.

Study 2: long-term examination of effects of STN-DBS in two patients

In a follow-on study, two of the five STN-DBS subjects described above were monitored over a 12 month post-operative period in relation to their general and high-level language abilities (Whelan et al., 2005). STN-DBS primarily affected clinically reliable fluctuations (i.e. both improvements and declines) in performance across subjects on tasks demanding cognitive-linguistic flexibility in the formulation and comprehension of complex language. Of additional interest, both subjects demonstrated a cumulative increase in the proportion of reliable post-operative improvements achieved over time.

The findings of this study again provided support for the hypothesis of a STN contribution to language processes. Bilateral STN-DBS affected alterations in language performance at both 3 and 12 months following electrode implantation and the commencement of active stimulation. Overall, a cumulative increase in the proportion of reliable improvements in performance was demonstrated by both subjects across testing phases, suggesting that bilateral STN-DBS may serve to enhance the proficiency of basal ganglia–thalamocortical linguistic circuits over time.

Of note, a greater number of high-level language in comparison to general language variables were subject to reliable change (including both improvements and decrements) during bilateral STN-DBS, at both 3 and 12 months following surgery, in both subjects. Furthermore, general language variables demonstrating reliable post-operative changes were typically representative of more high-level linguistic measures (e. g. verbal fluency, Token Test, sentence construction, etc.) enmeshed within a general language battery. Bilateral STN-DBS principally affected divergent language production proficiency (e.g. verbal fluency) and lexical semantic manipulation skills (e.g. TWT-R, Token Test), potentially implicating cognitive-linguistic basal ganglia–thalamocortical pathways involved in the enlistment and directed interplay of frontal and temporoparietal cortical activity. Despite individual differences between subjects, these results support an adaptation hypothesis with respect to the nature of neural network responses to continuous patterns of stimulation (Benazzouz and Hallet, 2000). A general trend towards improved linguistic performance over time implied the prospective enhancement of synaptic efficiency as a consequence of chronic bilateral STN-DBS. The findings again lent support to models of subcortical participation in language which specifically integrate the STN within a frontal lobe system of language processing.

Study 3: examination of subthalamic nucleus language dominance in two patients

The final study examined the effects of left versus right functional inhibition of the STN on language function in two cases (i.e. one patient with left ablative lesion of the STN and one patient with right STN-DBS) (Whelan et al., 2004). Neuropsychological reports have described higher proportions of post-operative deterioration among executive function-dependent variables such as planning, spatial working memory, verbal memory and attention in patients with left versus right ablative lesions of the STN (McCarter et al., 2000). Given that language is considered to be anastomosed with executive function (Denckla, 1996), the current authors proposed that functional inhibition of the left as opposed to right STN may serve to disturb linguistic processes disproportionately.

On inspection of individual profiles, variability with respect to magnitudes and directions of reliable change was demonstrated both between subjects and across assessment variables. Median values were subsequently employed as a measure of central tendency to accommodate the presence of potential outliers (Moore and McCabe, 1989). Overall, each of the subjects demonstrated a general reliable decline on tests of high-level language function, yet failed to demonstrate comparable declines on tests of general language function.

The results of the above study largely failed to provide support for the hypothesis of left STN dominance, relevant to the mediation of linguistic processes. Left subthalamic nucleotomy and right STN-DBS affected similar fluctuations in language performance in the two Parkinson's disease cases presented. Overall, surgically induced functional inhibition of the STN largely evoked declines in complex language function, suggesting that STN disruption has the potential to disturb frontally loaded cognitive-linguistic operations, regardless of hemispheric orientation. On the basis of these findings, a potential interhemispheric regulatory function for the STN was postulated, relative to higher-level linguistic processing mechanisms.

Indeed, the STN has been previously ascribed an interhemispheric regulatory function, challenging unilateralized models of functional basal ganglia organization (Perier et al., 2000). Of particular note, is the postulate that simultaneous bilateral alterations in basal ganglia activity have been hypothesized to arise as a result of interthalamic information transfer, as opposed to interhemispheric communications by the corpus callosum, anterior commissure or mesencephalic decussation (Leviel et al., 1981). Parafascicular cross talk by way of the NR has been specifically hypothesized to represent the anatomical substrate facilitating the bilateral regulation of the firing mode of STN neurones (Mouroux et al., 1995). Pharmacological depression of the parafascicular nucleus typically facilitates a reduction in ipsilateral STN activity, while simultaneously affecting an increase in contralateral STN firing rates (Mouroux et al., 1995). Reduced ipsilateral STN activity suggests a post-lesional impediment to parafascicular-STN excitatory outflow. The subsequent increase in discharge rates within STN neurones contralateral to the side of lesion indicates the existence of compensatory basal ganglia regulation mechanisms, potentially mediated via a STN-parafascicular-NR-NR-parafascicular-STN pathway.

On the strength of the above findings, surgically induced unilateral functional inhibition of the STN within the current investigation was also hypothesized to evoke asymmetrical changes in ipsilateral and contralateral STN activity relative to the side of lesion. Based on the premise that ablative basal ganglia lesions facilitate the depression of function at the lesion site, left subthalamic nucleotomy and associated interhemispheric compensation mechanisms were predicted to facilitate an increase in contralateral/right STN activity. Despite the therapeutic effects of functional inhibition, however, DBS has been associated with increased neuronal activity at stimulated target sites (Windels et al., 2000). As such, increased STN activity as a consequence of right STN-DBS may have facilitated a reduction in left STN discharge rates contralateral to the side of lesion. This neurophysiological dichotomy suggests that left STN nucleotomy and right STN-DBS may evoke comparable effects relevant to dominant hemisphere activity underpinning language processes; that is, a depression in left STN neuronal activity.

In relation to models of subcortical participation in language, Selective Engagement theory (Nadeau and Crosson, 1997) provided the most viable interpretation of the current findings. As mentioned previously, the original theory proposed a frontal-ITP-NR-CM system to regulate language functions by way of the NR and its inherent ability to modulate the firing mode of thalamic output neurones. Thalamic outputs were hypothesized to govern the enlistment or engagement of cortical language territories. Following on from the hypothesis of Mouroux *et al.* (1995), NR-CMPFC-STN and potentially STN-GPe-NR connections were postulated to facilitate interhemispheric basal ganglia cross talk pertaining to STN activity. STN-GPe disconnection as a consequence of surgically induced functional inhibition of the STN was postulated to alter the nature of GPe-NR interactions. Anomalous NR activity was predicted to result in the production of aberrant thalamic firing modes. Relevant thalamic nuclei project to language-dedicated cortical regions within the left hemisphere, consequently resulting in linguistic disturbances.

In relation to the current research, functional depression of neuronal activity within the left STN largely affected declines in complex or higher-level language function. Metacontrol systems have been defined as neural mechanisms involved in arbitrating the regulation of hemispheric control relative to information processing (Levy and Trevarthen, 1976). As the processing requirements of a task increase, enhancements in performance are reportedly achieved via the interhemispheric distribution of processing. Interhemispheric regulation of the basal ganglia by way of the thalamus, with respect to the mediation of high-level linguistic processes, may represent such a metacontrol system. High-level linguistic tasks have been hypothesized to demand divergent thought and production processes dependent upon spontaneous flexibility (Eslinger and Grattan, 1993). Spontaneous flexibility has been defined as a cognitive domain reliant upon frontal lobe integrity (Eslinger and Grattan, 1993). On the basis of these postulates, therefore, frontally loaded or complex language tasks would be potentially sustained by interhemispheric processing mechanisms.

Individual case study: left subthalamic nucleotomy

Case history

PB was a 67 year-old right-handed, English-speaking male with 13 years of formal education and a diagnosis of idiopathic Parkinson's disease. Age of disease onset was 59 years and primary symptom presentation at the time of assessment involved right-sided tremor. No previous history of head injury, cerebrovascular accident, cerebral tumour or abscess, coexisting neurological disease, substance abuse, psychiatric disorder, developmental language disorder or speech and/or language disturbance prior to the onset of Parkinson's disease was reported. PB was deemed by a neurologist an appropriate candidate for left subthalamic nucleotomy. Pre-operative magnetic resonance imaging (MRI) revealed nil focal brain abnormalities and extensive neuropsychological testing revealed executive functioning to be largely intact, with no evidence of comorbid dementing illness or indicators of anxiety or depression. See Figure 6.4 for a post-operative MRI scan of the lesion placement. The pre-operative medication regimen included levodopa/benserazide (1000 mg) and Selegiline (10 mg). Post-operative regimen included levodopa/benserazide (400 mg) and levodopa/carbidopa (1100 mg).

Language profile

PB was administered the general and high-level language-assessment battery summarized in Box 5.1, at both baseline and 3 month post-operative time points. Raw

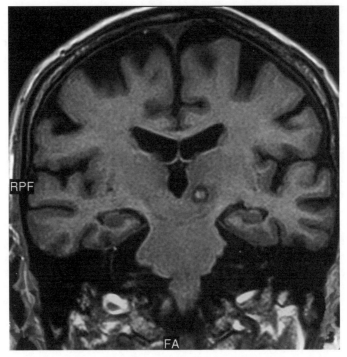

Figure 6.4 Post-operative MRI data for patient PB, illustrating a coronal view of the left ablative STN lesion.

language and reliable change scores demonstrated that PB predominantly exhibited post-operative changes in higher-level language skills, with a general tendency towards overall decline in these areas. On the general language battery, PB achieved negative (i.e. reduced) reliable changes on subtests of visual naming, digit reversal, word fluency and sentence construction. With the exception of visual naming, where PB produced semantically based errors (e.g. naming the item *paper clip* as 'drawing pin'), the remaining subtests were actually considered to be high level in nature. The Neurosensory Centre Comprehensive Examination for Aphasia (NCCEA), although a test of general language function, includes a range of subtests which tap higher-level language processes. Improvements in performance were also apparent on the Token Test, an assessment of complex comprehension/lexical-semantic manipulation; and written naming, attributed to improved motor function in the right hand. On the high-level language battery, reduced post-operative performance was observed on the following items: animal fluency (reduced number of items produced); the recreating sentences (e.g. when asked to combine the lexical units *without*, *difficult*, *again* within the context of *a track meeting*, PB responded 'Would you try again . . . and may not find the hill so difficult') and figurative language subtests of the Test of Language Competence-Expanded edition (TLC-E); the associations, semantic absurdity interpretation and definition formulation (e.g. when asked to identify and communicate the critical semantic elements of the word *skeleton* (i.e. bones), PB responded 'A frame for the body . . . it sustains the flesh') subtests of TWT-R and Test of Word Knowledge (TOWK); and the comparative, passive, temporal and spatial relationships on the Wiig–Semel Test of Linguistic Concepts (WSTLC). Improvements were noted on the antonym generation and multiple definition formulation subtests of the TLC-E.

Interpretation
From the above profile it may be interpreted that STN lesions or functional inhibition of the STN may produce deficits in cognitive flexibility impacting upon search strategies which underpin access to organized semantic knowledge and the generation of novel semantic categories (e.g. reduced visual naming, semantic and phonemic fluency, semantic associations) (N'Kaoua *et al.*, 2001). In addition, a reduced ability to interpret logical relationships relative to complex linguistic structures (e.g. WSTLC and TOWK) and reduced performance on divergent syntactic tasks such as recreating sentences (TLC-E) and definition formulation (TWT-R) suggest that STN lesions may interfere with the efficient organization, integration and production of specified lexical content within appropriate syntactic structures and/or produce concept-generation deficits and a lack of detail in verbal expression.

More generally, STN lesions may hinder the simultaneous integration of temporo-spatial patterns of activation and inhibition within the frontal lobes and other language-dedicated cortical regions (Eslinger and Grattan, 1993). For this reason, STN lesion/DBS patients should be assessed with measures that adequately tap higher-level language abilities, which extend beyond single-word naming tasks. Intervention may then also be designed accordingly.

Summary

Until recently, models of subcortical participation have neglected to include consideration of the STN as a component of the cortico-subcortico-cortical networks that regulate language function. Largely based on the findings of studies conducted by Whelan and colleagues into the effects of STN-DBS on language, there is now some evidence that the STN may play an interhemispheric regulatory role relative to higher-level linguistic processing mechanisms. A range of language alterations may result as a consequence of functionally inhibiting the STN. In particular, (1) both improvements and decrements in functioning may result, (2) higher-level language processes appear to be more sensitive than general language processes in relation to post-operative changes, (3) there is a general tendency towards improvements in performance over time and (4) there is no apparent evidence of STN hemispheric dominance effects.

As per ablative lesions (outlined in Chapter 5), of particular relevance to both the researcher and clinician is the evident variability in post-operative language profiles produced by patients following STN-DBS. Divergent profiles were presented across subjects in relation to affected subtests, as well as magnitudes and directions of change across variables. Such variability again warrants statistical and clinical caution, suggesting that STN-DBS patients may be best considered on a case-by-case basis. As a final note it must also be mentioned that the small sample sizes utilized in the previously summarized language research limit the generalization potential of results reported, yet provide valuable direction for future studies of the role of the STN in mediating language processes.

References

Albin, R.L., Young, A.B. and Penney, J.B. (1989). The functional anatomy of basal ganglia disorders. *Trends in Neuroscience* 12, 366–75.

Alegret, M., Junque, C., Valldeoriola, F., Vendrell, P., Pilleri, M. *et al.* (2001). Effects of bilateral subthalamic stimulation on cognitive function in Parkinson's disease. *Archives of Neurology* 58, 1223–7.

Alexander, G.E. (1994). Basal ganglia-thalamocortical circuits: their role in control of movements. *Journal of Clinical Neurophysiology* 11(4), 420–31.

Alexander, G.E. and Crutcher, M.D. (1990). Functional architecture of basal ganglia circuits: neural substrates of parallel processing. *Trends in Neuroscience* 13, 266–71.

Alexander, G.E., DeLong, M.R. and Strick, P.L. (1986). Parallel organisation of functionally segregated circuits linking basal ganglia and cortex. *Annual Review of Neuroscience* 9, 357–81.

Alexander, G.E., Crutcher, M.D. and DeLong, M.R. (1990). Basal ganglia-thalamocortical circuits: parallel substrates for motor, oculomotor, 'prefrontal' and 'limbic' functions. *Progress in Brain Research* 85, 119–46.

Ardouin, C.M., Pillon, B., Peiffer, E., Bejjani, P., Limousin, P. *et al.* (1999). Bilateral subthalamic or pallidal stimulation for Parkinson's disease affects neither memory nor executive functions: a consecutive series of 62 patients. *Annals of Neurology* 46(2), 217–23.

Asanuma, K., Tang, C., Ma, Y., Dhawan, V., Mattis, P. *et al.* (2006). Network modulation in the treatment of Parkinson's disease. *Brain* 129, 2667–78.

Benazzouz, A. and Hallet, M. (2000). Mechanism of action of deep brain stimulation. *Neurology* 55 (suppl. 6), S13–16.

Benazzouz, A., Ni, Z., Bouali-Benazzouz, R., Breit, S., Gao, D. A. *et al.* (2001). Physiology of subthalamic nucleus neurones in animal models of Parkinson's disease. In K. Kultas-Ilinsky and I. Ilinsky (eds), *Basal Ganglia and Thalamus in Health and Movement Disorders* (pp. 249–56). New York: Kluwer Academic/Plenum Publishers.

Berney, A., Vingerhoets, F. and Perrin, A. (2002). Effect on mood of subthalmic DBS for Parkinson's disease: a consecutive series of 24 patients. *Neurology* 59, 1427–9.

Broggi, G. (1998). Chronic deep brain stimulation: clinical results. In I. Germano (ed.), *Neurosurgical Treatment of Movement Disorders* (pp. 169–75). Park Ridge, IL: Thieme.

Ceballos-Baumann, A.O. (2003). Functional imaging in Parkinson's disease: activation studies with PET, fMRI and SPECT. *Journal of Neurology* 250 (suppl. 1), 15–23.

Crosson, B. (1985). Subcortical functions in language: a working model. *Brain and Language* 25, 257–92.

Crosson, B. (1992). *Subcortical Functions in Language and Memory*. New York: Guilford Press.

Crosson, B. and Early, T.A. (1990). *A Theory of Subcortical Functions in Language: Review and Critique*. Unpublished manuscript.

Daniele, A., Albanese, A., Contarino, M.F., Zinzi, P., Barbier, A. *et al.* (2003). Cognitive and behavioural effects of chronic stimualtn of the subthalamic nucleus in patients with Parkinson's disease. *Journal of Neurology, Neurosurgery and Psychiatry* 74, 175–82.

De Gaspari, D., Siri, C., Di Gioia, M., Antonini, A., Isella, V. *et al.* (2006a). Clinical correlates and cognitive underpinnings of verbal fluency impairment after chronic subthalamic stimulation in Parkinson's disease. *Parkinsonism and Related Disorders* 12, 289–95.

De Gaspari, D., Siri, C., Landi, A., Cilia, R., Bonetti, A. *et al.* (2006b). Clinical and neuropsychological follow up at 12 months in patients with complicated Parkinson's disease treated with subcutaneous apomorphine infusion or deep brain stimulation of the subthalamic nucleus. *Journal of Neurology, Neurosurgery and Psychiatry* 77, 450–3.

DeLong, M.R. (1990). Primate models of movement disorders of basal ganglia origin. *Trends in Neuroscience* 13, 281–5.

DeLong, M.R. and Georgopoulos, A.P. (1981). Motor functions of the basal ganglia. In J.M. Brookhart, V.B. Mountcastle and V.B. Brooks (eds), *Handbook of Physiology*, vol. 2 (pp. 1017–61). Bethseda, MD: American Physiology Society.

DeLong, M.R., Georgopoulos, A.P. and Crutcher, M.D. (1983). Cortico-basal ganglia relations and coding of motor performance. *Experimental Brain Research* 7, 30–40.

Denckla, M.B. (1996). A theory and model of executive function: a neuropsychological perspective. In G.R. Lyon and N.A. Krasnegor (eds), *Attention, Memory and Executive Function*. Baltimore, MD: Paul Brookes.

Dujardin, K., Defebvre, L., Krystkowiak, P., Blond, S. and Destee, A. (2001). Influence of chronic bilateral stimulation of the subthalamic nucleus on cognitive function in Parkinson's disease. *Journal of Neurology* 248, 603–11.

Eidelberg, D. and Edwards, C. (2000). Functional brain imaging of movement disorders. *Neurology Research* 22, 305–12.

Eslinger, P.J. and Grattan, L.M. (1993). Frontal lobe and frontal-striatal substrates for different forms of human cognitive flexibility. *Neuropsychologia* 31(1), 17–28.

Feger, J., Mouroux, M., Benazzouz, A., Boraud, T., Gross, C. *et al.* (1994). The subthalamic nucleus: a more complex structure than expected. In G. Percheron, J.S. McKenzie and J. Feger (eds), *The Basal Ganglia IV: New Ideas and Data on Structure and Function* (pp. 371–82). New York: Plenum Press.

Funkiewiez, A., Ardouin, C.M., Caputo, E., Krack, P., Fraix, V. *et al.* (2004). Long term effects of bilateral subthalamic nucleus stimulation on cognitive function, mood, and behaviour in Parkinson's disease. *Journal of Neurology, Neurosurgery and Psychiatry* 75, 834–9.

Garcia, L., D'Alessandro, G., Bioulac, B. and Hammond, C. (2005). High-frequency stimulation in Parkinson's disease: more or less? *Trends in Neuroscience* 28(4), 209–16.

Gironell, A., Kulisevsky, J., Rami, L., Fortuny, N., Garcia-Sanchez, C. *et al.* (2003). Effects of pallidotomy and bilateral subthalamic stimulation on cognitive function in Parkinson disease: a controlled comparative study. *Journal of Neurology* 250, 917–23.

Grafton, S.T., Turner, R.S., Desmurget, M., Bakay, R.A.E., DeLong, M.R. *et al.* (2006). Normalising motor related brain activity: subthalamic nucleus stimulation in Parkinson's disease. *Neurology* 66, 1192–9.

Groves, P.M. (1983). A theory of the functional organisation of the neostriatum and neostriatal control of voluntary movement. *Brain Research Review* 5, 109–32.

Guridi, J., Herrero, M.T., Luquin, M.R., Guillen, J., Ruberg, M. *et al.* (1996). Subthalamotomy in Parkinsonian monkeys: behavioural and biochemical analysis. *Brain* 119, 1717–25.

Haber, S.N., Lynd-Balta, E. and Spooren, W.P.J.M. (1994). Integrative aspects of basal ganglia circuitry. In G. Percheron, J.S. McKenzie and J. Feger (eds), *The Basal Ganglia IV: New Ideas and Data on Structure and Function* (pp. 71–80). New York: Plenum Press.

Hamada, I. and DeLong, M.R. (1992a). Excitotoxic acid lesions of the primate subthalamic nucleus result in reduced pallidal neuronal activity during active holding. *Journal of Neurophysiology* 68, 1859–66.

Hamada, I. and DeLong, M.R. (1992b). Excitotoxic acid lesions of the primate subthalamic nucleus result in transient dyskinesias of the contralateral limbs. *Journal of Neurophysiology* 68, 1850–58.

Hazrati, L.-N. and Parent, A. (1991). Projection from the external pallidum to the reticular thalamic nucleus in the squirrel monkey. *Brain Research* 550, 142–6.

Hazrati, L.-N. and Parent, A. (1992). Differential patterns of arborisation of striatal and subthalamic fibres in the two pallidal segments in primates. *Brain Research* 598, 311–15.

Hazrati, L.-N. and Parent, A. (1993). Striatal and subthalamic afferents to the primate pallidum: interactions between two opposite chemospecific neuronal systems. *Progress in Brain Research* 99, 89–104.

Hazrati, L.-N., Parent, A., Mitchell, S. and Haber, S.N. (1990). Evidence for interconnections between the two segments of the globus pallidus in primates: a PHA-L anterograde tracing study. *Brain Research* 533, 171–5.

Hutchinson, W.D., Allan, R.J., Opits, H., Levy, R., Dostrovsky, J.O. *et al.* (1998). Neurophysiological identification of the subthalamic nucleus in surgery for Parkinson's disease. *Annals of Neurology* 44, 622.

Jackson, A. and Crossman, A.R. (1981). Subthalamic nucleus efferent projection to the cerebral cortex. *Neuroscience* 6, 2367–77.

Jahanshahi, M., Ardouin, C.M., Brown, R.G., Rothwell, J.C., Obeso, J.A. *et al.* (2000). The impact of deep brain stimulation on executive function in Parkinson's disease. *Brain* 123, 1142–54.

Jones, E. (1985). *The Thalamus.* New York: Plenum Press.

Kita, H. (1994). Physiology of two disynaptic pathways from the sensorimotor cortex to the basal ganglia output nuclei. In G. Percheron, J.S. McKenzie and J. Feger (eds), *The Basal Ganglia IV: New Ideas and Data on Structure and Function* (pp. 263–75). New York: Plenum.

Kita, H. and Kitai, S.T. (1987). Efferent projections of the subthalamic nucleus in the rat: light and electron microscopic analysis with the PHA-L method. *Journal of Comparative Neurology* 260, 435–52.

Kopell, B.H., Rezai, A., Chang, J.-W. and Vitek, J.L. (2006). Anatomy and physiology of the basal ganglia: implications for deep brain stimulation for Parkinson's disease. *Movement Disorders* 21 (suppl. 14), 238–46.

Krack, P., Pollack, P., Limousin, P., Hoffman, D., Xie, J. *et al.* (1998). Subthalamic nucleus or internal pallidal stimulation in young onset Parkinson's disease. *Brain* 121, 451–7.

Lang, A.E. and Lozano, A.M. (1998). Medical progress: Parkinson's disease (Part II of II). *New England Journal of Medicine* 339(15), 1130–43.

Leviel, V., Chesselet, M.-F., Glowinski, J. and Cheramy, A. (1981). Involvement of the thalamus in the asymmetric effects of unilateral sensory stimuli on the two nigrostriatal dopaminergic pathways in the cat. *Brain Research* 223(2), 257–72.

Levy, J. and Trevarthen, C. (1976). Metacontrol of hemispheric function in human split brain patients. *Journal of Experimental Psychology: Human Perception and Performance* 2, 299–312.

Levy, J., Hutchison, W.D., Lozano, A.M. and Dostrovsky, J.O. (2002). Synchronised neuronal discharge in the basal ganglia of Parkinsonian patients is limited to oscillatory activity. *Journal of Neuroscience* 22(7), 2855–61.

Liu, X., Rowe, J., Nandi, D., Hayward, G., Parkin, S. *et al.* (2001). Localisation of the subthalamic nucleus using radionics image fusion TM and stereoplan TM combined with field potential recording. *Stereotactic and Functional Nuerosurgery* 76, 63–73.

Lozano, A.M. and Mahant, N. (2004). Deep brain stimulation surgery for Parkinson's disease: mechanisms and consequences. *Parkinsonism and Related Disorders* 10, 49–57.

Malapani, C., Pillon, B., Dubois, B. and Agid, Y. (1994). Impaired Simultaneous Cognitive Task Performance in Parkinson's disease: a dopamine-related dysfunction. *Neurology* 44, 319–26.

McCarter, R.J., Walton, N.H., Rowan, A.F., Gill, S.S. and Palomo, M. (2000). Cognitive functioning after subthalamic nucleotomy for refractory Parkinson's disease. *Journal of Neurology, Neurosurgery and Psychiatry* 69, 60–6.

McIntyre, C.C., Savasta, M., Walter, B.L. and Vitek, J.L. (2004). How does deep brain stimulation work? Present understanding and future questions. *Journal of Clinical Neurophysiology* 21, 40–50.

Miller, W.C. and DeLong, M.R. (1987). Altered tonic activity of neurons in the globus pallidus and subthalamic nucleus in the primate MPTP model of Parkinsonism. In M.B. Carpenter and A. Jayaraman (eds), *The Basal Ganglia II* (pp. 415–27). New York: Plenum Press.

Montgomery, E. and Baker, K.B. (2000). Mechanisms of deep brain stimulation and future technical developments. *Neurology Research* 22, 259–66.

Moore, D.S. and McCabe, G.P. (1989). *Introduction to the Practice of Statistics.* New York: W.H. Freeman and Company.

Moretti, R., Torre, E., Antonello, R.M., Capus, L., Zambito Marsala, S. *et al.* (2003). Neuropsychological changes after subthalamic nucleus stimulation: a 12 month follow-up in nine patients with Parkinson's disease. *Parkinsonism and Related Disorders* 10, 73–9.

Moro, E., Scerrati, M., Romito, L.M.A., Roselli, R., Tonali, P. *et al.* (1999). Chronic subthalamic nucleus stimulation reduces medication requirements in Parkinson's disease. *Neurology* 53, 85–90.

Moro, E., Esselink, R.J.A., Benabid, A.-L. and Pollak, P. (2002). Response to levodopa in Parkinsonian patients with bilateral subthalamic nucleus stimulation. *Brain* 125(11), 2408–17.

Morrison, C.E., Borod, J.C., Perrine, K., Beric, A., Brin, M.F. *et al.* (2004). Neuropsychological functioning following bilateral subthalamic nucleus stimulation in Parkinson's disease. *Archives of Clinical Neurophysiology* 19, 165–81.

Mouroux, M., Hassani, O.K. and Feger, J. (1995). Electrophysiological study of the excitatory parafascicular projection to the subthalamic nucleus and evidence for ipsi- and contralateral controls. *Neuroscience* 67(2), 399–407.

Nadeau, S.E. and Crosson, B. (1997). Subcortical aphasia. *Brain and Language* 58, 355–402.

Nauta, H.J.W. (1979). A proposed conceptual reorganisation of the basal ganglia and telencephalon. *Neuroscience* 4, 1875–81.

Nauta, H.J.W. and Cole, M. (1978). Efferent projections of the subthalamic nucleus: an autoradiographic study in monkey and cat. *Journal of Comparative Neurology* 180, 1–16.

N'Kaoua, B., Lespinet, V., Barsse, A., Rougier, A. and Claverie, B. (2001). Exploration of hemispheric specialisation and lexico-semantic processing in unilateral temporal lobe epilepsy with verbal fluency tasks. *Neuropsychologia* 39, 635–42.

Parent, A. and Hazrati, L.-N. (1993). Anatomical aspects of information processing in primate basal ganglia. *Trends in Neuroscience* 16, 111–16.

Parent, A. and Hazrati, L.-N. (1995a). Functional anatomy of the basal ganglia. I. The cortico-basal ganglia-thalamo-cortical loop. *Brain Research Reviews* 20, 91–127.

Parent, A. and Hazrati, L.-N. (1995b). Functional anatomy of the basal ganglia. II. The place of subthalamic nucleus and external pallidum in basal ganglia circuitry. *Brain Research Reviews* 20, 128–54.

Parent, A., Hazrati, L.-N. and Lavoie, B. (1991). The pallidum as a duel structure in primates. In G. Bernadi, M.B. Carpenter, G. DiChiara, M. Morelli and P. Stanzione (eds), *The Basal Ganglia III* (pp. 81–8). New York: Plenum Press.

Perier, C., Agid, Y., Hirsch, E.C. and Feger, J. (2000). Ipsilateral and contralateral subthalamic activity after unilateral dopaminergic lesion. *Neuroreport* 11(14), 3275–8.

Pillon, B., Ardouin, C.M., Damier, P., Krack, P., Houeto, J.L. *et al.* (2000). Neuropsychological changes between 'off' and 'on' STN or GPi stimulation in Parkinson's disease. *Neurology* 55(1), 411–18.

Rodriguez-Oroz, M.C., Gorospe, A., Guridi, J., Ramos, E., Linazasoro, G. *et al.* (2000). Bilateral deep brain stimulation of the subthalamic nucleus in Parkinson's disease. *Neurology* 55 (suppl. 6), S45–51.

Rouzaire-Dubois, B. and Scarnati, E. (1985). Bilateral corticosubthalamic nucleus projections: an electrophysiological study in rats with chronic cerebral lesions. *Neuroscience* 15, 69–75.

Rubenstein, H., Garfield, L. and Millikan, J. (1970). Homographic entries in the internal lexicon. *Verbal Learning and Verbal Behaviour* 9, 484–94.

Saint-Cyr, J.A., Trepanier, L.L., Kumar, R., Lozano, A.M. and Lang, A.E. (2000). Neuropsychological consequences of chronic bilateral stimulation of the subthalamic nucleus in Parkinson's disease. *Brain* 123, 2091–2108.

Schroeder, U., Kuehler, A., Lange, K.W., Haslinger, B., Tronnier, V.M. *et al.* (2003). Subthalamic nucleus stimulus affects frontotemporal network: a PET study. *Annals of Neurology* 54, 445–50.

Smeding, H.M.M., Speelman, J.D., Koning-Haanstra, M., Schuurman, P.R., Nijssen, P. *et al.* (2006). Neuropsychological effects of bilateral STN stimulation in Parkinson's disease: a controlled study. *Neurology* 66, 1830–6.

Smith, Y., Shink, E. and Sidibe, M. (1998). Neuronal circuitry and synaptic connectivity of the basal ganglia. *Neurosurgery Clinics of North America* 9(2), 203–22.

Starr, P.A., Vitek, J.L. and Bakay, R.A.E. (1998). Ablative surgery and deep brain stimulation for Parkinson's disease. *Neurosurgery* 43(5), 989–1015.

Trepanier, L.L., Kumar, R., Lozano, A.M., Lang, A E. and Saint-Cyr, J.A. (2000). Neuropsychological outcome of GPi pallidotomy and GPi or STN deep brain stimulation in Parkinson's disease. *Brain and Cognition* 42, 324–47.

Van Orden, G.C. and Goldinger, S.D. (1994). Interdependence of form and function in cognitive systems explains perception of printed words. *Journal of Experimental Psychology: Human Perception and Performance* 20, 1269–91.

Voon, V., Kubu, C.S., Krack, P., Houeto, J.L. and Troster, A. (2006). Deep brain stimulation: neuropsychological and neuropsychiatric issues. *Movement Disorders* 21 (suppl. 14), 305–26.

Wallesch, C.-W. (1997). Symptomatology of subcortical aphasia. *Journal of Neurolinguistics* 10(4), 267–75.

Wallesch, C.-W. and Papagno, C. (1988). Subcortical aphasia. In F.C. Rose, R. Whurr and M.A. Wyke (eds), *Aphasia* (pp. 256–87). London: Whurr Publishers.

Walter, B.L. and Vitek, J.L. (2004). Stereotactic surgery and deep brain stimulation for Parkinson's disease and movement disorders. In R.L. Watts and W.C. Koller (eds), *Movement Disorders: Neurologic Principles and Practices* (pp. 289–318). New York: McGraw-Hill.

Weiner, D.J. (1997). The connections of the primate subthalamic nucleus: indirect pathways and the open-interconnected scheme of basal ganglia-thalamocortical circuitry. *Brain Research Reviews* 23, 62–78.

Whelan, B.-M., Murdoch, B., Theodoros, D.G., Hall, B. and Silburn, P. (2003a). Building upon working theories of subcortical participation in language: integration of intrinsic basal ganglia circuitry. *Acta Neuropsychologia* 1(2), 174–93.

Whelan, B.-M., Murdoch, B., Theodoros, D.G., Hall, B. and Silburn, P. (2003b). Defining a role for the subthalamic nucleus (STN) within operative theoretical models of subcortical participation in language. *Journal of Neurology, Neurosurgery and Psychiatry* 74, 1543–50.

Whelan, B.-M., Murdoch, B., Theodoros, D.G., Hall, B. and Silburn, P. (2004). Re-appraising contemporary theories of subcortical participation in language: proposing an interhemispheric regulatory function for the subthalamic nucleus (STN) in the mediation of high-level linguistic processes. *Neurocase* 10(5), 345–52.

Whelan, B.-M., Murdoch, B., Theodoros, D.G., Hall, B. and Silburn, P. (2005). Beyond verbal fluency: investigating the long-term effects of bilateral subthalamic (STN) deep brain stimulation (DBS) on language function in 2 cases. *Neurocase* 11, 93–102.

Wichmann, T. and DeLong, M.R. (1998). Models of basal ganglia function and pathophysiology of movement disorders. *Neurosurgery Clinics of North America* 9, 223–36.

Wichmann, T. and DeLong, M.R. (2006). Deep brain stimulation for neurologic and neuropsychiatric disorders. *Neuron* 52, 197–204.

Wichmann, T., DeLong, M.R. and Vitek, J.L. (2000). Pathophysiological considerations in basal ganglia surgery: role of the basal ganglia in hypokinetic and hyperkinetic movement disorders. *Progress in Neurology and Surgery* 15, 31–57.

Williams, D., Tijssen, M., van Bruggen, G., Bosch, A., Insola, A. *et al.* (2002). Dopamine-dependent changes in the functional connectivity between basal ganglia and cerebral cortex in humans. *Brain* 125, 1558–69.

Windels, F., Bruet, N., Poupard, A., Urbair, N., Chouvet, G. *et al.* (2000). Effects of high frequency stimulation of subthalamic nucleus on extracellular glutamate and GABA in substantia nigra and globus pallidus in the normal rat. *European Journal of Neuroscience* 12, 4141–6.

Witt, K., Pulkowski, U., Herzog, J., Lorenz, D., Hamel, W. *et al.* (2004). Deep brain stimulation of the subthalamic nucleus improves cognitive flexibility but impairs response inhibition in Parkinson disease. *Archives of Neurology* 61, 697–700.

Wojtecki, L., Timmerman, L., Jorgens, S., Sudmeyer, M., Maarouf, M. *et al.* (2006). Frequency-dependent reciprocal modulation of verbal fluency and motor functions in subthalamic deep brain stimulation. *Archives of Neurology* 63, 1273–6.

Woods, S.P., Fields, J. and Troster, A. (2002). Neuropsychological sequelae of subthalamic nucleus deep brain stimulation in Parkinson's disease: a critical review. *Neuropsychology Review* 12(2), 111–26.

7 Influence of the cerebellum on language function

Introduction

Typically, damage to the cerebellum results in motor disturbances characterized by incoordination of the limbs (dysmetria), wide-based gait, disturbances of occular movements (nystagmus) and dysarthria. Consequently, the cerebellum has traditionally been viewed as part of the brain dedicated to the regulation and coordination of motor function, a view held since the early nineteenth century based on reports of the effects of ablation of the cerebellum in animals and reinforced by the first clinical reports of patients with cerebellar pathology by Babinski (1913) and Holmes (1917, 1922). Consistent with this view, the majority of cerebellar lesion studies reported throughout the twentieth century focused largely on investigations into the nature of associated motor impairments to the exclusion of the cerebellum's broader capabilities. Unfortunately, until recently, this preoccupation with cerebellar coordination of motor control overshadowed any consideration of a possible role for the cerebellum in cognitive and language processing. This oversight is even more surprising given some of the anatomical and functional features of the cerebellum, including: the population of neurones in the cerebellum exceeding that of any other part of the human nervous system, including the cerebral cortex; its speed of operation, allowing it to respond rapidly to information it receives; its massive neural connections with the cerebral cortex, which sends more fibres to the cerebellum than any other part of the nervous system; and the extensive connections of its output fibres, which pass to many other parts of the nervous system, including areas of the cerebral cortex well beyond motor areas.

Since the mid-1980s, however, methodological and conceptual advances of contemporary neuroscience have brought about a substantial modification of the traditional view of the cerebellum as a mere coordinator of autonomic and somatic motor functions. These advances have included realization of the importance of parallels in the phylogenetic development of the neocerebellum and associated areas of the cerebral cortex, greater understanding of the neuroanatomy of the cerebellum and its connections with the cerebral cortex, introduction of advanced neuroimaging techniques, including functional neuroimaging, capable of detecting activation of the cerebellum during performance of language tasks, and advances in neuropsychological/linguistic testing capable of detection of subtle changes in cognitive/linguistic function in patients with cerebellar pathology. Collectively these advances in neuroscience have established the view that the cerebellum participates in a much wider range of functions than conventionally accepted, including cognitive and linguistic functions, among others, in addition to regulation and coordination of motor function.

Bloedel and Bracha (1997) outlined five periods in the conceptual growth and development of insights into cerebellar functioning. First, the role of the cerebellum was considered to be coordination of voluntary movements and orientation of the body and head in space. Next, an additional function of the cerebellum was considered to be the regulation and integration of sensory information for reflex organization. Thirdly, the cerebellum was believed to also be responsible for regulating vestibulo-ocular movements and posture of the head. Fourthly, the cerebellum was recognized as an essential structure for learning conditioned responses. Lastly and most currently, various investigations have indicated a possible role for the cerebellum in the regulation of linguistic, cognitive and affective functions. (For a more detailed description of cerebellar functioning from a historical perspective see Chapter 1 of the present volume.)

Currently, it is thought that, in addition to its contribution to motor control, the cerebellum (particularly the right cerebellum) is responsible for modulating non-motor language processes and cognitive functions of those parts of the brain to which it is reciprocally connected (Lalonde and Botez-Marquard, 2000; Silveri and Misciagna, 2000; Marien et al., 2001). Thus the particular role of the cerebellum in this domain is to modulate rather than generate language and cognition, the latter function being considered to be specific to supratentorial structures, particularly the cerebral cortex (Silveri and Misciagna, 2000). Silveri and Misciagna (2000) described this role of the cerebellum as representing the interface between cognition and execution, coordinating information coming from the supratentorial structures responsible for the precise cognitive process and its executive level. This proposed role for the cerebellum in modulating language has major implications for the assessment and rehabilitation of patients with cerebellar lesions and challenges conventional localizationist theories which promote cerebral cortical exclusivity in relation to language processing in the brain.

Several reasons possibly underly why the recently recognized role for the cerebellum in language and cognition was overlooked for several centuries. According to some authors, a primary explanation lies in the modulatory role of the cerebellum in language and cognition, which results in linguistic and cognitive impairments that are both qualitatively and quantitatively different from those produced by lesions of supratentorial structures (Silveri and Misciagna, 2000). Akin to models of motor control that define a role for the cerebellum in the refinement and coordination of movement (Fabbro, 2000), cerebellar contributions to cognition have been postulated as being high level in nature (Chafetz et al., 1996; Marien et al., 2001). In relation to language, it has been proposed that cerebellar lesions may evoke a form of linguistic incoordination or crudity, potentially manifesting as high-level language deficits (Cook et al., 2004). Complex or high-level language measures have been described as tasks that demand frontal lobe support in the manipulation of novel situations, lexical-semantic operations, the development of language strategies and the organization and monitoring of responses (Copland et al., 2000). Detection of these high-level linguistic impairments with routine language tests may have been difficult in previous investigations, as standard language test batteries may not have been sensitive or extensive enough to identify such subtle deficits that may follow cerebellar damage (Cook et al., 2004; Murdoch and Whelan, 2007). Consequently the presence of subtle, high-level language problems, although present, would most likely have been masked by the severity of any motor impairment in patients with cerebellar pathology. Based on the findings of Cook et al. (2004), it would appear that linguistic disturbances subsequent to cerebellar lesions may be more accurately detected and characterized by high-level assessments that evaluate the proficiency of more complex language processes beyond single-word hierarchies.

The present chapter will review the neuroanatomical, neuroimaging and clinical evidence suggestive of a role for the cerebellum in language. Further, the possible neuropathophysiological substrates of language impairment associated with cerebellar pathology will be explored and the nature of linguistic deficits caused by disease or destruction of the cerebellum described.

Neuroanatomical evidence for a cerebellar role in language

Over the past two decades, attempts to understand the cognitive/linguistic function of the cerebellum have relied on evidence from many different methodologies, including neuroanatomical, neuroimaging and clinical studies. The primary factor, and hence the cornerstone, in the development of the concept of a cerebellar role in language was the discovery of major reciprocal neural pathways between the cerebellum and frontal areas of the language dominant hemisphere, including Broca's area and the supplementary motor area. In particular the work of Leiner *et al.* (1986, 1987, 1991, 1993) was fundamental to this development in that they were the first to draw attention to the possibility that expanded connections from the cerebellum to the cerebral cortex and from the cortex to the cerebellum present in human brains, but not those of other species, provided a potential neural substrate for the cerebellum to participate in cognitive/linguistic functions in addition to motor functions. Specifically, Leiner *et al.* (1986, 1987, 1989, 1991) drew attention to long-neglected evidence that the lateral portion of the cerebellar hemispheres and dentate nuclei (particularly the ventrolateral phylogenetically newer part referred to as the neodentate) had enlarged significantly greater than any other part of the brain with the exception of the cerebral cortex, during the phylogenetic evolution of the human brain. Importantly this expansion in size had not occurred in parallel with the cerebral cortex as a whole, but rather specifically in parallel with the cerebral association areas (Leiner *et al.*, 1986). In the course of human evolution these expanded parts of the cerebellum became linked to newly enlarged areas of the cerebral cortex to form a phylogenetically new cerebro-cerebellar system in humans. Of particular relevance to enabling the cerebellum to contribute to cognitive/linguistic processes, these newly formed links between the neocerebellum and the frontal lobe included not only the frontal motor areas (Brodmann areas 4 and 6) but also other areas of the frontal cortex including Broca's area (Brodmann areas 44 and 45), which in turn send back new connections to the cerebellum. This reciprocal connectivity forms a series of segregated neural loops that are hypothesized to facilitate cognitive/linguistic function in the same way that the cerebellum enhances motor functions (Leiner *et al.*, 1989).

It has been proposed that the cerebrocortico-cerebellar loops that connect the lateral parts of the cerebellar hemispheres to the frontal lobe consist of a feedforward, afferent limb and a feedback, efferent limb (Leiner *et al.*, 1986; Schmahmann, 1996). The feedforward limb comprises two pathways, one of which passes from the cerebral cortex to the pontine nuclei in the brainstem (cerebrocortico-pontine pathways) and from there connects via mossy fibre projections to the cortex of the lateral portion of the cerebellar hemispheres (ponto-cerebellar pathways). The second feedforward limb passes from the cerebral cortex to the red nucleus, from where the central tegmental tract leads to the inferior olivary nucleus and then via climbing fibres to the lateral cerebellar cortex (Schmahmann, 1996). The feedback limb passes from the dentate nucleus, the primary outflow nucleus of the cerebellum to the nucleus ventralis intermedius and nucleus ventralis anterior of the thalamus via the cerebello-thalamic pathways and from there to various areas in the contralateral frontal lobe (including Brodmann areas 6, 44 and 45) via the thalamo-cortical pathways (Schmahmann, 1996; Engelborghs *et al.*, 1998). Therefore, although the cerebellum is a relay for many circuits involved in the control process of several physiological functions (e.g. vestibulo-cerebello-vestibular loops regulate equilibrium and ocular motility; reticulo-cerebello-reticular loops are involved in muscle tone, control of posture and regulation of several vegetative functions; spino-cerebello-rubro-spinal loops participate in regulation of motor function at the spinal level; hypothalamo-cerebello-hypothalamic loops regulate visceral functions) the primary loops involved in the regulation of voluntary movements and cognitive/linguistic functions are the cerebrocortico-ponto-cerebellocortico-dentato-thalamo-cerebrocortical loops (Bloedel and Bracha, 1997; Middleton and Strick, 1997; Schmahmann and Pandya, 1997) and the cerebro-cortico-rubro-olivo-neodentato-cerebrocortical loops (Leiner *et al.*, 1991, 1993). Importantly, in both loops each cerebellar hemisphere sends information to, and receives it from the contralateral cerebral hemisphere. Therefore the right cerebellar hemisphere is connected to the left cerebral hemisphere and vice versa. A diagramatic representation of major cerebrocortico-cerebellar loops in the human brain proposed by Leiner *et al.* (1989) is shown in Figure 7.1.

Several neuroanatomical studies of the cerebellum have provided critical evidence that the proposed circuits connecting the cerebellum and non-motor cortical areas do exist. For example, Middleton and Strick (1994) reported retrograde transneuronal transport of a retroviral tracer from the dorsolateral prefrontal cortex to the dentate nucleus. More recently, the same authors also using a retrograde transneuronal transport technique demonstrated the presence of cerebello-thalamo-cortical pathways in primates (Middleton and Strick, 2000).

In summary, anatomically cerebello-cerebrocortical pathways lend themselves to a neuroregulatory role apropos non-motor and motor functions, via associative as well as motor cortex terminations. More specifically, the prefrontal, parietal, temporal and paralimbic cortices demonstrate topographically organized feedforward projections to the cerebellum which are siphoned through cortico-pontine and cortico-rubro-olivary pathways and transmitted via deep cerebellar nuclei (particularly the dentate nucleus) to thalamic nuclei and then back to the cerebral cortex (Schmahmann, 1996; Middleton and Strick, 2000). It has been proposed that this configuration provides a neural substrate whereby the cerebellum may be actively and directly involved in the organization, construction and execution of higher-order behaviours, including language.

The reciprocal neuroanatomical connections between the cerebellum and cerebral cortex that are proposed to enable cerebellar input into cognitive linguistic functions have a number of parallel features to equivalent pathways involved in the coordination and modulation of motor function. Indeed, models of motor control have been lent in the translation of cerebellar cognitive disturbances. The term 'cerebellar cognitive affective syndrome' was coined by Schmahmann and Sherman (1998) to describe a syndrome typically characterized by impaired executive function, spatial cognition, linguistic processing and affective regulation, and has been defined operationally as 'dysmetria of thought' (Schmahmann, 1991, 1996). Analogous to the overshooting and undershooting of ataxic limb movements, dysmetria of thought has been hypothesized to involve either the inadequate or overly elaborate planning or misinterpretation of stimuli. In relation to cognition, the intact cerebellum has been described as

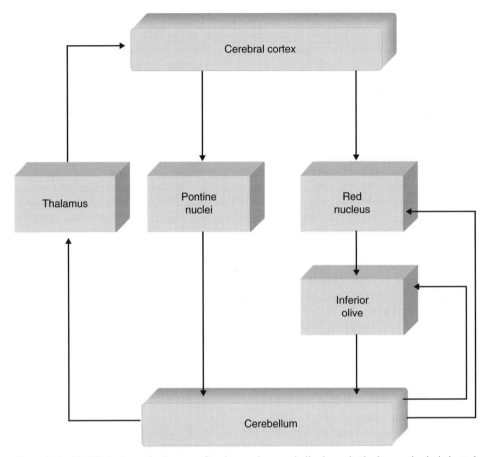

Figure 7.1 Modified schematic diagram of major cerebro-cerebellar loops in the human brain (adapted from Leiner *et al.*, 1989).

capable of detecting, preventing and correcting mismatches between the intended outcomes and the perceived outcomes of an organism's interaction with the environment (Schmahmann, 1998). Therefore, in the same way as the cerebellum regulates the rate, force, rhythm and accuracy of movement, it may also control the speed, capacity, consistency and appropriateness of cognitive and linguistic processing.

Evidence from functional neuroimaging studies for a cerebellar role in language

In addition to the neuroanatomical evidence outlined above, data supporting participation of the cerebellum in language has in recent years also come from a number of functional neuroimaging studies that have utilized techniques such as positron emission tomography (PET), functional magnetic resonance imaging (fMRI) and single-photon emission computed tomography (SPECT). These techniques are important because they represent the only relatively non-invasive means of monitoring neuronal activity in humans by directly measuring associated changes in blood flow and oxygenation. In general these studies have shown that the right lateral cerebellum (neo-cerebellum) is activated during cognitive processing of words, while anatomically distinct from areas activated during performance of motor tasks.

Petersen *et al.* (1988, 1989) were among the first to report cerebellar changes in blood flow as measured by PET during a word-generation task. Specifically these authors reported right lateral cerebellar activation when subjects were asked to produce appropriate verbs in response to visually presented nouns (e.g. 'bark' in response to 'dog') but not when they read the nouns aloud. Since their subjects produced spoken words in both tasks, the increase in blood flow observed in the right lateral cerebel-lum, which projects to the left prefrontal language areas, was interpreted as support for the hypothesis of cerebellar involvement in non-motor language. Although sub-sequent studies have varied the original task design, activation of the right lateral cerebellum during word-generation tasks has been consistently reproduced (Raichle *et al.*, 1994; Martin *et al.*, 1995; Grabowski *et al.*, 1996). Leiner *et al.* (1989) interpreted the simultaneous activation of the right lateral cerebellum and Broca's area during word generation as a reflection of accelerated transmission of signals between these two centres during word finding.

In an examination of human visual information processing, Shulman *et al.* (1997) analysed nine PET studies to determine the consistency of brain blood-flow increases during active relative to passive viewing of the same stimulus array. While no con-sistent blood-flow increases were found in the cerebral cortex outside of the visual cortex, increases were observed in the thalamus and cerebellum. More specifically, a left cerebellar and a medial cerebellar focus reflected motor-related processes, whereas blood-flow increases in the right cerebellar region were considered to be not motor-related. The right thalamic focus exhibited sensitivity to variables related to focal attention, suggesting involvement of this region in the attentional engagement of visual stimuli (Shulman *et al.* 1997). The left thalamic focus, however, was completely uncorrelated with the right region, indicating involvement in separate functions. The results of the study indicated that both the left thalamus and right cerebellum yielded larger blood flow increases when subjects performed a complex rather than a simple language task which, according to Shulman *et al.* (1997) possibly reflected a language-related pathway. Based on their observations, Shulman *et al.* (1997) concluded that the left-frontal cortex, left thalamus and right cerebellum may form a circuit in certain language tasks.

In contrast to the several PET studies suggesting a contribution of the lateral aspects of the right cerebellar hemisphere to the cognitive aspects of speech production, Ackermann *et al.* (1998) report that, in their study of 18 subjects who underwent fMRI during continuous silent automatic speech (recitation of names of the months of the year), observed cerebellar activation appeared to be related to the articulatory level of speech. During the study, activation in the right cerebellar hemisphere together with an asymmetric activation pattern occurred towards the left side at the level of the motor strip in the cerebral cortex. These authors argued that this was attributable to the fact that highly overlearned word strings supposedly posed few demands on the controlled response selection, together with the fact that the projections of the right cerebellar hemisphere to the left precentral gyrus also participate in motor control.

Desmond *et al.* (1998) used fMRI to examine the distinctive contributions of the right cerebellar regions and left-frontal cerebral cortex using a word-stem completion task. Subjects were asked to complete three-letter word stems that had either many possible completions (e.g. STA-) or few possible completions (e.g. PSA-). Findings revealed that conspicuous increases in activation were observed in the left middle frontal gyrus and left caudate nucleus in the condition which had many word-stem completions, compared to the condition with few possible word-stem completions. Conversely, portions of the right cerebellar hemisphere (posterior quadrangular lobule and superior semilunar lobule) and cerebellar vermis exhibited increases in the 'few' condition, in comparison to the 'many' condition. The authors believed that this double dissociation suggested that the frontal and cerebellar regions make distinctive contributions to cognitive performance, with left-frontal (and striatal) activations reflecting response selection (which increases in difficulty when there are many appropriate responses), and right cerebellar activations illustrating the search for responses (which increases in difficulty when even a single appropriate response is hard to retrieve). Desmond et al. (1998) concluded that these results did not challenge previous findings that the left-frontal and right cerebellar regions regularly interact in verbal performance, but rather believed that such findings demonstrated that these two regions make distinctive contributions to that interaction, providing insight into the nature of such unique contributions. In addition to the increased need for working-memory resources required for the search for responses, the 'few' condition may also require more error correction in order to reject similar but incorrect matches that would likely occur more often for the 'few' condition. Desmond et al. (1998) therefore suggested that the right cerebellar activations may also reflect such error-correction operations.

Further support for a role for the right cerebellar hemisphere in the non-motor aspects of language was provided by the work of Papthanassiou et al. (2000) and Schlosser et al. (1998). Based on a PET study, Papthanassiou et al. (2000) reported right cerebellar cortex activation during both speech comprehension and production, which was particularly evident during a verb-generation task. These authors believed that the findings were indicative of cerebellar control of the neural computations involved during word semantic processing. Using fMRI, Schlosser et al. (1998) reported areas of activation in the left prefrontal cortex and right cerebellum in subjects during performance of a verbal fluency task.

Based on a review of functional neuroimaging studies reporting changes in cerebellar activation during cognitive tasks, Desmond and Fiez (1998) concluded that the cerebellum is involved in basic cognitive processes such as working memory, implicit and explicit learning and memory, and language. These authors also concluded that unlike damage to the left-hemisphere perisylvian regions, damage to the cerebellum is not firmly related to central disturbances of language and reading as in the acquired aphasias and dyslexias, suggesting rather that the cerebellum is not integral to the access and representation of orthographic, phonological, semantic and syntactic information, and that it exerts a more indirect influence. For example, the verb-generation task often used to highlight involvement of the cerebellum in language processing (e.g. in studies such as Petersen et al. 1988, 1989) has features associated with implicit learning tasks, such that performance improves rapidly with practice (Desmond and Fiez, 1998). Additionally, the cerebellum may participate in the search for valid responses from semantic memory, possibly forming the basis for improved performance observed with repeated exposure of the same items (Desmond and Fiez, 1998).

Functional neuroimaging studies have also provided support for neuroanatomical data that suggests crossed reciprocal connections between the cerebellum and higher-order cortical association areas (Silveri et al., 1994; Marien et al., 1996, 2000; Hubrich-Ungureanu et al., 2002). Hubrich-Ungureanu et al. (2002) used fMRI to examine one left- and one right-handed volunteer during performance of a silent verbal fluency task. Their findings indicated that cerebellar activation is contralateral to the activation of the frontal cortex even under conditions of different language dominance. Silveri *et al.* (1994) described a 67 year-old right-handed patient who presented with a right-sided cerebellar syndrome, ataxic dysarthria and transient expressive agrammatism subsequent to a right cerebellar stroke. Although repeated structural neuroimaging examinations were unable to identify any supratentorial abnormality to account for the observed language deficits, a SPECT examination evidenced a relative hypoperfusion in the entire left cerebral hemisphere, but particularly involving the left posterior temporal region. During follow-up examinations, the perfusion defects were noted to parallel the clinical course of improvements in motor and linguistic symptoms.

Silveri *et al.* (1994) ascribed the agrammatism of their patient to a delay in the processes underlying sentence construction. More specifically, they proposed that the cerebellum has no direct influence on linguistic processing but rather plays an important role in the timing of linguistic functions represented at the level of the cerebral cortex. According to this so-called timing hypothesis, patients with cerebellar damage will experience great difficulty in temporal modulation, required for several linguistic processes such as phonological processing, sentence construction and comprehension and application of syntactic rules. They proposed that in the case they presented, the on-line application of syntactic rules may have been slowed, causing the representation of morphemes to decay from working memory and leading to a disturbance in sentence integration. According to Silveri *et al.* (1994) therefore, language deficits following right cerebellar lesions are not really aphasic disorders but are due to the impairment of some cognitive components (e.g. working memory) that are involved in language processing.

A different hypothesis was proposed by Marien *et al.* (1996) who maintained that cerebellar lesions may provoke an aphasic syndrome. Marien *et al.* (1996, 2000) also reported the case of a 73 year-old right-handed patient who presented with a predominantly expressive aphasic syndrome and agrammatism subsequent to an ischaemic infarct in the territory of the right arteria cerebellaris superior. Specifically the aphasic disorder resembled a transcortical motor aphasia and was characterized by an impairment of syntax, reduced spontaneous speech, reduced verbal output, perseverations, word-finding difficulties, reduced speech rate, lack of content words, disturbances in mental spelling and comprehension of oral spelling, as well as an expressive and receptive agrammatism. Although the neuroanatomical correlates of this type of aphasia are reported to focus on the frontal lobe of the dominant cerebral hemisphere, repeated structural neuroimaging examinations involving computed tomography (CT) or MRI were unable to identify a lesion in the expected supratentorial areas. Repeated SPECT studies did, however, yield positive findings to account for the language symptoms. In addition to a marked hypoperfusion of the right cerebellar hemisphere, SPECT revealed a left frontoparietal hypoperfusion which involved the gyrus frontalis medius and inferior as well as the gyrus precentralis and postcentralis. As in the case reported by Silveri *et al.* (1994) improvements in linguistic performance paralleled reduction in the level of hypoperfusion.

Marien *et al.* (2000) believed that the co-occurrence of a right cerebellar lesion and an aphasic syndrome possibly illustrated the pathophysiological hypothesis of a deactivation of prefrontal left cerebral hemisphere language functions due to loss of excitatory impulses passing via the cerebello-ponto-thalamo-cerebrocortical pathways. This phenomenon, called crossed cerebello-cerebral diaschisis, was first documented in a patient with cerebellar infarction by Broich *et al.* (1987). If, as proposed by Marien *et al.* (1996, 2000), the possible explanation for language disturbances following right cerebellar damage is a reduction of excitatory impulses through the cerebello-ponto-thalamo-cerebrocortical pathways (Sönmezoglu *et al.*, 1993), it would follow that aphasia in cerebellar pathology does not imply representation of language functions at the level of the cerebellum but rather reflects a diaschisis phenomenon involving diminished or abolished function of the supratentorial 'language zones' due to reduced input via cerebellocortical pathways (Marien *et al.*, 2001).

The case of a 17 year-old left-handed man with a right cerebellar hemisphere infarction associated with ataxic dysarthria and subtle language dysfunction was described by Hassid (1995). Moderate anomia was demonstrated in all modalities along with mild difficulties in auditory reception and reading, with severe difficulties in writing and mathematics. Although structural neuroimaging by way of CT and MRI scans only revealed a right-sided wedge-shaped cerebellar infarction, a SPECT scan indicated reduced blood flow in the right cerebellum and the left temporal, frontal and parietal lobes consistent with right cerebellar infarction induced crossed cerebello-cerebral diaschisis. Hassid (1995) suggested that complex cerebellar-cerebral connections are therefore capable of influencing both motor and cognitive functions, with the anatomic substrates of each of these functions distinct, both in the cerebellum and thalamus.

Following an extensive review of contemporary investigations, Marien *et al.* (2001) concluded that the cerebellum is topographically organized in subserving a wide range of cognitive, linguistic and affective functions. These authors proposed that within a framework of topographical functional representation, a substantial amount of clinical and experimental evidence supported that the specific modulatory role of the cerebellum in language processes, such as lexical retrieval, syntax and language dynamics, are represented in a highly restricted way in the fourth cerebellar area that Marien and colleagues termed the 'lateralized linguistic cerebellum'. Marien *et al.* (2001) also outlined that the right hemisphere of the cerebellum is crucially involved in the integrated subsystem of working memory that subserves several language processes, articulatory planning, a variety of linguistic operations implicated in semantic and phonological word retrieval, syntactic processing and the dynamics of language processing. Thus Marien *et al.* (2001) advanced the concept of a functionally lateralized linguistic cerebellum with a modulatory role in apraxia of speech, classic aphasia syndromes and aphasia in atypical populations. Additionally, these authors postulated that linguistic deficits following cerebellar pathology do not imply representation of linguistic functions at the cerebellar level, but reflect functional deactivation of the supratentorial language areas due to reduced input via cerebello-cerebrocortical pathways, thereby placing emphasis on diaschisis processes as the relevant neuropathological mechanism for cerebellum-induced language disorders.

Evidence from clinical studies for a cerebellar role in language

Further evidence for a role for the cerebellum in language has been derived from the evaluation of the performance of patients with various cerebellar pathologies (including cerebellar atrophy and focal lesions caused by strokes or tumours) on a range of linguistic and neuropsychological tests. The results from several clinical studies converge with the neuroanatomical and neuroimaging studies described above to implicate the cerebellum in various aspects of language function. Fiez *et al.* (1992) examined a patient with a vascular lesion of the right cerebellar hemisphere on a word-genera-tion task. Although the patient had high-level conversational skills and normal per-formance on standard neuropsychological assessments, he had difficulty storing information and failed in various semantic word-generation tasks. For instance, when asked to generate verbs in response to nouns, he produced many associated but incor-rect errors (e.g. although associated, many errors were not verbs, such as 'red' in response to *brick*) and failed to learn the task normally. Fiez *et al.* (1992) theorized that the deficits evident in this case indicated that the right cerebellar hemisphere was involved in error-detection tasks and control of some semantic and syntactic aspects of language production. Patients with cerebellar lesions have also been reported to have difficulty learning new verbal associations by other researchers. For instance, Bracke-Tolkmitt *et al.* (1989) reported that a group of patients with cerebellar damage were significantly impaired compared to matched controls at learning random asso-ciations between six words and six colours.

Three aetiologically distinct patient groups with cerebellar pathology were studied by Leggio *et al.* (1995) using both phonological and semantic fluency tests. The pho-nological tasks required the subjects to produce as many words as possible with the initial phonemes F, A and S within 1 min. The semantic verbal fluency tasks consisted of the generation of as many words as possible belonging to the semantic categories *birds* and *furniture*. Two of the groups had restricted focal lesions (lateral part of the left or right cerebellar hemisphere) while the third group had atrophic lesions (mainly involving the vermis or paravermal region). Leggio *et al.* (1995) reported that as a group the subjects with cerebellar lesions performed at a lower level than matched controls on both the phonological and semantic fluency tasks. In addition the atrophic patients obtained better results than those with focal lesions despite having more severe ataxic impairments. The patients with atrophic lesions performed significantly poorer than controls only on the phonological task and patients with lesions involving the right lateral cerebellum performed slightly worse than those with focal lesions to the left cerebellar hemisphere. Overall these findings provided further evidence in support of a functional role for the cerebellum in language and suggested a strong association, first between damage to the lateral cerebellum, especially the right cere-bellar hemisphere and verbal fluency deficits and secondly between medial cerebellar lesions and the prevalence of motor deficits. These findings were later confirmed by Leggio *et al.* (2000) who also demonstrated that the observed deficits in verbal fluency were not the outcome of motor speech impairment. These latter authors also proposed that cerebellar lesions affect phonological processes to a greater extent than semantic processes because phonological tasks depend on unusual novel and less automatized search strategies than semantic tasks.

According to Silveri and Misciagna (2000), patients with cerebellar damage show differing degrees of impairment in the various cognitive domains. In fact, different impairments are recognized at different levels of linguistic organization, from the articulatory level to sentence production. The cerebellum is active, according to Silveri and Misciagna (2000), in tasks requiring single-word selection and production. However, as noted in the findings of neuroimaging studies discussed above (e.g. Silveri *et al.*, 1994), one of the most interesting findings in patients with cerebellar lesions is agrammatic speech (a disorder in speech production characterized by sim-plification of the syntactic structures, reduced sentence length and omission and substitution of grammatical morphemes) (Silveri and Misciagna, 2000). Several other researchers have also reported agrammatism in association with right cerebellar lesions (Zettin *et al.*, 1997; Gasparini *et al.*, 1999). Occasionally, production of content words is impaired to different degrees, such that verbs, for example, may be produced with more difficulty than nouns (Silveri and Misciagna, 2000).

The language abilities of four patients with focal cerebellar lesions of differing aetiologies and localized in different areas of the cerebellum were investigated by Fabbro *et al.* (2000) to determine whether linguistic difficulties existed and whether these deficits were stable or evolved following surgery. All four patients exhibited mild language impairments, particularly affecting morphosyntactic features and lexical access. The first patient, who presented with an arachnoid cyst compressing the superior portion of the vermis, exhibited some morphosyntactic errors in preoperative spontaneous speech, while a few months post-surgery no errors were found. While propositioning had reportedly improved from the pre-surgical assessment, the most compromised linguistic level was found to be syntax. Difficulties in some word-generation tasks were also reported, particularly synonym and attribute generation. The second case presented with a hemangioblastoma compressing the right cerebellar hemisphere. While spontaneous speech remained fluent, some of the morphosyntactical errors exhibited pre- and post-surgery resolved 10 months following surgery, as did deficits in syntactic comprehension, reading and writing. Improvement of propositionizing skills and morphological and syntactic levels also occurred, although difficulties in mental arithmetic and synonym generation did not change. The third patient was diagnosed with an astrocytoma in the vermis and exhibited cerebellar dysarthria, non-fluent spontaneous speech and morphosyntactic errors following surgery. An assessment of language revealed difficulties in grammatical comprehension, antonyms, morphological opposites, reading and writing, with the most compromised tasks including propositionizing and lexical access. Of most significance were impairments in morphology, syntax and semantics. Fabbro *et al.* (2000) suggested that findings from this case particularly supported involvement of both the right cerebellar hemisphere and the vermis in language processing. The final patient, with an astrocytoma involving the left cerebellar hemisphere, exhibited fluent spontaneous speech with some morphosyntactic errors, poor grammatical comprehension and arithmetic, significantly poor performance in both propositionizing and reading, and significantly impaired syntax. While two of the patients (one with an arachnoid cyst compressing the superior portion of the vermis, and the other with a hemangioblastoma compressing the right cerebellar hemisphere) showed partial recovery of linguistic deficits following surgery, the remaining two (both with cerebellar tumours) did not experience an improvement in language function.

Fabbro *et al.* (2000) believed that the mild linguistic deficits shown by their four cases with focal cerebellar lesions demonstrated an alteration of language-control processes rather than to a structural impairment of specific components of the language system. In their view, the vermis and portions of the cerebellar hemispheres operate within a large functional language network as an organizational control mechanism via the frontal lobe system. The rapid recovery of linguistic disturbances noted in two of the four patients following acute cerebellar damage was attributed to partial functional reactivation of linguistic centres after regression of diaschisis phenomena. Also of note is that while the findings of Fabbro *et al.* (2000) generally supported the view that the cerebellar structures involved in language are essentially the right cerebellar hemisphere and some structures of the vermis, one of their four cases demonstrated linguistic deficits subsequent to a tumour in the left cerebellar hemisphere that were similar to those observed in the three cases with right cerebellar lesions.

Although the concept of 'crossed aphasia' in relation to cortical-based language disorders is well documented, to date only two other studies in addition to Fabbro *et al.* (2000) have reported the occurrence of language problems in right-handed individuals in association with left cerebellar hemisphere lesions (Cook *et al.*, 2004; Murdoch and Whelan, 2007). Cook *et al.* (2004) outlined the linguistic profiles of five individuals with left primary cerebellar lesions of vascular origin. All five of their participants demonstrated deficits on measures of word fluency, sentence construction within a set context, producing word definitions and producing multiple definitions of the same words. Cook *et al.* (2004) also reported deficits for several of their participants on measures of understanding figurative language, forming word associations, identifying and correcting semantic absurdities and producing synonyms and antonyms. The findings of Murdoch and Whelan (2007) supported those of Cook *et al.* (2004) that left cerebellar lesions may disrupt language processing, particularly in the area of complex or high-level language skills, including phonemic fluency, sentence formulation and lexical-semantic manipulation tasks. Such tasks, involving the manipulation of novel situations, lexical-semantic operations, the development of language strategies and the organization and monitoring of responses, have been hypothesized to demand frontal lobe support in their manipulation (Copland *et al.*, 2000). Murdoch and Whelan (2007) therefore suggested that frontal lobe hypoperfusion as a consequence of ipsilateral cortical diaschisis provided one plausible explanation for the language deficits exhibited by their ten patients with primary left cerebellar vascular lesions. Ipsilateral cerebellar-cerebral diaschisis has been reported as a consequence of cerebellar lesions (Beldarrain *et al.*, 1997). In an investigation of the relationship between neuropsychological deficits (including language) and SPECT scan perfusion patterns in the cerebral hemispheres subsequent to cerebellar lesions, Beldarrain *et al.* (1997) noted that of the nineteen participants in their study who underwent a SPECT scan, six showed contralateral diaschisis and seven ipsilateral diaschisis with the remaining six subjects showing no evidence of diaschisis. On the basis of their findings, Murdoch and Whelan (2007) suggested that cerebellar involvement in language may be bilateral. Collectively the findings of Cook *et al.* (2004), Fabbro *et al.* (2000) and Murdoch and Whelan (2007) highlight the need for further investigation of language disorders associated with both left and right cerebellar lesions to further elucidate the extent and nature of language lateralization in the cerebellum.

Cerebellar lesions and language function in childhood

Although the majority of evidence supporting a role for the cerebellum in language processing comes from studies of adults, an increasing body of support is also being derived from studies of children with acquired cerebellar lesions primarily resulting from treatment for posterior cranial fossa tumours (Levisohn *et al.*, 2000; Riva, 2000; Docking *et al.*, 2007). Overall, evidence from childhood studies suggests that cerebellar contributions to language and cognition in children reflect observations in adults. Deficits observed in frontal lobe functions following cerebellar lesions in paediatric populations confirm the existence of connections between the cerebellum and frontal lobes via the thalamus (Steinlin *et al.*, 1999; Riva, 2000). Additionally it has been suggested that the earlier cerebellar damage occurs during development, the greater the subsequent impact on language and cognitive function (Riva, 2000).

Studies examining the role of the cerebellum in children have indicated that damage to specific areas of the cerebellum exerts impact on a distinct range of functions, indicating that functional specialization is present at a very early age. The right cerebellar hemisphere has been recently considered to maintain substantial responsibility for language processing (Riva and Giorgi, 2000a, 2000b; Scott *et al.*, 2001). Particularly, clinical manifestations resulting from damage to this specific region in children include disturbances in auditory sequential memory, alterations in verbal intelligence, decreased competence in complex language processing, significantly reduced syntactic comprehension, reduced abilities in verbal sequencing and categorical memory and an interruption to literacy skills. In the absence of functional neuroimaging in their study, Riva and Giorgi (2000a, 2000b) suggested that it was not possible to determine whether these language deficits were the direct outcome of the cerebellar lesion, or due to diaschisis arising from the interruption of the reciprocal connections between the cerebellum and cerebral cortex. Conversely, damage to the left cerebellar hemisphere has been associated with visual and spatial memory, non-verbal information processing, non-verbal intelligence and impairments in prosody (Schatz *et al.*, 1998; Riva and Giorgi, 2000a, 2000b; Scott *et al.*, 2001). Other authors have also noted the presence of high-level language deficits, global impairment, and declines in expressive language and syntax as an outcome of treatment for posterior cranial fossa tumours in childhood (Hudson and Murdoch, 1992; Murdoch and Hudson-Tennent, 1994; Docking *et al.*, 2007).

In addition to the role of the right and left cerebellar hemispheres, the impact of a lesion in the vermis was also analysed by Riva and Giorgi (2000a, 2000b). These authors reported two different presentations subsequent to lesions in this region: namely post-surgical mutism and behavioural disturbances. With respect to the profile distinguished by post-surgical mutism, this reportedly either evolved into a classical speech disorder, or a language disorder characterized by agrammatism with intact comprehension. The second profile involved affective and social behavioural alterations, ranging in severity from irritability to a more autistic manifestation. The relationship between vermal lesions and expressive language and behavioural dysfunction has also been reported by other studies (Oki *et al.*, 1999).

Riva and Giorgi (2000b) also presented data for a patient with viral cerebellitis who demonstrated a complex neuropsychological profile with deficits in language processing and general sequential function. In support of the findings of agrammatism in adults with cerebellar lesions (e.g. Silveri *et al.*, 1994), language was also considered telegraphic, commonly without function words, and reflected a breakdown in linguistic content. Riva and Giorgi (2000b) attributed responsibility for such findings to the diaschisis of the cerebello-frontal loops in activating those strategies that are significant to processing and programming verbal and sequential activities.

It has also been documented that the intimate relationship between proposed functions of the cerebellum and the observed deficits in children with dyslexia strongly suggests that children with dyslexia experience a mild dysfunction of the cerebellum and that this cerebellar deficit is at least partly responsible for many of their symptoms (Nicholson *et al.*, 1995). A study by Fawcett *et al.* (1996) supported that cerebellar impairment was indeed associated with dyslexia following an examination of 55 children with dyslexia and their matched controls. The children with dyslexia were found to exhibit highly significant impairment across all cerebellar tasks, which included clinical cerebellar tests of balance, time estimation, muscle tone and coordination.

Summary

In summary, the results of recent neuroanatomical, neuroimaging and clinical studies have demonstrated that the role of the cerebellum is not limited to motor functions but appears to be involved in the modulation of a broad spectrum of linguistic functions such as verbal fluency, word retrieval, syntax, reading, writing and metalinguistics abilities. Based on neural evidence and information-processing theory, Leiner *et al.* (1986) showed that the phylogenetically newest part of the cerebellum (particularly the lateral portions of the cerebellar hemispheres and dentate nuclei) might interact with the frontal association cortex to allow for skilled manipulation of information or ideas. In support of this proposal, neuroanatomical studies have demonstrated reciprocal connections linking the cerebellum with centres in the cerebral cortex, including areas crucially involved in high-level linguistic functions (Middleton and Strick, 2000). The existence of a reciprocal functional connectivity has been clearly demonstrated by functional neuroimaging studies that show cerebellar activation during a range of linguistic tasks which require no motor response (e.g. Petersen *et al.*, 1989). Further clinical investigations of both adults and children with cerebellar pathology using sensitive linguistic tests capable of detecting subtle, high-level language impairments (e.g. Docking *et al.*, 2007; Murdoch and Whelan, 2007) have demonstrated the presence of a variety of linguistic impairments in association with cerebellar pathology.

Several different theories have been proposed relating to possible neuropathological mechanisms involved in the occurrence of language disorders subsequent to cerebellar lesions. First, it has been suggested that crossed cerebello-cerebrocortical diaschisis reflecting a functional depression of supratentorial language areas due to reduced input to the cerebral cortex via cerebello-cerebrocortical pathways may represent the neuropathological mechanism responsible for linguistic deficits associated with cerebellar pathology (Broich *et al.*, 1987; Marien *et al.*, 2001). In support of this suggestion, functional neuroimaging studies based on SPECT, PET or fMRI have consistently revealed regions of contralateral cortical hypoperfusion in relation to the orientation of the cerebellar lesion (e.g. Silveri *et al.*, 1994; Beldarrain *et al.*, 1997). According to the cerebello-cerebrocortical diaschisis model, therefore, the cerebellum is not involved in the generation of language (which remains a supratentorial activity) but rather modulates language function via segregated, multi-component neural circuits the major pathways of which include the cerebrocortico-ponto-cerebellocortico-dentato-thalamic-cerebrocortical loop and the cerebrocortico-rubro-olivo-neodentato-cerebrocortical loop. In this way the cerebellum acts as an important relay in the neural circuits responsible for language in much the same way as other subcortical structures, such as the basal ganglia, form important components of the segregated, multi-component neural circuits that enable those structures to also influence frontal lobe activities.

A second theory proposed to explain cerebellar involvement in linguistic function is the timing hypothesis which proposes that the cerebellum has no direct influence on linguistic processes but plays an important role in the timing of linguistic functions represented on a supratentorial level (Keele and Ivry, 1991; Silveri *et al.*, 1994). A third hypothesis relating to the role of the cerebellum in language proposes a direct cerebellar contribution via the topographically organized reciprocal connections with the cerebral cortex. According to this theory, the cerebellum does not act as a sole modulator of language but is actively involved in the organization, construction and execution of linguistic processes. As yet, however, the precise role of the cerebellum in language is not clear. Further studies that rely on a combination of neuroanatomical, neuroimaging and neurolinguistic investigations are needed to further elucidate the nature of the role of this complex and somewhat neglected and underestimated part of the brain in language function.

References

Ackermann, H., Wildgruber, D., Daum, I. and Grodd, W. (1998). Does the cerebellum contribute to cognitive aspects of speech production? A functional magnetic resonance (fMRI) study in humans. *Neuroscience Letters* 247, 187–90.

Babinski, J. (1913). *Exposé des travaux scientifiques: syndrome céerebelleux.* Paris: Masson.

Beldarrain, M.G., Garcia-Monco, J.C., Quintana, J.M., Llorens, V. and Rodeno, E. (1997). Diaschisis and neuropsychological performance after cerebellar stroke. *European Neurology* 37(2), 82–9.

Bloedel, J.R. and Bracha, V. (1997). Duality of cerebellar motor and cognitive functions. In J.D. Schmahmann (ed.), *International Review of Neurobiology: the Cerebellum and Cognition*, vol. 41 (pp. 613–34). San Diego, CA: Academic Press.

Bracke-Tolkmitt, R., Linden, A., Canavan, A.G.M., Rockstroh, B., Scholz, E. *et al.* (1989). The cerebellum contributes to mental skills. *Behavioral Neuroscience* 103, 442–6.

Broich, K., Hartmann, A., Biersack, H.J. and Horn, R. (1987). Crossed cerebello-cerebral diaschisis in a patient with cerebellar infarction. *Neuroscience Letters* 83, 7–12.

Chafetz, M.D., Friedman, A.L., Kevorkain, C.G. and Levy, J.K. (1996). The cerebellum and cognitive function. Implications for rehabilitation. *Archives of Physical Medicine and Rehabilitation* 77(12), 1303–8.

Cook, M., Murdoch, B.E., Cahill, L. and Whelan, B.-M. (2004). Higher-level language deficits resulting from left primary cerebellar lesions. *Aphasiology* 18(9), 771–84.

Copland, D.A., Chenery, H.J. and Murdoch, B.E. (2000). Persistent deficits in complex language function following dominant nonthalamic subcortical lesions. *Journal of Medical Speech-Language Pathology* 8(1), 1–14.

Desmond, J.E. and Fiez, J.A. (1998). Neuroimaging studies of the cerebellum: language, learning, and memory. *Trends in Cognitive Sciences* 2, 355–62.

Desmond, J.E., Gabrieli, J.D.E. and Glover, G.H. (1998). Dissociation of frontal and cerebellar activity in a cognitive task: evidence for a distinction between selection and search. *Neuroimage* 7, 368–76.

Docking, K.M., Murdoch, B.E. and Suppiah, R. (2007). The impact of a cerebellar tumour on language function in childhood. *Folia Phoniatrica et Logopaedica* 59, 190–200.

Engelborghs, S., Marien, P., Martin, J.J. and DeDeyn, P.P. (1998). Functional anatomy, vascularization and pathology of the human thalamus. *Acta Neurologica Belgica* 98, 252–65.

Fabbro, F. (2000). Introduction to language and cerebellum. *Journal of Neurolinguistics* 13(2–3), 83–94.

Fabbro, F., Moretti, R. and Bava, A. (2000). Language impairments in patients with cerebellar lesions. *Journal of Neurolinguistics* 13(2–3), 173–88.

Fawcett, A.J., Nicholson, R.I. and Dean, P. (1996). Impaired performance of children with dyslexia on a range of cerebellar tasks. *Annals of Dyslexia* 46, 259–83.

Fiez, J.A., Petersen, S.E., Cheney, M.K. and Raichle, M.E. (1992). Impaired non-motor learning and error detection associated with cerebellar damage. *Brain* 115, 155–78.

Gasparini, M., Di Piero, V., Ciccarelli, O., Cacioppo, M.M., Pantano, P. *et al.* (1999). Linguistic impairment after right cerebellar stroke: a case report. *European Journal of Neurology* 6, 353–6.

Grabowski, T.J., Frank, R.J., Brown, C.K., Damasio, H., Boles-Ponto, L.L. *et al.* (1996). Reliability of PET activation across statistical methods, subject groups, and sample sizes. *Human Brain Mapping* 4, 23–46.

Hassid, E.I. (1995). A case of language dysfunction associated with cerebellar infarction. *Journal of Neurological Rehabilitation* 9, 157–60.

Holmes, G. (1917). The symptoms of acute cerebellar injuries due to gunshot injuries. *Brain* 40, 401–534.

Holmes, G. (1922). Clinical symptoms of cerebellar disease and their interpretation. *Lancet* 2, 59–65.

Hubrich-Ungureanu, P., Kaemmerer, N., Henn, F.A. and Braus, D.F. (2002). Lateralized organization of the cerebellum in a silent verbal fluency task. A functional magnetic resonance imaging study in healthy volunteers. *Neuroscience Letters* 319, 91–4.

Hudson, L.J. and Murdoch, B.E. (1992). Chronic language deficits in children treated for posterior fossa tumour. *Aphasiology* 6(2), 135–50.

Keele, S.W. and Ivry, R. (1991). Does the cerebellum provide a common computation for diverse tasks? A timing hypothesis. In A. Diamond (ed.), *The Developmental and Neural Basis of Higher Cognitive Functions* (pp. 179–211). New York: New York Academy of Sciences.

Lalonde, R. and Botez-Marquard, T. (2000). Neuropsychological deficits of patients with chronic or acute cerebellar lesions. *Journal of Neurolinguistics* 13(2–3), 117–28.

Leggio, M.G., Solida, A., Silveri, M.C., Gainotti, G. and Molinari, M. (1995). Verbal fluency impairments in patients with cerebellar lesions. *Society of Neuroscience Abstracts* 21, 917.

Leggio, M.G., Silveri, M.C., Petrosini, L. and Molinari, M. (2000). Phonological grouping is specifically affected in cerebellar patients: a verbal fluency study. *Journal of Neurology, Neurosurgery and Psychiatry* 69, 102–6.

Leiner, H.C., Leiner, A.L. and Dow, R.S. (1986). Does the cerebellum contribute to mental skills? *Behavioral Neuroscience* 100, 443–54.

Leiner, H.C., Leiner, A.L. and Dow, R.S. (1987). Cerebro-cerebellar learning loops in apes and humans. *Italian Journal of Neurological Sciences* 8, 425–36.

Leiner, H.C., Leiner, A.L. and Dow, R.S. (1989). Reappraising the cerebellum: what does the hindbrain contribute to the forebrain. *Behavioral Neuroscience* 103, 998–1008.

Leiner, H.C., Leiner, A.L. and Dow, R.S. (1991). The human cerebro-cerebellar system: its computing, cognitive and language skills. *Behavioral Brain Research* 24, 113–28.

Leiner, H.C., Leiner, A.L. and Dow, R.S. (1993). Cognitive and language functions of the human cerebellum. *Trends in Neurosciences* 16, 444–7.

Levisohn, L., Cronin-Golomb, A. and Schmahmann, J.D. (2000). Neuropsychological consequences of cerebellar tumour resection in children: cerebellar cognitive affective syndrome in a paediatric population. *Brain* 123, 1041–50.

Marien, P., Saerens, J., Nanhoe, R., Moens, E., Nagels, G. *et al.* (1996). Cerebellar induced aphasia: case report of cerebellar induced prefrontal aphasic language phenomena supported by SPECT findings. *Journal of the Neurological Sciences* 144, 34–43.

Marien, P., Engelborghs, S., Pickut, B.A. and DeDeyn, P.P. (2000). Aphasia following cerebellar damage: fact or fallacy? *Journal of Neurolinguistics* 13, 145–71.

Marien, P., Engelborghs, S., Fabbro, F. and DeDeyn, P.P. (2001). The lateralized linguistic cerebellum: a review and a new hypothesis. *Brain and Language* 79, 580–600.

Martin, A., Haxby, J.V., Lalonde, F.M., Wiggs, C.L. and Ungerleider, L.G. (1995). Discrete cortical regions associated with knowledge of color and knowledge of action. *Science* 270, 102–5.

Middleton, F.A. and Strick, P.L. (1994). Anatomical evidence for cerebellar and basal ganglia involvement in higher cognitive function. *Science* 266, 458–61.

Middleton, F.A. and Strick, P.L. (1997). Dentate output channels: motor and cognitive components. *Progress in Brain Research* 114, 555–68.

Middleton, F.A. and Strick, P.L. (2000). Basal ganglia output and cognition: evidence from anatomical, behavioural and clinical studies. *Brain and Cognition* 42, 183–200.

Murdoch, B.E. and Hudson-Tennent, L.J. (1994). Differential language outcomes in children following treatment for posterior fossa tumours. *Aphasiology* 8(6), 507–34.

Murdoch, B.E. and Whelan, B-M. (2007). Language disorders subsequent to left cerebellar lesions: a case for bilateral cerebellar involvement in language? *Folia Phoniatrica et Logopaedica* 59, 184–9.

Nicholson, R.I., Fawcett, A. and Dean, P. (1995). Time estimation deficits in developmental dyslexia: evidence of cerebellar involvement. *Proceedings of the Royal Society of London Series B Biological Sciences* 259, 43–7.

Oki, J., Takahashi, S., Miyamoto, A. and Tachibana, Y. (1999). Cerebellar hypoperfusion and developmental dysphasia in a male. *Pediatric Neurology* 21, 745–8.

Papthanassiou, D., Etard, O., Mellet, E., Zago, L., Mazoyer, B. and Tzourio-Mazoyer, W. (2000). A common language network for comprehension and production: a contribution to the definition of language epicenters with PET. *Neuroimage* 11, 347–57.

Petersen, S.E., Fox, P.T., Posner, M.I., Mintum, M. and Raichle, M.E. (1988). Positron emission tomographic studies of the cortical anatomy of single-word processing. *Nature* 331, 585–9.

Petersen, S.E., Fox, P.T., Posner, M.I., Mintum, M. and Raichle, M.E. (1989). Positron emission tomographic studies of the processing of single words. *Journal of Cognitive Neuroscience* 1, 153–70.

Raichle, M.E., Fiez, J.A., Videen, T.O., MacLeod, A.M., Pardo, J.V. *et al.* (1994). Practice-related changes in human brain functional anatomy during nonmotor learning. *Cerebral Cortex* 4, 8–26.

Riva, D. (2000). Cerebellar contribution to behaviour and cognition in children. *Journal of Neurolinguistics* 13(2–3), 215–25.

Riva, D. and Giorgi, C. (2000a). The contribution of the cerebellum to mental and social functions in developmental age. *Human Physiology* 26(1), 21–5.

Riva, D. and Giorgi, C. (2000b). The cerebellum contributes to higher functions during development: evidence from a series of children surgically treated for posterior fossa tumours. *Brain* 123, 1051–61.

Schatz, J., Hale, S. and Myerson, J. (1998). Cerebellar contribution to linguistic processing efficiency revealed by focal damage. *Journal of the International Neuropsychological Society* 4, 491–501.

Schlosser, R., Hutchinson, M., Joseffer, S., Rusinek, H., Saarimak, A. *et al.* (1998). Functional magnetic resonance imaging of human brain activity in a verbal fluency task. *Journal of Neurology, Neurosurgery and Psychiatry* 64, 492–8.

Schmahmann, J.D. (1991). An emerging concept: the cerebellar contribution to higher function. *Archives of Neurology* 48, 1178–87.

Schmahmann, J.D. (1996). From movement to thought: anatomic substrates of the cerebellar contribution to cognitive processing. *Human Brain Mapping* 4, 174–98.

Schmahmann, J.D. (1998). Ataxia of thought: clinical consequences of cerebellar dysfunction on cognition and affect. *Trends in Cognitive Sciences* 2, 362–71.

Schmahmann, J.D. and Pandya, D.N. (1997). The cerebro-cerebellar system. *International Review of Neurobiology* 41, 31–60.

Schmahmann, J.D. and Sherman, J.C. (1998). The cerebellar cognitive affective syndrome. *Brain* 121, 561–79.

Scott, R.B., Stoodley, C.J., Anslow, P., Paul, C., Stein, J.F. *et al.* (2001). Lateralized cognitive deficits in children following cerebellar lesions. *Developmental Medicine and Child Neurology* 43, 685–91.

Shulman, G.L., Corbetta, M., Buckner, R.L., Fiez, J.A., Miezin, F.M. *et al.* (1997). Common blood flow changes across visual tasks: I. Increases in subcortical structures and cerebellum but not in visual cortex. *Journal of Cognitive Neuroscience* 9(5), 624–47.

Silveri, M.C. and Misciagna, S. (2000). Language, memory and the cerebellum. *Journal of Neurolinguistics* 13(2–3), 129–43.

Silveri, M.C., Leggio, M.G. and Molinari, M. (1994). The cerebellum contributes to linguistic production: a case of agrammatic speech following a right cerebellar lesion. *Neurology* 44, 2047–50.

Sönmezoglu, K., Sperling, B., Henriksen, T., Tfelt-Hansen, P. and Lassen, N.A. (1993). Reduced contralateral hemispheric flow measured by SPECT in cerebellar lesions. Crossed cerebral diaschisis. *Acta Neurologica Scandinavia* 87, 275–80.

Steinlin, M., Styger, M. and Boltshauser, E. (1999). Cognitive impairments in patients with congenital nonprogressive cerebellar ataxia. *Neurology* 53, 966–73.

Zettin, M., Cappa, S.F., D'Amico, A., Rago, R., Perino, C. *et al.* (1997). Agrammatic speech production after a right cerebellar haemorrhage. *Neurocase* 3, 375–80.

8 Degenerative subcortical syndromes: aetiology, clinical features, medical treatment and associated language disorders

Introduction

As previously outlined in Chapter 2, subcortical syndromes are typically associated with movement disorders which are classified according to a binary taxonomy of hyper- or hypokinetic subtypes. The hallmark of hyperkinetic syndromes is an excess of spontaneous movement, and in contrast, hypokinetic syndromes entail a lack of spontaneous movement. Manifestations of specific symptoms arise as a result of unique disease- or damage-driven imbalances in activity within basal ganglia circuitry (for a full description of the basal ganglia circuitry see Chapter 2). More specifically, hypokinetic symptoms typically arise as a consequence of overactive indirect pathway activity and excessive inhibitory output from the internal segment of the globus pallidus (GPi) (Valls-Sole, 2007), and include difficulty initiating and coordinating the size and speed of movements. Alternatively, hyperkinetic symptoms occur as a result of impoverished indirect pathway activity, and depleted inhibitory output from the GPi (Valls-Sole, 2007), and include chorea, tremor, dystonia, ballismus, athetosis, dyskinesia, tics and myoclonus. For the purposes of the present chapter, the ensuing discussion will focus upon the syndromes of Parkinson's disease, Huntington's disease, dystonia, essential tremor and tardive dyskinesia, given that these conditions are considered among those movement disorders more commonly encountered within the setting of clinical speech pathology.

Degenerative subcortical syndromes

Hypokinetic disorders

As mentioned above, hypokinetic syndromes arise as a result of basal ganglia dysfunction, instigated by an increase in indirect basal ganglia pathway activity and hence an increase in inhibitory output of the GPi (see Figure 10.2, p. 224). It is hypothesized that excessive GPi output results in the disproportionate inhibition of thalamocortical neurones, producing the hypokinetic symptoms common to Parkinson's disease, such as bradykinesia (i.e. slowness of movement), akinesia (i.e. difficulty initiating movement), muscle rigidity and rest tremor (DeLong, 1990).

Parkinson's disease

Parkinson's disease arises from nigrostriatal dopaminergic cell degeneration (Obeso *et al.*, 1997), which produces an activity imbalance within dopamine-regulated pathways of the basal ganglia; namely an increase in indirect pathway activity and a decrease in direct pathway activity (Wichmann and DeLong, 1998) (see Figure 10.2). Aetiological influences remain undetermined but the current consensus espouses environmental influences in tandem with a genetic susceptibility as the potential underlying cause of Parkinson's disease (Guttman *et al.*, 2003).

A clinical presentation of bradykinesia plus one of rigidity, tremor or postural instability confirms the diagnosis of Parkinson's disease (Valls-Sole, 2007). As previously defined, bradykinesia refers to abnormal reductions in the amplitude and velocity of voluntary movement (DeLong, 1990); rigidity refers to a general increase in muscle tone, or resistance to passive movement (Adams and Jog, 2008); Parkinsonian tremor is typically present at rest; and postural instability is characterized by an unsteadiness in gait and poor balance (Adams and Jog, 2008). Parkinson's disease is also commonly associated with hypokinetic dysarthria (for a detailed description of the clinical features of hypokinetic dysarthria see Chapter 11). Non-motor symptoms including depression, cognitive decline, anxiety and sleep disorders, however, have also been commonly reported in Parkinson's disease (Braak *et al.*, 2003). As mentioned in Chapter 5 the medical management of Parkinson's disease has conventionally involved the administration of dopamine-replacement (e.g. levodopa) and dopamine-enhancement (e.g. dopamine receptor agonists) drug therapies (Schapira, 2005), with the modulation of depleted dopamine stores producing an improvement in motor function, at least for the short term. Recognized limitations in relation to dopaminergic pharmacotherapy, such as the development of dyskinesias and on/off states, however, prompted the recent re-evaluation and more general application of neurosurgical techniques such as pallidotomy, thalamotomy and deep-brain stimulation to treat the Parkinsonian symptom complex (Obeso *et al.*, 1997) (see Chapters 5 and 6 for a more detailed discussion of surgical techniques).

Hyperkinetic disorders

In concert with hypokinetic syndromes, hyperkinetic syndromes also arise as a result of basal ganglia dysfunction, but are generally instigated by a decrease in indirect basal ganglia pathway activity and hence a decrease in inhibitory output of the GPi (see Figure 10.3, p. 226). It is hypothesized that reduced GPi output results in the disproportionate disinhibition of thalamocortical neurones, producing hyperkinetic symptoms such as choreic movements (i.e. irregular/jerky movements of the face and/or extremities), tremor (i.e. rhythmic movement of hands, limbs, head or articulators), dystonia (i.e. sustained muscle contractions involving twisting or repetitive movements) or dyskinesia (i.e. involuntary movements of articulators, trunk and/or extremities).

Huntington's disease

Huntington's disease is an autosomal dominant neurodegenerative genetic condition which causes pathological changes in the striatum (in particular, head of the caudate nucleus) (Martin and Gusella, 1986), namely the loss of γ-aminobutyric acid (GABA) neurones (Albin *et al.*, 1989). In relation to basal ganglia circuitry, the preferential loss of GABAergic striatal neurones in the indirect pathway (Hedreen and Folstein, 1995) results in the disinhibition of inhibitory GPe projections to the subthalamic nucleus, and consequently reduced inhibitory output from the GPi-substantia nigra pars reticulata (SNr) and superfluous excitation of thalamocortical projection neurones (DeLong, 1990) (see Figure 10.3). Clinical symptoms typically present after 30 years of age and characteristically include choreic body movements (i.e. involuntary writhing movements), which may produce flow-on effects of abnormal gait, dysarthria and swallowing difficulties (Enderby, 2008). Ataxia, dystonia, bruxism, myoclonus, tics, Tourettism and Parkinsonism have also been observed in Huntington's disease, and cognitive, psychiatric and behavioural disturbances are common as well (Adam and Jankovic, 2008). Motor symptoms may be further divided into impaired accessory/ involunatry (e.g. chorea, dystonia, rigidity) and voluntary movements (e.g. speech, gait and swallowing), with evidence of a disproportionate exacerbation in voluntary versus involuntary movement impairments over the course of the disease, associated with greater levels of functional disability (Folstein, 1989).

Medical management of Huntington's disease has conventionally involved the symptomatic treatment of chorea and dystonia, with neuroleptic (e.g. haloperidol, pimozide, fluphenazine, thioridazine, sulpiride, tiapride, olanzapine) and dopamine-depleting (e.g. tetrabenazine) medications (Jankovic, 2006a; Bonelli and Hoffman, 2007). Of particular note, it has been observed that effective antichoreic medications may exacerbate voluntary movement impairments such as speech and/or swallowing (Bonelli et al., 2003), with evident implications for management of speech pathology. (For a detailed description of the effects of Huntington's disease on motor speech function see Chapter 11.)

Essential tremor

Essential tremor has been described as the most prevalent of all movement disorders (Duffy, 1995). Essential tremor is typically characterized by the presentation of a bilateral, symmetric postural (i.e. against gravity) tremor within the upper limbs, made worse by voluntary movement or upon reaching a movement target (Deuschl et al., 1998). The tremor has also been documented to ascend to the head and articulators (Evidente, 2000). Isolated tremors of certain body parts, including vocal tremor, may be diagnosed as essential tremor by some experts (Evidente, 2000). Symptoms are usually exacerbated by fatigue, excitement, anxiety, hunger, temperature extremes (Singer et al., 1994) and certain drugs (e.g. nicotine, caffeine, psychostimulants) (Evidente, 2000), and alleviated by alcohol consumption (Charles et al., 1999).

Essential tremor may be of idiopathic or familial origin, with estimated prevalence rates of equal proportion in each subgroup (Duffy, 1995). Onset is most common in the second and sixth decades of life (Charles et al., 1999), and progression is typically protracted (Evidente, 2000). Familial and idiopathic essential tremor have been described as indistinguishable, although the familial subtype is generally associated with an earlier age at onset (Evidente, 2000). Familial essential tremor has been identified as an autosomal dominant genetic disorder with variable penetrance (Evidente, 2000). A functional disturbance of the oliviocerebellar circuit provides the hypothetical pathophysiological substrate for essential tremor (Deuschl and Bergman, 2002), supported by observations of tremor eradication following lesions of the cerebellum (Dupuis et al., 1989), pons (Nagaratnam and Kalasabail, 1997) or thalamus (Duncan et al., 1988); as well as evidence of increased PET activity within the cerebellum, red nucleus, thalamus and inferior olives in essential tremor patients (Deuschl et al., 1998).

Pharmacotherapeutics provide the primary treatment regimen for essential tremor. A range of antitremor agents have been shown to be effective (Evidente, 2000), including β-blockers (e.g. propanolol, metropolol, nodolol), anticonvulsants (e.g. primidone), benzodiazepines (e.g. diazepam, clonazepam, alprazolam), carbonic anhydrase inhibitors, particularly methazolamide in the case of head and voice tremor (Muenter *et al.*, 1991), and botulinum toxin injections, again, particularly in the case of hand, voice and head involvement (Wasielewski *et al.*, 1998). Similarly to Parkinson's disease, however, in the case of drug-resistant or severe essential tremor, thalamotomy or thalamic deep-brain stimulation have been reported to successfully alleviate tremor (Schuurman *et al.*, 2000). The effect of essential tremor on speech production is described and discussed in Chapter 11.

Dystonia

Dystonia is a hyperkinetic disorder affecting movement control which typically manifests as twisting movements and/or abnormalities in posture as a result of involuntary contractions of muscles (Fahn, 1988). Dystonia may involve extremity, axial or branchial musculature (Albin *et al.*, 1989), and is generally classified as either a primary or secondary subtype. Primary dystonia occurs spontaneously in the absence of any known cause, and with the exception of tremor and myoclonus is not associated with any other neurological symptoms (Fahn, 1988). The primary subtype is more commonly associated with a genetic component and symptoms generally demonstrate a progressive course over time (Fahn, 1988). Genetic inheritance is autosomal dominant with reduced penetrance, suggesting that additional genetic and environmental factors may be necessary for the development of this condition (Geyer and Bressman, 2006). Late-onset as opposed to early-onset primary dystonias are most common, and are more focal in nature, such as blephorospasm, oromandibular dystonia, cervical dystonia, hand dystonia and spastic dysphonia (i.e. laryngeal dystonia) (Fahn, 1988). In contrast, secondary dystonias usually develop as a result of neurological disease or brain injury (Geyer and Bressman, 2006), and are commonly associated with conditions such as Huntington's disease, juvenile Parkinson's disease, cortical atrophy, Wilson's disease and Rett syndrome (Fahn, 1988), the use of certain medications (e.g. neuroleptics), toxicity (e.g. wasp sting, carbon monoxide poisoning) and brain damage attributed to vascular or traumatic injury, viral infection and demyelination (Geyer and Bressman, 2006). Secondary dystonias have been informative in relation to determining the neurophysiological substrates of dystonia in general. For example, basal ganglia injury typically produces dystonia; however, damage to the thalamus, cerebellum, brainstem and parietal lobe may also produce dystonic symptoms (Geyer and Bressman, 2006). In relation to motor circuitry, dystonia has been likened to Parkinson's disease with evidence of excessive indirect pathway activity, yet differs in that direct pathway activity is also excessive, producing an overall reduction in GPi output (Starr *et al.*, 2005) (see Figure 10.4, p. 227).

Medical management of dystonia typically involves the administration of dopaminergic, anticholinergic and GABA agonist medications (Jankovic, 2006b) which alter GABA-mediated inhibition, and dopaminergic and muscarinic cholinergic neurotransmission within dystonic brains (Breakefield *et al.*, 2008). In addition, intramuscular injections of botulinum toxin within effected muscles may also provide relief in more focal cases by blocking the release of acetylcholine from motor neurones, thereby reducing excessive muscle activity (Breakefield *et al.*, 2008). Similarly to Parkinson's disease, deep-brain stimulation of the GPi, providing functional manipulation of dystonic motor circuits, has also been successful in alleviating some cases of dystonia

(Breakefield *et al.*, 2008). A description of the effects of dystonia on motor speech function is presented in Chapter 11.

Dyskinesia

Dyskinesias constitute a fourth category of hyperkinetic movement disorders that typically arise following the use of dopaminergic replacement or antipsychotic medications. Dyskinesias represent abnormal involuntary motor acts that may involve repetitive twisting, writhing, extension or flexion movements, with or without the presence of tremor (Murdoch, 1990). Indeed, levodopa-induced dyskinesias as a consequence of dopamine excess are common in Parkinsonian patients (DeLong, 1990) and typically entail choreic movements of the trunk, neck and face; dystonia; blepharospasm; and/or repetitive movements of the limbs (Luquin *et al.*, 1992). In relation to basal ganglia circuitry, excessive dopamine-driven inhibition of GABAergic striatal neurones constituting the indirect pathway and stimulation of GABAergic neurones innervating the direct pathway leads to a net reduction in inhibitory GPi output, and the subsequent overactivation of motor cortical regions via excitatory thalamocortical projections (DeLong, 1990) (See Figure 10.5, p. 228).

Perhaps of most interest to the speech pathologist, however, is the condition known as tardive dyskinesia. Associated with a history of neuroleptic (i.e. antipsychotic) drug use, patients with tardive dyskinesia generally present with involuntary movements of the orofacial musculature, including the tongue, lips, palate, mandible, pharynx and face (Drummond, 2008). Commonly observed symptoms include facial tics, tongue and lip smacking, as well as eye blinking (Drummond, 2008). Tardive dyskinesia has also been described as buccolingual-masticatory syndrome, but may also be associated with limb dyskinesia, rest tremor, chorea and myoclonus (Drummond, 2008). Akin to levodopa-induced dyskinesias, tardive dyskinesia arises as a result of increased dopaminergic, as well as noradrenergic activity within the striatum (Drummond, 2008).

In relation to medical management, the subcutaneous injections of botulinum toxin into effected facial muscles has been successful in relieving the associated dystonia (Drummond, 2008), yet the greatest improvements in speech symptoms have been identified upon the termination of antipsychotic treatment (Drummond and Fitzpatrick, 2004). (For a description of the effects of tardive dyskinesia on speech see Chapter 11.)

Language disorders in Parkinson's disease

As outlined above, Parkinson's disease is a progressive, degenerative neurological condition resulting from nigrostriatal dopamine depletion and characterized primarily by motor symptoms such as tremor, bradykinesia, rigidity and postural instability. When James Parkinson first described Parkinsonism in 1817, he claimed that there were no mental manifestations of the disease. Today, however, it is widely acknowledged that even in the absence of global intellectual decline or dementia, some individuals with Parkinson's disease will experience subtle deficits in a range of cognitive domains including memory, visuospatial abilities, executive planning, attention and language function (Cooper *et al.*, 1991; Dubois *et al.*, 1991; Levin and Katzen, 1995).

Support for the proposal that language may be compromised in Parkinson's disease comes from distributed processing models of neural function as well as proposals that implicate subcortical structures in both cognitive and linguistic functions (for models of subcortical participation in language see Chapter 3). Whereas the potential role of dopamine as an important neuroregulator of cognitive functioning has been recognized (Nieoullon, 2002), disruption to the functioning of the striatum and the dopamine connections to the frontal lobes may also be expected to influence cognitive functioning. Consistent with this proposal, it has been suggested that cognitive deficits in Parkinson's disease may be consistent with a disturbance in frontostriatal function (Bondi *et al.*, 1993). Accordingly, given the role of dopamine and the striatum in cognitive function, it is highly likely that language function is also impaired in Parkinson's disease. Indeed, there have been some isolated reports of abnormal performance by persons with Parkinson's disease on language tasks such as naming, sentence repetition and auditory comprehension (Cummings *et al.*, 1988; Beatty and Monson, 1989; Blonder *et al.*, 1989; Lewis *et al.*, 1998).

Early investigations of language disorders in Parkinson's disease

Of all the cognitive domains, language deficits remain the most controversial and the least well defined in Parkinson's disease. Comprehensive investigations of language function in Parkinson's disease are limited. More common are studies that have focused on the impact of Parkinson's disease on specific aspects of language performance, such as sentence comprehension and verbal fluency. Early investigations of language functioning reported equivocal results of language assessment in Parkinson's disease. Studies of single-word use and sentence processing based on traditional aphasiologic measures at times described mild deficits (Cummings *et al.*, 1988; Geyer and Grossman, 1994). Confrontation naming difficulties and compromised category-naming fluency have been reported by some investigators (Matison *et al.*, 1982; Cooper *et al.*, 1991; Auriacombe *et al.*, 1993). Even in the absence of dementia, persons with Parkinson's disease exhibit subtle difficulties in processing semantic language, as shown by impaired performance on off-line tests of verbal fluency and naming (Beatty and Monson, 1989; Blonder *et al.*, 1989; Raskin *et al.*, 1992; Bayles *et al.*, 1993; Frank *et al.*, 1996).

Lewis *et al.* (1998) identified subtle language impairments across a range of complex linguistic functions in a group of 20 subjects with idiopathic Parkinson's disease on a battery of measures selected to be sensitive to frontal lobe language function. More specifically, as a group the Parkinsonian group examined by Lewis *et al.* (1998) presented with impaired naming and definitional abilities and difficulties in interpreting ambiguity and figurative language. Further, Lewis *et al.* (1998) reported that, when the subjects with Parkinson's disease were divided into groups based on their score on a cognitive rating scale, those individuals with below-normal cognitive status presented with a larger range of language impairments than those persons with normal cognitive status. The former group presented with deficits in naming, definition and multi-definition abilities, as well as problems in interpreting ambiguity and figurative language, sentence construction and semantic verbal fluency. In contrast, the subjects with Parkinson's disease and normal cognitive status presented with problems in providing definitions and in sentence construction alone. Based on their findings, Lewis *et al.*, (1998) concluded that the difficulties inherent in idiopathic Parkinson's disease go well beyond the motoric sphere that affects ambulation and motor speech production.

Individuals with Parkinson's disease are, in general, able to perform basic receptive and expressive language functions such as the recognition and repetition of single words and simple sentences, and the naming of common objects, in a normal manner.

However, language deficits are frequently observed on those tasks that place increasing demands on both the semantic and the syntactic subcomponents of the linguistic system. Indeed, researchers have demonstrated that the integrity of semantic processing may be compromised in Parkinson's disease (Bayles *et al.*, 1993; Randolph *et al.*, 1993). As previously mentioned, there is considerable evidence to suggest that verbal fluency and complex sentence comprehension is impaired in Parkinson's disease (Grossman, 1999; Gurd *et al.*, 2001). A number of researchers have reported reductions in the grammatical complexity and informative content of the sentences and discourse produced by non-demented persons with Parkinson's disease (Cummings *et al.*, 1988; Illes *et al.*, 1988; Murray, 1998). In addition, Parkinson's disease-related performance decrements have been identified on tasks of verbal and semantic reasoning (Bayles, 1990; Cohen *et al.*, 1994; Lewis *et al.*, 1998; Portin *et al.*, 2000).

Relationship between language impairment and cognitive status in Parkinson's disease

The relationship between language impairment and cognitive status in Parkinson's disease has been explored by a relatively small number of researchers. In general their results indicate that the deficits exhibited by non-demented persons with Parkinson's disease on cognitively demanding language-oriented tasks may be linked to mild reductions in cognitive status (Lewis *et al.*, 1998). Generally, however, reductions in cognitive status appear to be associated with more severe decrements that occur over a greater range of language-based tasks (Bayles, 1990; Bayles *et al.*, 1997; Lewis *et al.*, 1998). For example, as outlined above, Lewis *et al.* (1998) found that their patients with Parkinson's disease with reduced cognitive status exhibited worse performance than both their group of subjects with Parkinson's disease with normal cognitive status and their control group across a wide range of tasks that included the Boston Naming Test, the definitions and multiple contexts subtests of the Test of Word Knowledge, and the ambiguous sentences, recreating sentences and figurative language subtests of the Test of Language Competence-Expanded edition.

Based on the observations that Parkinson's disease is associated with a wide range of non-linguistic cognitive deficits and that the language-based tasks on which persons with Parkinson's disease exhibit impairments have a significant non-linguistic processing component, Bayles (1990) suggested that what appears as a language problem may, in fact, be the result of dysfunction in domains such as memory, attention or executive function. Accordingly, the author reasoned, the part played by non-linguistic cognitive deficits in impaired performance on language-based tasks must be evaluated before it can be concluded that Parkinson's disease impacts on linguistic dysfunction. As demonstrated by two studies undertaken by Bayles and colleagues, however, isolating the purely linguistic components of off-line language performance is not straightforward.

In the first of these studies, Bayles (1990) assessed a group of non-demented persons with Parkinson's disease on a range of language-based tasks including receptive vocabulary, object description, similarities and story retelling. To provide a measure of non-linguistic cognitive impairment, participants also completed a test of visuospatial construction, namely the block design subtest of the Wechsler Adult Intelligence Scale. The results of the language battery indicated that the performance of the Parkinson's disease group differed from that of their control counterparts only with respect to the test of similarities. After controlling the effects of non-linguistic cognitive deficits, however, the significance of the group difference was reduced to being 'borderline' (Bayles, 1990, p. 177).

Whereas the findings of Bayles (1990) tended to suggest a specific role for linguistic dysfunction in the abnormal performance exhibited by persons with Parkinson's disease on language-based tasks, the author advised a cautious approach. Bayles observed that group differences were only borderline and perhaps would have been eliminated entirely if control measures had been employed for deficits in non-linguistic cognitive domains that were not assessed by the block design subtest. Alternatively, as virtually all non-linguistic assessments involve some aspect of verbal performance, by controlling for block design performance, the effects of legitimate linguistic deficits may have been masked. Accordingly, the results were interpreted as being indicative of the intricate and complex relationship between language dysfunction and cognitive impairments in Parkinson's disease.

More recently, Bayles *et al.* (1997) evaluated 'linguistic competence', or the knowledge of linguistic rules, and 'linguistic performance', or the ability to use linguistic knowledge to communicate. Tasks used to evaluate linguistic competence involved the judgement and correction of semantically anomalous and ungrammatical sentences. Language performance, on the other hand, was assessed using more basic language-based tasks such as confrontation naming, repetition and reading. The authors reasoned that a linguistic competence deficit would reflect specific linguistic dysfunction. A linguistic performance deficit, on the other hand, would reflect cognitive resource limitations. The study's participants with Parkinson's disease exhibited impairments on only one experimental task, namely the linguistic performance task of verbal fluency. Based on these findings, Bayles and colleagues concluded that language decrements in Parkinson's disease occur on tasks that require greater cognitive effect and as such, are representative of performance deficits rather than impaired linguistic knowledge.

An examination of the test battery of Bayles *et al.* (1997) suggests, however, that the tasks employed to assess linguistic competence were just as cognitively demanding as those designed to assess linguistic performance. That is, competence and performance tasks alike required the conscious manipulation of semantic and syntactic information. The successful completion of both types of task relied, therefore, on linguistic and non-linguistic performance factors. Hence, it is proposed that, rather than isolating and evaluating linguistic knowledge in Parkinson's disease-related verbal fluency deficits, they do not allow any strong claims to be made regarding the effects of Parkinson's disease on linguistic dysfunction.

Semantic priming experiments in Parkinson's disease

As discussed previously, earlier investigations into the integrity of lexical-semantic processes in Parkinson's disease were largely directed at measures of language processes, such as verbal fluency paradigms. A more recent and significant advancement in the investigation into the semantic deficits reported in association with Parkinson's disease has emerged through the application of on-line semantic priming procedures to the investigation of the processing components underlying semantic deficits in Parkinson's disease. In a semantic priming procedure, word/non-word judgements are made on target stimuli which are usually preceded by a semantically related or semantically unrelated prime word. Semantic priming is said to occur when participant responses to real-word targets are faster for related word pairs (e.g. *cat, dog*) as opposed to unrelated conditions (e.g. *cat, book*). A generally accepted theory postulates that during a semantic priming task the presentation of the prime causes an automatic spreading of activation, which partially activates other related concepts, thereby speeding lexical decisions to semantically related target words (Collins and Loftus, 1974). Thus, by manipulating the stimulus-onset asynchrony (SOA) (i.e. the time lapse between presentation of the prime and target), the time course over which automatic semantic activation occurs can be estimated. It is also important to note that attentional or controlled processes can induce semantic priming effects, but these processes typically emerge when longer SOAs are used and when the proportion of related word pairs is high (Neely, 1991). Certainly, disruptions to fast-acting/automatic as opposed to controlled semantic processing may be most expected in Parkinson's disease, as it is proposed that dopamine and the striatum have a substantial influence on the integrity and speed of information processing.

Investigations into semantic priming effects in Parkinson's disease first emerged over a decade ago. In the earliest semantic priming investigation undertaken in Parkinson's disease, Hines and Volpe (1985) reported normal semantic priming effects for non-demented persons with Parkinson's disease at 500 ms SOA and concluded that the automatic access of semantic information is unimpaired in Parkinson's disease. More recently, Spicer *et al.*, (1994) used a variant of Neely's (1977) instructional manipulation procedures to dissociate the automatic and controlled aspects of semantic activation. They identified the presence of 'hyperpriming', or an abnormally large degree of facilitation, in patients with Parkinson's disease, at SOAs of 300, 600 and 900 ms. Spicer *et al.* (1994) concluded that the automatic aspects of semantic activation were unaffected by Parkinson's disease. Although unable to provide supportive evidence, they proposed that hyperpriming could be explained by the fact that patients with Parkinson's disease have difficulty retrieving information from semantic memory, and, as a consequence benefit more from semantic cues (such as the prime) than controls. Consequently, patients with Parkinson's disease show hyperpriming because they are slower (because of their semantic deficit) than controls in unrelated trials, and their attention to the prime word produced larger benefits in the related trials.

Later, in a study designed to further explore the origin of hyperpriming in Parkinson's disease, McDonald *et al.* (1996) adopted Spicer *et al.*'s (1994) variant of Neely's (1977) paradigm. Unlike Spicer *et al.*, however, McDonald and colleagues included only one short 300 ms SOA in their experimental procedures. Twenty-eight medicated persons with Parkinson's disease participated in the study. As in Spicer *et al.*'s study, Parkinson's disease-related hyperpriming was identified. McDonald *et al.* (1996) reiterated Spicer and colleagues' earlier claims regarding the robustness of automatic semantic activation in Parkinson's disease and proposed that observed hyperpriming in Parkinson's disease was related to problems shifting the cognitive set in the neutral condition. Specifically, McDonald *et al.* (1996) and later Brown *et al.* (1999) argued that target stimuli that were preceded by the neutral prime 'blank' were drawn from a wider range of semantic categories than target stimuli that followed category word primes. The researchers contended that their participants with Parkinson's disease experienced difficulties shifting the cognitive set from post-lexical semantic matching strategies in category word prime conditions to strategies suitable for accessing words in the absence of semantic context; that is, in the neutral condition. Accordingly, it was claimed that persons with Parkinson's disease exhibited selective slowing in the neutral or baseline condition, which in turn, led to inflated measures of facilitation (hyperpriming).

In reviewing semantic priming in Parkinson's disease, Arnott and Chenery (1999, 2001) highlighted key differences between the actual priming effects exhibited by Spicer *et al.*'s (1994) and McDonald *et al.*'s (1996) control participants and those predicted by the model of information processing (Posner and Snyder, 1975) upon which Neely's (1977) original paradigm had been based. They argued that the controls' results suggested that key changes to Neely's original paradigm had resulted in multiple processing mechanisms being evoked. Arnott and Chenery (1999, 2001) concluded that hyperpriming in Parkinson's disease may be the result of subtle deficiencies in a number of processes but there remained insufficient evidence to determine which mechanism (or mechanisms) was impaired. More recently, Mari-Beffa *et al.* (2005) provided evidence to support the view that the hyperpriming effect typically shown by persons with Parkinson's disease is the result of impaired inhibitory processes required to control word activation during reading.

Aspects of the experimental methodologies employed in the semantic priming studies outlined above suggest that each was biased towards being an assessment of attentional processing routines (i.e. these studies focused only on the manner in which semantic information is accessed). Further, by employing experimental methodologies that actively encourage the involvement of conscious processing, it has been suggested that the various researchers failed to address the more automatic aspects of lexical access (i.e. to determine the impact of Parkinson's disease on the lexical access stage of language processing) (Arnott and Chenery, 1999, 2001). Milberg *et al.* (1999) demonstrated the need for researchers in brain injury to examine the temporal aspects of semantic activation. In an attempt to remediate this situation, Arnott *et al.* (2001) directly investigated the automatic and controlled mechanisms of semantic priming and explored the time course of semantic priming in Parkinson's disease. Participants with Parkinson's disease presented with delayed time course of semantic activation during automatic (short SOA) semantic priming and impaired inhibitory processes when controlled semantic priming was elicited. Differing patterns of semantic priming as a function of SOA in participants with Parkinson's disease have also been reported in semantic priming paradigms measuring ambiguity priming (Copland, 2003) and semantic priming via multi-priming paradigms (Angwin *et al.*, 2003, 2005).

Dopamine and language impairment in Parkinson's disease

Over the past decade, traditional views of dopamine as an excitatory/inhibitory neurotransmitter have been revised. It is now thought that, in addition to its role as a neurotransmitter, dopamine acts as a non-specific neuromodulator. According to Cepeda and Levine (1998), a neuromodulator is ineffective alone but, when used with other substances, such as glutamate and GABA, is able to alter the actions of the substances to produce normal brain function. Neuromodulators, therefore, allow neurotransmitter systems to function in a normal manner.

Dopaminergic innervation of the cerebral cortex is widespread (Agid *et al.*, 1987; Previc, 1999). The basal ganglia system is linked to frontal areas by five circuits, namely the motor, oculomotor, dorsolateral prefrontal, orbitofrontal and anterior cingulate loops (Chow and Cummings, 1998). In addition, via mesocortical pathways, dopaminergic neurones project directly from the ventral tegmental area to much of the prefrontal cortex. Both the dorsolateral prefrontal circuit, sometimes called the complex loop, and the mesocortical pathway have been associated with cognitive function (Delis and Massman, 1992; Chow and Cummings, 1998). In particular, the prefrontal cortex is purported to be responsible for the integration of semantic memory function (Gabrieli *et al.*, 1998). Indeed Previc (1999) has proposed an integral role for dopamine in language processing.

The degeneration of midbrain dopaminergic neurones in Parkinson's disease causes massive depletion of neural dopamine. It has been estimated that by the time the motor symptoms of Parkinson's disease become apparent, dopamine concentrations are reduced by approximately 80% in the striatum and 40–60% in the ventral tegmentum (Agid *et al.*, 1987; Jellinger, 1991). Given that drug treatment acts to restore the dopamine levels of persons with Parkinson's disease and that, via the nigrostriatal and mesocortical dopaminergic systems, dopamine has recently been linked with the processing of both the semantic and syntactic aspects of language (Kischka *et al.*, 1996; Ullman *et al.*, 1997), biochemical changes to dopaminergic neurotransmitter systems may indeed represent the neuropathological basis for language decrements in Parkinson's disease.

With respect to the precise mechanisms by which dopamine availability may influence language processing in Parkinson's disease, it has been proposed that the function of dopaminergic modulating systems is to dampen weak signals (noise) while at the same time amplifying stronger signals (excitatory or inhibitory) in neural areas (Servan-Shreiber *et al.*, 1990) (i.e. in its role as a neuromodulator, dopamine regulates neural signal-to-noise ratios). Furthermore, Cepeda and Levine (1998) suggested that dopamine is able to increase the signal-to-noise ratio in the neostriatum by integrating relevant information and screening out less relevant information. It could be expected, therefore, that changes to dopaminergic functioning would change the signal-to-noise of information processing and subsequently influence language function.

The findings of semantic priming studies suggesting that dopamine may have a neuromodulatory influence on semantic processing are supportive of this argument. Several researchers have attributed aberrant lexical-semantic processing in Parkinson's disease to the neuromodulatory influence of dopamine depletion, resulting in a decreased signal-to-noise ratio in semantic networks or altering the time course of semantic processing (Kischka *et al.*, 1996; Arnott *et al.*, 2001; Angwin *et al.*, 2004). Kischka *et al.* (1996) examined the influence of dopamine on semantic activation by administering levodopa to healthy young adults. The results led the researchers to suggest that dopamine may modulate automatic semantic activation by increasing the signal-to-noise ratio in semantic networks. In considering the neuroanatomical/neurophysiological bases for their results, Kischka *et al.* (1996) proposed that dopaminergic projections arising from the ventral tegmental area and terminating in the prefrontal cortex modulate signal-to-noise ratios in semantic memory systems by either dampening background noise or enhancing excitatory or inhibitory signals. This increase in signal-to-noise ratio leads to a more focused activation of semantic concepts. Hence, increased dopaminergic activity results in decreased spreading activation.

Similar research by Angwin *et al.* (2004) also aimed to examine the influence of dopamine on the time course of semantic activation. The results revealed an earlier onset and decay of semantic activation in participants who had ingested levodopa, as measured by tests of direct (e.g. *tiger, stripes*) and indirect (e.g. *lion, stripes*) priming. On the basis of their findings, Angwin *et al.* (2004) suggested that dopamine may influence the time course of semantic processing. In a similar way, researchers have also suggested that the striatum is a key area of the brain that may support information processing speed (Harrington *et al.*, 1998; Poldrack *et al.*, 2001). Thus there is converging evidence to suggest that both dopamine and the striatum influence the speed of information processing, which may subsequently affect language function.

Summary of language disorders in Parkinson's disease

Evidence is available to show that some non-demented persons with Parkinson's disease exhibit impaired performance on more cognitively demanding assessments of language function such as verbal fluency, sentence comprehension and verbal reasoning. Further, these impairments reflect abnormalities in the use of both semantic and syntactic linguistic knowledge and may be exacerbated by mild reductions in cognitive status. Although some language difficulty is evident, however, patients with Parkinson's disease do not exhibit a language disorder that resembles one of the classic aphasia syndromes seen after stroke. Over the past decade a limited number of studies based on on-line semantic priming tasks have demonstrated the presence of impaired lexical-semantic processing in individuals with Parkinson's disease possibly resulting from disruption to the neuromodulatory role of dopamine as an outcome of neural dopamine depletion. Collectively these findings suggest that enlightened clinical management of individuals with Parkinson's disease should include an awareness, a sensitivity and perhaps an appropriate clinical intervention plan for the cognitive linguistic deficits that these individuals are likely to present.

Language disorders in Huntington's disease

As indicated previously, Huntington's disease is an autosomal dominant, neurodegenerative disorder associated with neuropathological changes that are most marked in the head of the caudate nucleus, and to a lesser extent the putamen and globus pallidus (Zakzanis, 1998), suggesting that at least part of any language impairments found in patients with this condition may result from non-thalamic subcortical pathology. The cause of the language impairment in Huntington's disease, however, has been a point of contention (Podoll et al., 1988; Wallesch and Fehrenbach, 1988). Specifically it has been suggested that language deficits in Huntington's disease are the result of the general cognitive impairment and/or dementia associated with the disease and it has been questioned whether the language disturbances in Huntington's disease are a consequence of damage to the subcortical structures. At a cognitive level, Huntington's disease is characterized by impaired performances on tests of delayed recall, measures of memory acquisition, cognitive flexibility and abstraction, manual dexterity, attention/concentration, performance skill and verbal skill (Zakzanis, 1998). Investigations of more specific cognitive deficits that may arise in Huntington's disease have highlighted problems in areas such as:

■ spatial working memory and visual recognition and planning (Lawrence et al., 1998),
■ cognitive flexibility and complex integration (Hanes et al., 1995),
■ attentional set-maintenance and the control processes assumed to prepare or to switch cognitive 'sets' in order to perform one or another task (termed set-shifting) (Lawrence et al., 1998),
■ problems with slower thought processes (termed bradyphrenia) (Hanes et al., 1995).

In one of the earliest studies of language function in individuals with Huntington's disease, Podoll *et al.* (1988) reported a loss of conversational initiative, visual confrontation naming deficits that were closely related to visual misperception of the picture, and reduced syntactic structure of spontaneous speech. Difficulties in reading aloud and dysgraphia were also prominent features exhibited by the subjects with Huntington's disease, but were suggested to be a consequence of dysarthria and choreiform movement disorder. Podoll *et al.* (1988) concluded that 'there are no primary language changes in Huntington's disease, [but rather] a variety of language impairments develop secondary to other neurological and neuropsychological changes' (p. 1475). Further to this, it has been suggested that the syntactic deficits observed in spontaneous speech and comprehension, along with poorer naming scores, are the result of the dementia associated with Huntington's disease (Wallesch and Fehrenbech, 1988). These results contrasted with those of an earlier study reported by Caine *et al.* (1986) who ensured that none of their subjects with Huntington's disease included in their study was pervasively demented. These latter authors reported a pattern of defective naming, impaired repetition and decreased language output in written narratives by patients with Huntington's disease who were very early in the course of their illness, and suggested that a subtle but 'definite language dysfunction' (Caine *et al.*, 1986, p. 253) appears during the earliest stage of the disease.

Recent language investigations have tended to focus on circumscribed aspects of linguistic function, particularly lexical-semantic functioning, with few studies attempting comprehensively to profile the spared and disturbed language function in people with Huntington's disease. Barr and Brandt (1996) investigated word-list generation using both initial-letter and category cues and reported that subjects with Huntington's disease with more severe impairment (as determined by scores on the Quantified Neurological Examination; Folstein *et al.*, 1983), exhibited greater impairment on semantic rather than phonemic generation tasks. These authors raised the possibility that a disturbance in the organization of semantic memory may occur early in the course of Huntington's disease but that increasing disease severity and associated greater generalized retrieval difficulties may obscure this specific semantic impairment. In contrast, Hodges *et al.* (1991) found no evidence to support a semantic basis to the naming deficit they observed in individuals with Huntington's disease on the basis of a confrontation naming task. Rather, visuoperceptual and visuospatial deficits were thought to contribute to the higher proportion of visually based errors by the subjects with Huntington's disease.

An important factor to be considered in determination of the possible causes of language disorders associated with Huntington's disease is whether the language changes observed form a pattern of deficits consistent with subcortical pathology. As stated previously, the neuropathological changes in Huntington's disease are most marked in the head of the caudate nucleus and, to a lesser extent, the putamen and globus pallidus, suggesting that the language changes found in people with Huntington's disease may share some features with those observed in people with lesions to the striatum resulting from subcortical stroke. As individuals with acute vascular lesions in the striatum are assumed to not have dementia, any similarities between the language impairments observed in these latter cases and persons with Huntington's disease are, therefore, more likely to arise from a common dysfunction in subcortico-frontal language mechanisms.

Although it is now accepted that language impairment can result from damage to the striatocapsular region of the brain, the means by which this language dysfunction occurs continues to be debated (Mega and Alexander, 1994; Crosson *et al.*, 1997;

Wallesch, 1997). The present literature does not reveal a clear, coherent pattern of symptoms resulting from striatocapsular lesions of vascular origin; rather it documents a wide range of types and severities of language impairments (Crosson, 1992; Kennedy and Murdoch, 1993; Nadeau and Crosson, 1997), including impairments in, for example, auditory comprehension (D'Esposito and Alexander, 1995), lexical-semantic processing (Vallar *et al.*, 1988) and complex language tasks (Copland *et al.*, 2000). The core language profile of patients with striatocapsular infarction was described by Mega and Alexander (1994) as including deficits in executive language functions such as word fluency, sentence generation and discourse compared with relatively spared responsive language, namely comprehension, repetition and, in some milder cases, naming. (For a full description of language disorders associated with striatocapsular lesions see Chapter 4.)

To test the hypothesis that a signature profile of impaired language functions is found in patients with either focally induced or degenerative lesions in striatocapsular structures, Chenery *et al.* (2002) compared the language profiles of a group of patients with Huntington's disease with those of a group of persons with striatocapsular lesions due to cerebrovascular accidents. Both groups of subjects were administered a comprehensive battery of standardized language tests that assessed both primary and more complex language abilities. They reported that patients with Huntington's disease exhibited deficits on complex language tasks primarily involving lexico-semantic operations, on both single-word and sentence-level generative tasks, and on tasks which required interpretation of ambiguous, figurative and inferential meaning. Further, Chenery *et al.* (2002) reported that the difficulties that patients with Huntington's disease experienced with tasks assessing complex language abilities were strikingly similar, both qualitatively and quantitatively, to the language profile produced by subjects with striatocapsular vascular lesions. They concluded that their results provided evidence to suggest that a signature language profile is associated with damage to the striatocapsular region of the brain resulting from either focal neurological insult or a degenerative condition such as Huntington's disease. In a follow-up study designed to investigate the impact of subcortical disturbances on complex language-formulation tasks, Jensen *et al.* (2006) also reported that the language profiles of patients with Huntington's disease and subjects with striatocapsular lesions of vascular origin were similar in nature and severity, with the only difference being the presence of a syntactic impairment in the group with Huntington's disease. These latter authors suggested that the syntactic deficit in the patients with Huntington's disease may have reflected a compensatory syntactic strategy related to the presence of dysarthria or generalized cognitive deficits associated with Huntington's disease rather than a primary language disturbance but conceded that this explanation requires confirmation.

Summary of language disorders in Huntington's disease

Several studies have documented the presence of language impairments in patients with Huntington's disease particularly involving lexical-semantic functioning. Whether these disorders are the product of the associated general cognitive impairment or the outcome of damage to the striatocapsular subcortex, however, remains uncertain and controversial. Recent studies involving investigation of complex language tasks have demonstrated that the language profile in Huntington's disease is essentially the same as that observed in persons with striatocapsular lesions of vascular origin, suggesting that a signatory language impairment is associated with damage to the striatocapsular region of the brain irrespective of whether such damage results from acute focal lesions or degenerative conditions such as Huntington's disease.

Summary

A range of subcortical syndromes, including both hypo- and hyperkinetic movement disorders, are commonly associated with speech and/or language disorders. The more common subcortical syndromes encountered clinically by speech-language pathologists include the hypokinetic syndrome of Parkinson's disease, and the hyperkinetic syndromes of Huntington's disease, dystonia, dyskinesia and essential tremor. The aetiology, site of lesion, presenting symptomatology and medical treatment relevant to each of these conditions is outlined in this chapter.

In the past, a major argument against a role for subcortical brain structures in language processing has been an apparent lack of documented language impairments in progressive degenerative subcortical disorders such as Parkinson's disease and Huntington's disease. On the basis of reports in the literature primarily published over the last decade or so, it is now well documented that both Parkinson's disease and Huntington's disease are associated with language disorders particularly involving the more complex aspects of language function. The documented language profiles of both of these progressive degenerative subcortical conditions are described in the present chapter. Despite evidence to show that language problems do accompany both Parkinson's disease and Huntington's disease, the precise neuropathological mechanisms that underlie the occurrence of language impairments in each of these conditions remains uncertain and whether or not the observed language disorders are the outcome of the subcortical damage *per se* or the product of associated decline in general cognitive abilities remains a point of controversy.

References

Adam, O.R. and Jankovic, J. (2008). Symptomatic treatment of Huntington disease. *Neurotherapeutics: the Journal of the American Society for Experimental Neurotherapeutics* 5, 181–97.

Adams, S.G. and Jog, M. (2008). Parkinson's disease. In M.R. McNeil (ed.), *Clinical Management of Sensorimotor Speech Disorders*, 2nd edn (pp. 365–8). New York: Thieme.

Agid, Y., Javoy-Agid, F. and Ruberg, M. (1987). Biochemistry of neurotransmitters in Parkinson's disease. In C.D. Marsden and S. Fahn (eds), *Movement Disorders*, 2nd edn (pp. 166–230). London: Butterworth and Co.

Albin, R.L., Young, A.B. and Penney, J.B. (1989). The functional anatomy of basal ganglia disorders. *Trends in Neuroscience* 12, 366–75.

Angwin, A.J., Chenery, H.J., Copland, D.A., Murdoch, B.E. and Silburn, P.A. (2003). Summation of semantic priming effects in Parkinson's disease and healthy individuals. *Brain and Language* 87, 96–7.

Angwin, A.J., Chenery, H.J., Copland, D.A., Arnott, W.L., Murdoch, B.E. *et al.* (2004). Dopamine and semantic activation: an investigation of masked direct and indirect priming. *Journal of the International Neuropsychological Society* 10, 15–25.

Angwin, A.J., Chenery, H.J., Copland, D.A., Murdoch, B.E. and Silburn, P.A. (2005). Summation of semantic priming and complex sentence comprehension in Parkinson's disease. *Cognitive Brain Research* 25, 78–89.

Arnott, W.L. and Chenery, H.J. (1999). Lexical decision in Parkinson's disease: a comment on Spicer, Brown, and Gorell (1994), and McDonald, Brown and Gorell (1996). *Journal of Clinical and Experimental Neuropsychology* 21, 289–300.

Arnott, W.L. and Chenery, H.J. (2001). Lexical decision in Parkinson's disease: a reply to Brown, McDonald, and Spicer (1999). *Journal of Clinical and Experimental Neuropsychology* 23, 250–1.

Arnott, W.L., Chenery, H.J., Murdoch, B.E. and Silburn, P.A. (2001). Semantic priming in Parkinson's disease: evidence for delayed spreading activation. *Journal of Clinical and Experimental Neuropsychology* 23, 502–19.

Auriacombe, S., Grossman, M., Carvell, S., Gollomp, S., Stern, M.B. *et al.* (1993). Verbal fluency deficits in Parkinson's disease. *Neuropsychology* 7, 182–92.

Barr, A. and Brandt, J. (1996). Word-list generation deficits in dementia. *Journal of Clinical and Experimental Neuropsychology* 6, 810–22.

Bayles, K.A. (1990). Language and Parkinson's disease. *Alzheimer Disease and Associated Disorders* 4, 171–80.

Bayles, K.A., Trosset, M.W., Tomoeda, C.K., Montgomery, E.G. and Wilson, J. (1993). Generative naming in Parkinson's disease patients. *Journal of Clinical and Experimental Neuropsychology* 15, 547–62.

Bayles, K.A., Tomoeda, C.K., Wood, J.A., Montgomery, E.B., Cruz, R.F. *et al.* (1997). The effect of Parkinson's disease on language. *Journal of Medical Speech Language Pathology* 5, 157–66.

Beatty, W.W. and Monson, N. (1989). Lexical processing in Parkinson's disease and multiple sclerosis. *Journal of Geriatric Psychiatry and Neurology* 2, 145–52.

Blonder, L.X., Gur, R.E., Ruben, C.G., Saykin, A.J. and Hurtig, H.I. (1989). Neuropsychological functioning in hemiparkinsonism. *Brain and Cognition* 9, 244–57.

Bondi, M.W., Kaszniak, A.W., Bayles, K.A. and Vance, K.T. (1993). Contributions of frontal system dysfunction to memory and perceptual abilities in Parkinson's disease. *Neuropsychology* 7, 89–102.

Bonelli, R. and Hoffman, P. (2007). A systematic review of the treatment studies in Huntington's disease since 1990. *Expert Opinion in Pharmacotherapy* 8, 141–53.

Bonelli, R., Wenning, G.K. and Kapfhammer, H.P. (2003). Huntington's disease: present treatments and future therapeutic modalities. *International Clinical Psychopharmacology* 19, 51–62.

Braak, H., Del Tredici, K., Rub, U., deVos, R.A., Jansen Steur, E.N. *et al.* (2003). Staging of brain pathology related to sporadic Parkinson's disease. *Neurobiology and Aging* 24, 197–211.

Breakefield, X.O., Blood, A.J., Li, Y., Hallet, M., Hanson, P.I. and Standaert, D.G. (2008). The pathophysiological basis of dystonias. *Nature Reviews: Neuroscience* 9, 222–34.

Brown, G.G., McDonald, C. and Spicer, K. (1999). Lexical priming on Neely's (1977) paradigm in Parkinson's disease: where do we stand? *Journal of Clinical and Experimental Neuropsychology* 21, 301–11.

Caine, E.D., Bamford, K.A., Schiffer, R.B., Shoulson, I. and Levy, S. (1986). A controlled neuropsychological comparison of Huntington's disease and multiple sclerosis. *Archives of Neurology* 43, 249–54.

Cepeda, C. and Levine, M.S. (1998). Dopamine and N-Methyl-D-Asparate receptor interactions in the neostriatum. *Developmental Neuroscience* 20, 1–18.

Charles, P.D., Esper, G.J. and Davis, T.L. (1999). Classification of tremor and update on treatment. *American Family Physician* 59(6), 1565–72.

Chenery, H.J., Copland, D.A. and Murdoch, B.E. (2002). Complex language function and subcortical mechanisms: evidence from Huntington's disease and patients with non-thalamic subcortical lesions. *International Journal of Language and Communication Disorders* 37, 459–74.

Chow, T.W. and Cummings, J.L. (1998). Frontal-subcortical circuits. In B.L. Miller and J.L. Cummings (eds), *The Human Frontal Lobes: Function and Disorders* (pp. 3–26). New York: Guilford Press.

Cohen, H., Baichard, S., Scherzer, P. and Whitaker, H. (1994). Language and verbal reasoning in Parkinson's disease. *Neuropsychiatry, Neuropsychology and Behavioral Neurology* 7, 166–75.

Collins, A.M. and Loftus, E.F. (1974). A spreading activation theory of semantic processing. *Psychological Reviews* 82, 407–28.

Cooper, J.A., Sagar, H.J., Jordan, N., Harvey, N.S. and Sullivan, E.V. (1991). Cognitive impairment in early, untreated Parkinson's disease and its relationship to motor disability. *Brain* 114, 2095–2122.

Copland, D. (2003). The basal ganglia and semantic engagement: potential insights from semantic priming in individuals with subcortical vascular lesions, Parkinson's disease and cortical lesions. *Journal of the International Neuropsychological Society* 9. 1041–52.

Copland, D., Chenery, H.J. and Murdoch, B.E. (2000). Persistent deficits in complex language function following dominant nonthalamic subcortical lesions. *Journal of Medical Speech Language Pathology* 8, 1–14.

Crosson, B. (1992). *Subcortical Functions in Language and Memory*. New York: Guilford Press.

Crosson, B., Zawacki, T., Brinson, G., Lu, L. and Sadek, J.R. (1997). Models of subcortical functions in language: current status. *Journal of Neurolinguistics* 10, 277–300.

Cummings, J.L., Darkins, A., Mendez, M., Hill, M.A. and Benson, D.F. (1988) Alzheimer's disease and Parkinson's disease: comparison of speech and language alternations. *Neurology* 38, 680–4.

Delis, D.C. and Massman, P.J. (1992). The effects of dopamine fluctuation on cognition and affect. In S.J. Huber and J.L. Cummings (eds), *Parkinson's Disease: Neurobehavioral Aspects* (pp. 288–302). New York: Oxford University Press.

DeLong, M.R. (1990). Primate models of movement disorders of basal ganglia origin. *Trends in Neuroscience* 13, 281–5.

D'Esposito, M. and Alexander, M.P. (1995). Subcortical aphasia: distinct profiles following left putaminal hemorrhage. *Neurology* 45, 38–41.

Deuschl, G. and Bergman, H. (2002). Pathophysiology of non-parkinsonian tremor. *Movement Disorders* 17 (suppl. 3), S41–8.

Deuschl, G., Bain, P. and Committee, A.H.S. (1998). Consensus statement of the movement disorder society on tremor. *Movement Disorders* 13 (suppl. 3), 2–23.

Drummond, S. (2008). Tardive dyskinesia. In M.R. McNeil (ed.), *Clinical Management of Sensorimotor Speech Disorders*, 2nd edn (pp. 396–7). New York: Thieme.

Drummond, S. and Fitzpatrick, A. (2004). Speech and swallowing performances in tardive dyskinesia: a case study. *Journal of Medical Speech Language Pathology* 12, 9–19.

Dubois, B., Boller, F., Pillon, B. and Agid, Y. (1991). Cognitive deficits in Parkinson's disease. In F. Boller and J. Grafman (eds), *Handbook of Neuropsychology*, vol. 5 (pp. 195–239). New York: Elsevier.

Duffy, J.R. (1995). *Motor Speech Disorders: Substrates, Differential Diagnosis and Management*. Baltimore: Mosby-Year Book.

Duncan, R., Bone, I. and Melville, I.D. (1988). Essential tremor cured by infarction adjacent to the thalamus. *Journal of Neurology, Neurosurgery and Psychiatry* 51, 591–2.

Dupuis, M.J., Delwaide, P.J., Boucquey, D. and Gonsette, R.E. (1989). Homolateral disappearance of essential tremor after cerebellar stroke. *Movement Disorders* 4, 183–7.

Enderby, P. (2008). Huntington's disease. In M.R. McNeil (ed.), *Clinical Management of Sensorimotor Speech Disorders*, 2nd edn (pp. 331–333). New York: Thieme.

Evidente, V.G.H. (2000). Understanding essential tremor: differential diagnosis and options for treatment. *Postgraduate Medicine* 108(5), 138–9.

Fahn, S. (1988). Concept and classification of dystonia. *Advances in Neurology* 50, 1–8.

Folstein, S.E. (1989). *Huntington's Disease: a Disorder of Families*. The Johns Hopkins Series in Contemporary Medicine and Public Health. Baltimore, MD: Johns Hopkins University Press.

Folstein, S.E., Jensen, B., Leigh, R.J. and Folstein, M.F. (1983). The measurement of abnormal movement: methods developed for Huntington's disease. *Neurobehavioural Toxicology and Teratology* 5, 605–9.

Frank, E.M., McDade, H.L. and Scott, W.K. (1996). Naming in dementia secondary to Parkinson's, Huntington's and Alzheimer's diseases. *Journal of Communication Disorders* 29, 183–97.

Gabrieli, J.D.E., Poldrack, R.A. and Desmond, J.E. (1998). The role of left prefrontal cortex in language and memory. *Proceedings of the National Academy of Sciences USA* 95, 906–13.

Geyer, H.L. and Bressman, S.B. (2006). The diagnosis of dystonia. *Lancet Neurology* 5, 780–90.

Geyer, H.L. and Grossman, M. (1994). Investigating the basis for the sentence comprehension deficit in Parkinson's disease. *Journal of Neurolinguistics* 8, 191–205.

Grossman, M. (1999). Sentence processing in Parkinson's disease. *Brain and Cognition* 40, 387–413.

Gurd, J.M., Master, N. and Oliveira, R.M. (2001). A method for investigating the relationship between cognitive and motor functions in Parkinson's disease. *Journal of Neurolinguistics* 14, 45–57.

Guttman, M., Kish, S.J. and Furukawa, Y. (2003). Current concepts in the diagnosis and management of Parkinson's disease. *Canadian Medical Association Journal* 168, 293–301.

Hanes, K.R., Andrewes, D.G. and Pantelis, C. (1995). Cognitive flexibility and complex integration in Parkinson's disease, Huntington's disease and schizophrenia. *Journal of the International Neuropsychological Society* 1, 545–53.

Harrington, D.L., Haaland, K.Y. and Hermanowicz, N. (1998). Temporal processing in the basal ganglia. *Neuropsychology* 12, 3–12.

Hedreen, J.C. and Folstein, S.E. (1995). Early loss of neostriatal striosome neurons in Huntington's disease. *Journal of Neuropathology and Experimental Neurology* 54, 105–20.

Hines, T.M. and Volpe, B.T. (1985). Semantic activation in patients with Parkinson's disease. *Experimental Aging Research* 11, 105–7.

Hodges, J.R., Salmon, D.P. and Butter, N. (1991). The nature of the naming deficit in Alzheimer's and Huntington's disease. *Brain* 114, 1547–58.

Illes, J., Metter, E.J., Hanson, W.R. and Iritani, S. (1988). Language production in Parkinson's disease: acoustic and linguistic considerations. *Brain and Language* 33, 146–60.

Jankovic, J. (2006a). Huntington's disease. In J.H. Noseworthy (ed.), *Neurological Therapeutics: Principles and Practice*, 2nd edn (pp. 2869–81). London: Informa Healthcare.

Jankovic, J. (2006b). Treatment of dystonia. *Lancet Neurology* 5, 864–72.

Jellinger, K.A. (1991). Pathology of Parkinson's disease: changes other than the nigrostriatal pathway. *Molecular and Chemical Neuropathology* 14, 153–97.

Jensen, A.M., Chenery, H.J. and Copland, D.A. (2006). A comparison of picture description abilities in individuals with vascular subcortical lesions and Huntington's disease. *Journal of Communication Disorders* 39, 62–77.

Kennedy, M. and Murdoch, B.E. (1993). Chronic aphasia subsequent to striatocapsular and thalamic lesions in the left hemisphere. *Brain and Language* 44, 284–95.

Kischka, U., Kammer, T., Maier, S., Weisbrod, M., Thimm, M. *et al.* (1996). Dopaminergic modulation of semantic network activation. *Neuropsychologia* 34, 1107–13.

Lawrence, A.D., Sahakian, B.J. and Robbins, T.W. (1998). Cognitive functions and corticostriatal circuits: insights from Huntington's disease. *Trends in Cognitive Sciences* 2, 379–88.

Levin, B.E. and Katzen, H.L. (1995). Early cognitive changes and nondementing behavioral abnormalities in Parkinson's disease. *Behavioral Neurology of Movement Disorders* 65, 85–95.

Lewis, F.M., La Pointe, L.L., Murdoch, B.E. and Chenery, H.J. (1998). Language impairment in Parkinson's disease. *Aphasiology* 12, 193–206.

Luquin, M.R., Scipioni, O., Vaamonde, J., Gershanik, O. and Obeso, J.A. (1992). Levodopa-induced dyskinesias in Parkinson's disease: clinical and pharmacological classification. *Movement Disorders* 7(2), 117–24.

Mari-Beffa, P., Hayes, A.E., Machado, L. and Hindle, J.V. (2005). Lack of inhibition in Parkinson's disease: evidence from a lexical decision task. *Neuropsychologia* 43, 638–46.

Martin, J.B. and Gusella, J.F. (1986). Huntington's disease: pathogenesis and management. *New England Journal of Medicine* 315(20), 1267–76.

Matison, R., Mayeux, R., Rosen, J. and Fahn, S. (1982). 'Tip of the tongue' phenomenon in Parkinson's disease. *Neurology* 32, 567–70.

McDonald, C., Brown, G.G. and Gorell, J.M. (1996). Impaired set-shifting in Parkinson's disease: new evidence from a lexical decision task. *Journal of Clinical and Experimental Neuropsychology* 18, 793–809.

Mega, M.S. and Alexander, M.P. (1994). Subcortical aphasia: the core profile of capsulostriatal infarction. *Neurology* 44, 1824–9.

Milberg, W., McGlinchey-Berroth, R., Duncan, K.M. and Higgins, J.A. (1999). Alterations in the dynamics of semantic activation in Alzheimer's disease: evidence for the gain/decay hypothesis of a disorder of semantic memory. *Journal of the International Neuropsychological Society* 5, 641–58.

Muenter, M.D., Daube, J.R. and Caviness, J.N. (1991). Treatment of essential tremor with methazolamide. *Mayo Clinic Proceedings* 66(10), 991–7.

Murdoch, B. (1990). *Acquired Speech and Language Disorders: a Neuroanatomical and Functional Neurological Approach*. London: Chapman and Hall.

Murray, L. (1998). Productive syntax in adults with Huntington's or Parkinson's disease: preliminary analyses. *Brain and Language* 65, 36–9.

Nadeau, S.E. and Crosson, B. (1997). Subcortical aphasia. *Brain and Language* 58, 355–402.

Nagaratnam, N. and Kalasabail, G. (1997). Contralateral abolition of essential tremor following pontine stroke. *Journal of Neurological Science* 149, 195–6.

Neely, J.H. (1977). Semantic priming and retrieval from lexical memory: roles of inhibitionless spreading activation and limited-capacity attention. *Journal of Experimental Psychology: General* 106, 226–54.

Neely, J.H. (1991). Semantic priming effects in visual word recognition: a selective review of current findings and theories. In D. Besner and G.W. Humphreys (eds), *Basic Processes in Reading: Visual Word Recognition* (pp. 264–336). Hillsdale, NJ: Lawrence Erlbaum.

Nieoullon, A. (2002). Dopamine and the regulation of cognition and attention. *Progress in Neurobiology* 67, 53–83.

Obeso, J.A., Guridi, J. and DeLong, M.R. (1997). Surgery for Parkinson's disease. *Journal of Neurology, Neurosurgery and Psychiatry* 62(1), 2–8.

Podoll, K., Caspary, P., Lange, H.W. and Noth, J. (1988). Language functions in Huntington's disease. *Brain* 111, 1475–1503.

Poldrack, R.A., Temple, E., Protopapas, A., Nagarajan, S., Tallal, P. *et al.* (2001). Relationships between the neural bases of dynamic auditory processing and phonological processing: evidence from fMRI. *Journal of Cognitive Neuroscience* 13, 687–97.

Portin, R., Laatu, S., Revonsuo, A. and Rinne, U.K. (2000). Impairment of semantic knowledge in Parkinson's disease. *Archives of Neurology* 57, 1338–43.

Posner, M.I. and Snyder, C.R.R. (1975). Attention and cognitive control. In R.L. Solso (ed.), *Information Processing and Cognition: the Loyola Symposium* (pp. 55–85). Hillsdale, NJ: Lawrence Erlbaum.

Previc, F.H. (1999). Dopamine and the origins of human intelligence. *Brain and Cognition* 41, 299–350.

Randolph, C., Braun, A.R., Goldberg, T.E. and Chase, T.N. (1993). Semantic fluency in Alzheimer's, Parkinson's and Huntington's disease: dissociation of storage and retrieval failures. *Neuropsychology* 7, 83–8.

Raskin, S.A., Sliwinski, M. and Borod, J.C. (1992). Clustering strategies on tasks of verbal fluency in Parkinson's disease. *Neuropsychologia* 30, 95–9.

Schapira, A.H.V. (2005). Present and future drug treatment for Parkinson's disease. *Journal of Neurology, Neurosurgery and Psychiatry* 76, 1472–8.

Schuurman, P.R., Bosch, D.A. and Bossuyt, P.M. (2000). A comparison of continuous thalamic stimulation and thalamotomy for suppression of severe tremor. *New England Journal of Medicine* 342(7), 461–8.

Servan-Schreiber, D., Printz, H. and Cohen, J.D. (1990). A network model of catecholamine effects: gain, signal-to-noise ratio, and behaviour. *Science* 249, 892–6.

Singer, C., Sanchez-Ramos, J. and Weiner, W.J. (1994). Gait abnormality in essential tremor. *Movement Disorders* 9(2), 193–196.

Spicer, K.B., Brown, G.G. and Gorell, J.M. (1994). Lexical decision in Parkinson's disease: lack of evidence for generalized bradyphrenia. *Journal of Clinical and Experimental Neuropsychology* 16, 457–71.

Starr, P.A., Rau, S. and Davis, V. (2005). Spontaneous neuronal activity in human dystonia: comparison with Parkinson's disease and normal macaque. *Journal of Neurophysiology* 93, 3165–76.

Ullman, M.T., Corkin, S., Coppola, M., Hickok, G., Growdon, J.H. *et al.* (1997). A neural dissociation within language: evidence that the mental dictionary is part of declarative memory and that grammatical rules are processed by the procedural system. *Journal of Cognitive Neurosurgery* 9, 266–76.

Vallar, G., Papagno, C. and Cappa, S. (1988). Latent dysphasia after left hemisphere lesions: a lexical-semantic and verbal memory deficit. *Aphasiology* 2, 463–78.

Valls-Sole, J. (2007). Neurophysiology of motor control and movement disorders. In J. Jankovic and E. Tolosa (eds), *Parkinson's Disease and Movement Disorders* (pp. 7–22). Philadelphia: Lippincott Williams and Wilkins.

Wallesch, C.W. (1997). Symptomatology of subcortical aphasia. *Journal of Neurolinguistics* 10, 267–75.

Wallesch, C.W. and Fehrenbach, R.A. (1988). On the neurolinguistic nature of language abnormalities in Huntington's disease. *Journal of Neurology, Neurosurgery and Psychiatry* 51, 367–73.

Wasielewski, P.G., Burns, J.M. and Koller, W.C. (1998). Pharmacologic treatment of tremor. *Movement Disorders* 13 (suppl. 3), 90–100.

Wichmann, T. and DeLong, M.R. (1998). Models of basal ganglia function and pathophysiology of movement disorders. *Neurosurgery Clinics of North America* 9(2), 223–36.

Zakzanis, K.K. (1998). The subcortical dementia of Huntington's disease. *Journal of Clinical and Experimental Neuropsychology* 20, 565–78.

9 Assessment and treatment of subcortical language disorders

Introduction

As highlighted in previous chapters, disturbances in language function may occur as a consequence of subcortical lesions of vascular or surgically induced origin or as an outcome of neurodegenerative conditions. Subsequently, the appropriate evaluation of these populations is deemed critical to the establishment of efficacious treatment programmes to remediate these disturbances. In a manner somewhat similar to other neurological populations, such as traumatic brain injury (Hinchliffe *et al.*, 2001a), results from recent studies suggest that subcortical language disorders are intrinsically related to frontal lobe or cognitive dysfunction (Lethlean and Murdoch, 1997; Whelan *et al.*, 2000, 2002, 2003, 2004a, 2004b, 2005a, 2005b; Whelan and Murdoch, 2005), as opposed to deficits of primary or more general language function. Language profiles subsequent to subcortical lesions characteristically involve deficits of higher-level function, or rather, language abilities which have been hypothesized to demand frontal lobe support in their mediation (Copland *et al.*, 2000). See Chapters 4–6 for specific language features, such as cognitive-linguistic inflexibility.

Assessment of subcortical language disorders

As outlined in Chapters 4–8, patients with subcortical language disorders typically present normal profiles on tests of primary language function, yet demonstrate difficulty on tasks which assess metacognitive and metalinguistic processes. When intact, these processes permit the conscious and effective manipulation of the semantic system via the interaction of primary language, cognitive and executive processes (Hinchliffe *et al.*, 2001a). Failure to adequately evaluate these skills within this population, by way of the exclusive application of traditional aphasia assessments which appraise primary comprehension and production abilities, may serve to mask more complex language deficits that exist as a result of subcortical lesions.

Previous studies examining the effects of traumatic brain injury on language function have employed language-assessment batteries that evaluate function across a range of modalities as well as a hierarchy of structure, complexity and predictability (Hinchliffe *et al.*, 1998). This selection of tests was based on a conceptual model which defined communicative competence as the endpoint of the efficient interaction of language with other cognitive processes. Assessments included clinically available tests of primary language function as well as linguistically complex/higher-level language abilities. A number of these assessments have been subsequently applied to the study of subcortical language disorders, some of which are listed in Box 5.1 (p. 122). The following section provides a summary of recommended assessments, demonstrated as sensitive to the language disturbances caused by subcortical lesions, as well as a description of component subtests.

Recommended language assessments for the evaluation of subcortical language disorders

In previous subcortical studies (Whelan *et al.*, 2000, 2002, 2003, 2004a, 2005a, 2005b; Whelan and Murdoch, 2005) language tests have been divided into two principal batteries: (1) a general language battery, consisting of assessments of primary language functions, and (2) a high-level language battery, consisting of assessments of more complex language functions. The general language battery included the Neurosensory Centre Comprehensive Examination for Aphasia (NCCEA) (Spreen and Benton, 1977) and the Boston Naming Test (BNT) (Kaplan *et al.*, 1983), including an analysis of error types (Chenery *et al.*, 1996). The high-level linguistic assessment battery included the Test of Language Competence-Expanded edition (TLC-E) (Wiig and Secord, 1989), The Word Test-Revised (TWT-R) (Huisingh *et al.*, 1990), Test of Word Knowledge (TOWK) (Wiig and Secord, 1992), Wiig–Semel Test of Linguistic Concepts (WSTLC) (Wiig and Semel, 1974) and semantic fluency tasks.

General language battery
Neurosensory Centre Comprehensive Examination for Aphasia (NCCEA)
The NCCEA constitutes a detailed assessment of language functions (Spreen and Benton, 1977), incorporating subtests which evaluate primary as well as high-level linguistic abilities (Murdoch and Leathlean, 1996). Principally designed for the assessment of aphasic individuals, the NCCEA comprises 20 language tasks which specifically evaluate the status of immediate verbal memory, verbal production and fluency, receptive language, reading, writing and basic articulatory proficiency (Spreen and Benton, 1977). Overall, the assessment provides a descriptive versus taxonomic classification of linguistic abilities (Spreen and Benton, 1977). Refer to Box 9.1 for a description of individual NCCEA subtests.

Boston Naming Test (BNT)
The BNT is a reliable measure of confrontation naming abilities (Guilford and Nawojczk, 1988) and provides information about the effectiveness of semantic and phonemic cues in facilitating word retrieval (Kaplan *et al.*, 1983). Subjects are instructed to name 60 constituent black and white line drawings of various objects ranging in frequency from *bed* to *abacus* and are permitted up to 20 s to respond to each item. A semantic cue is given if the subject provides a response that represents a misinterpretation of the target or a lack of recognition. A phonemic cue is provided subsequent to any failure to respond or incorrect response to a semantic cue, or in the event of recognition of the item but an inability to produce its name.

Error responses may also be transcribed on-line and later coded for analysis. Errors may be classified according to a system devised by Chenery *et al.*, (1996), based on the naming error taxonomies of Kushner *et al.* (1987), LeDorze and Nespoulous (1989), Smith *et al.* (1989) and LaBarge *et al.* (1992). A summary of error types and examples has been given in Table 9.1.

Box 9.1 Description of individual Neurosensory Centre Comprehensive Examination for Aphasia (NCCEA) subtests (Spreen and Benton, 1977).

1 Visual object naming (VN): requires subjects to verbally label objects presented on a tray.
2 Description of object use (DOU): requires subjects to provide a description of use pertaining to a range of presented objects following the probe 'What do you use this for?'
3 Tactile naming right hand (TNR): a range of objects are individually placed into the subject's right hand under a covering screen, and the subject is instructed to name the objects accordingly.
4 Tactile naming left hand (TNL): as per TNR, however, objects are placed in left hand.
5 Sentence repetition (SR): requires subjects to repeat spoken sentences of increasing length but of minimal grammatical complexity.
6 Repetition of digits (REPD): requires subjects to repeat a series of spoken digit strings ranging from three to seven numbers.
7 Reversal of digits (REVD): subjects are instructed to reverse a series of spoken digit strings ranging from three to seven numbers.
8 Phonemic fluency (WF): requires subjects to generate as many words as possible beginning with the letters F, A and S, each within 60 s time intervals.
9 Sentence construction (SC): subjects are instructed to produce grammatically correct sentences incorporating two or three stimulus words provided by the examiner.
10 Object identification by name (IDNAME): subjects are instructed to point to a range of objects on command.
11 Token test (TT): subjects are required to point to or move a number of coloured tokens relative to a series of spoken instructions of increasing length and grammatical complexity.
12 Oral reading of names (ORNAME): subjects are instructed to read object names from a series of flash cards.
13 Oral reading of sentences (ORSENT): subjects are instructed to read sentences of increasing difficulty extracted from the token test, from a series of flash cards.
14 Reading names for meaning (RNM): typically administered after subtest 12 (ORNAME), subjects are required to point to range of objects corresponding to written names on a series of flash cards.
15 Reading sentences for meaning (RSM): typically administered after subtest 13 (ORSENT), subjects are required to follow simple commands written on a series of flash cards.
16 Visual graphic naming (VGN): subjects are instructed to write the names of a range of presented objects.
17 Written naming (WN): relates to performance on the VGN task. Items are scored according to accuracy of writing and spelling.
18 Writing to dictation (WD): subjects are required to write their name and two dictated sentences.
19 Writing to copy (WC): subjects are instructed to copy two sentences presented on flash cards.
20 Articulation (ART): subjects are required to repeat a series of real words and non-words containing a variety of consonant/vowel blends.

High-level language battery
The Test of Language Competence-Expanded edition (TLC-E)
The TLC-E is an assessment of language proficiency and metalinguistic ability, consisting of a range of subtests which probe the semantic system, semantic–syntactic interfaces and pragmatics (Wiig and Secord, 1989). Designed and standardized on two levels (i.e. Level 1: children 5–9 years; Level 2: pre-adolescents and adolescents aged 9–18+ years), the TLC-E assesses language competence by way of complex tasks that demand divergent language production, cognitive-linguistic flexibility and plan-

Table 9.1 Classification system for errors produced on the Boston Naming Test (BNT) adapted from Chenery *et al.* (1996).

Error type	Description	Example
1. Semantic		
Semantic paraphasia	Single word with a semantic relationship to the target	*leash* for *muzzle*
Definitional circumlocution	Informative multi-word response with a semantic relationship to the target	*remembrance flowers to go to a memorial* for *wreath*
Vague circumlocution	Multi-word response lacking specific definitional information but with a tangential relationship to the target	*the person who is going to be murdered* for *noose*
Semantic negation	Response indicating what the target is not	*not an otter* for *beaver*
Semantically related whole/part-part/whole	Response named a part of target that formed part of its semantic specification	*bedstead* for *bed*
2. No relationship		
Wild paraphasia	Single-word response with no relationship to target	*cup* for *scroll*
Neutral (i) deixis	Target labelled by non-specific pronoun	*the thing* for *dart*
Neutral (ii) empty syntax	Non-informative utterance used to describe target	*it's a funny thing too* for *mask*
Deviant circumlocution	Inappropriate multi-word response referring to attributes not typically associated with target	*nice piece of elephant* for *cactus*
Don't know	Statement of inability to label target	*I don't know the name of it* for *palette*
No response		
Question to examiner	Acknowledgment of examiner with enquiry as to whether response was correct or incorrect	*is that right?* for *octopus*
Self-centred	Relation of target to self/ possessions or a phase or sentence relating personal experience to word meaning	*I bought that with the . . .* for *mushroom*
Incomplete	Response comprising incomplete carrier phrase or sentence	*thing around making the . . .* for *compass*
Meta task	A comment about the task or target	*I should know that one* for *wreath*
3. Perceptual		
Perceptually related	Response involved label that was visually similar to target	*snake* for *pretzel*
Perceptually related: part/ whole or whole/part	Response labelled part of the target that was perceptually misinterpreted	*it's a bicycle* for *wheelchair*

Table 9.1 *Continued*

Error type	Description	Example
4. Phonological		
Phonemic paraphasia	Real word that shares some phonological elements of the target	*corn* for *accordion*
Literal paraphasia	Non-word that shares more than half the phonemes of the target word	*mush* for *mushroom*
Neologistic	Jargon non-word	*squizzle* for *octopus*
Phonemic letter cue	Response specified target letter beginning name	*it starts with 'c' for camel*
5. Unrecognized correct		*it's not a beaver* for *beaver*

ning for production. The TLC-E Level 2 was utilized for the purposes of our research, including: ambiguous sentences (AS), listening comprehension: making inferences (MI), oral expression: recreating sentences (RS), figurative language (FL) and remembering word pairs (RWP) subtests.

The ambiguous sentences subtest assesses the ability to identify and interpret the alternative meanings of lexical and structural ambiguities (Wiig and Secord, 1989). Lexically, ambiguous sentences contain lexical elements with more than one possible meaning (e.g. *He bought the glasses*, where glasses may refer to *eyeglasses* or *drinking glasses*). Structural ambiguities may be classified as either surface or deep subtypes. Surface-structure-level ambiguities contain adjacent words that may be grouped in two or more distinct ways (e.g. *Mary likes small dogs and cats*, where *small dogs and cats* may refer to *all small dogs* and *small cats* or rather *small dogs* and *cats in general*, regardless of size). Deep-structure-level ambiguities contain more than one logical relationship between words and phrases (e.g. *The turkey is ready to eat*, where the *turkey* may be *ready to eat something* or *ready to be eaten*). Subjects are presented with a series of ambiguous sentences in both spoken and written form and instructed to provide two distinct interpretations for each item. Responses are scored quantitatively according to essential meaning criteria.

The making inferences subtest assesses a subject's ability to utilize causal relationships or chains in short paragraphs to make logical inferences (Wiig and Secord, 1989). Subjects are provided with a series of paired propositions including a lead-in (e.g. *Jack went to a Mexican restaurant*) and concluding sentence (e.g. *He left without giving a tip*). On the basis of this information they are then instructed to make logical inferences pertaining to the event chain, by selecting two plausible intervening clauses from four possible choices; for example, (a) *The restaurant closed when he arrived*, (b) *He only had enough money to pay for the meal*, (c) *The food and service were excellent* or (d) *He was dissatisfied with the service*. All test stimuli are provided in spoken as well as written form. The correct responses for the above example would be (b) and (d).

The recreating sentences subtest evaluates the ability to formulate grammatically complete sentences utilizing key semantic elements within defined contexts (Wiig and Secord, 1989). Subjects are provided with a situational context (e.g. *At the ice-cream store*) and three words (e.g. *some, and, get*) in spoken and written/pictorial form, and instructed to generate a complete sentence that reflects the relevant situational context, utilizing all three words. Responses are scored according to holistic scoring rules pertaining to semantic, syntactic and pragmatic accuracy, as well as the number of target words used successfully.

The figurative language subtest evaluates the ability to interpret metaphorical expressions and to correlate structurally related metaphors according to shared meanings (Wiig and Secord, 1989). Subjects are provided with a series of metaphorical expressions (e.g. *She sure casts a spell over me*) accompanied by defined situational contexts (e.g. *A boy talking about a girl at a school dance*), and instructed to provide a novel verbal interpretation of the metaphor. Once the subject has explained the metaphor in his/her own words, they are then instructed to identify a match for the sample metaphor from four possible choices. Response choices include: a metaphoric match (e.g. *She is totally bewitching to me*), an oppositional foil (e.g. *I am out from under her spell*), a literal foil (e.g. *She spells much better than I*) and a non-related foil (e.g. *In her life, every day is Halloween*). All test stimuli are presented in spoken as well as written form. Metaphorical explanations are recorded verbatim and scored according to specified interpretation rules. The final score represents a composite of the verbal interpretation score and the match selection score.

The remembering word pairs supplemental subtest assesses the ability to recall paired word associates (Wiig and Secord, 1989). Associations are classified as one of four possible categories, including paradigmatic (e.g. *coat-sock*), spatial (e.g. *plane-cloud*), temporal (e.g. *moon-bed*) and unrelated (e.g. *antler-egg*). Subjects are provided with two presentations (i.e. elicitation lists A and B) of 16 spoken word pairs, considered to be representative of common and familiar vocabulary. Subsequent to the oral presentation of each elicitation list, the examiner provides one of the words from each pair. Subjects are then instructed to recall its associate. The sum of correctly recalled pairs relative to elicitation lists A and B represents the total score.

The Word Test-Revised (TWT-R)
The Word Test-Revised (TWT-R) represents an assessment of expressive vocabulary and semantics (Huisingh *et al.*, 1990), originally designed for use with school-age children. The TWT-R specifically probes the ability to identify and express critical semantic features of the lexicon by way of tasks that involve categorization, definition, verbal reasoning and lexical selection. For the purposes of the current research, all subtests of the TWT-R were administered, including: associations (ASS), synonyms (SYN), semantic absurdities (SEMAB), antonyms (ANT), definitions (DEF) and multiple definitions (MULDEF).

The associations subtest requires subjects to identify a semantically unrelated word within group of four spoken words and to provide an explanation for the selected word in relation to the category of semantically related words. For example, from the group of words *knee, shoulder, bracelet* and *ankle* the word *bracelet* is considered semantically unrelated *because it is not a body part*. Responses are scored according to word choice as well as criteria pertaining to acceptable and unacceptable explanations.

The synonyms subtest requires subjects to generate synonyms for verbally presented stimuli (Huisingh *et al.*, 1990). Answers are again scored in reference to acceptable and unacceptable response criteria. For example, in response to the stimulus *donate*, acceptable responses include words with similar sets of semantic features such as *give/contribute*, whereas unacceptable responses include *offer/fund*.

The semantic absurdities subtest evaluates a subject's ability to identify and repair semantic incongruities (Huisingh *et al.*, 1990). Subject's are presented orally with a series of semantically absurd sentences (e.g. *My grandfather is the youngest person in my family*) and instructed to repair the evident incongruity by generating a semantically appropriate sentence. Scoring is again based upon acceptable and unacceptable response criteria. Acceptable responses demand the simultaneous identification of the resident semantic incongruity, the replacement of inappropriate with appropriate vocabulary and the maintenance of the integrity of essential elements within the generated sentence (e.g. *My grandfather is the oldest person in my family*). Incorrect repairs (e.g. *My grandfather is the biggest person in my family*), explanation of the semantic absurdity despite prompting (e.g. *My grandfather can't possibly be the youngest person in my family*) or semantic negation (e.g. *My grandfather is not the youngest person in my family*) are all classified as unacceptable responses.

The antonyms subtest requires subjects to generate antonyms for verbally presented stimuli (Huisingh *et al.*, 1990). Answers are scored in reference to acceptable and unacceptable response criteria. In response to the stimulus *first*, *last* would be classified as an acceptable response as it encapsulates reversible critical semantic dimensions of the stimulus word, whereas *second* would be classified as an unacceptable response.

The definitions subtest evaluates a subject's ability to identify and describe the critical semantic features of a word (Huisingh *et al.*, 1990). Subjects are provided with a series of stimulus words and instructed to explain their meaning. Answers are again scored according to acceptable and unacceptable response criteria, in relation to specific critical semantic elements. For example, in providing a definition for the word *house*, the attributes *person+lives* are defined as critical semantic elements. *Where my family lives* therefore, would be classified as a complete/acceptable definition; however, *Where you play* would be classified as an incomplete/unacceptable response.

The multiple definitions subtest requires subjects to provide two distinct meanings for a series of spoken homophonic words in relation to specific referents, probing flexibility in vocabulary use (Huisingh *et al.*, 1990). Scoring is again based upon acceptable and unacceptable response criteria. For example, germane definition references pertaining to the word *rock* include a *stone*, *music* or an *action*. Acceptable task responses would include *It's a hard piece of earth*, *Music you play* or *Moving back and forth*. *A hard thing* or *A thing you throw*, however, would be classified as unacceptable responses, as they fail to incorporate specified semantic referents.

Test of Word Knowledge (TOWK)

The conjunctions and transitions subtest of the TOWK has been employed in a number of research projects investigating subcortical language disorder as an additional probe of semantic integrity, involving the evaluation of logical relationships between clauses and sentences (i.e. coherence) (Wiig and Secord, 1992). This task consists of a series of written paragraphs, each two sentences in length. The first sentence defines the relevant context and is syntactically complete (e.g. *It is too cold to play outside now*). The second sentence is incomplete, missing a conjunction or transition (e.g. *We will play outside __ it gets warmer*). The absent word defines a logical semantic relationship between the sentences and is provided in multiple-choice format as one of four possible choices; for example, (a) *until*, (b) *when*, (c) *where* or (d) *while*. Subjects are subsequently instructed to select the linguistic marker that most adequately defines the underlying semantic relationship. In relation to the previous example, the correct answer is (b) *when*.

Wiig–Semel Test of Linguistic Concepts (WSTLC)

The WSTLC assesses the auditory comprehension of complex linguistic structures (Wiig and Semel, 1974). Consisting of 50 yes/no questions, correct responses are contingent upon the undertaking of logical semantic operations in the manipulation of a range of complex linguistic relationships, including passive (PASS), comparative (COMP), temporal (TEMP), spatial (SPAT) and familial (FAM) structures.

Semantic fluency

Semantic fluency tasks involve the generation of as many item names as possible within specified semantic categories, in 60 s time intervals. In the majority of subcortical language studies conducted by the current authors the categories of *animals* and *tools* were selected. An animate/inanimate fluency dichotomy was chosen to assess the status of knowledge processing relevant to frequently dissociated semantic categories following brain injury (Tranel et al., 1997; Ilmberger et al., 2002).

Strengths and weaknesses of recommended assessments

The application of tests of metalinguistic competence, language integration and lexical-semantic system manipulation to populations with subcortical lesions has provided unprecedented insight into the nature of resultant language deficits. It is now known that tests which focus exclusively on the status of primary language functions, such as traditional aphasia assessments, fail to adequately capture the true nature of subcortical language disorders which exist at the interface of language and cognition. More complex language measures, such as those listed within the high-level language battery above, provide more sensitive indices of language dysfunction within this population and, as such, should be administered accordingly.

An inherent limitation of these assessments (with the exception of semantic fluency), however, is that they were originally designed for use with pediatric populations. Consequently, they have no accompanying standardized data relevant to normal adult or brain-injured populations. Despite this weakness, however, these measures have been identified as sensitive to language disorders within subcortical lesion populations within a research context (i.e. when research subjects were paired with age and education matched controls). A direction for future research lies with the compilation of adult norms for the relevant tests summarized within this chapter, or the development of similar assessments for which norms have been compiled on non-neurologically impaired adults as well as adult brain-injured populations. Current clinical recommendations for the application of these tests to adult populations, however, would be the adoption of maximal or ceiling score criteria as a benchmark for normal performance.

An additional limitation of the assessments recommended above is that they focus primarily on the evaluation of language abilities from an impairment perspective (i.e. they identify the presence of language deficits but fail to ascertain the impact of these deficits on functional communication skills) (Hinchliffe et al., 2001b). Alternatives or adjuncts to the assessments outlined above include measures of communication activity limitation and participation restriction. As defined by Hinchliffe et al. (2001b), assessments of communication activity limitation encompass measures of functional and pragmatic communication abilities, which enable the evaluation of a patient's ability to plan, deliver and understand communication content within a

Table 9.2 Suggested functional and pragmatic communication assessments that may be applied to the management of subcortical language disorders.

Assessment	Reference
Functional assessments	
Functional communication profile	Sarno (1975)
Everyday Communication Needs Assessment (ECNA)	Worrall (1999)
Functional Assessment of Communication Skills for Adults (ASHA FACS)	Frattali *et al.* (1995)
Communicative Effectiveness Index (CETI)	Lomas *et al.* (1989)
Communicative Adequacy in Daily Situations	Clark and White (1995)
The Communication Profile	Payne (1994)
Pragmatic assessments	
The Profile of Communicative Appropriateness	Penn (1985)
The Edinburgh Functional Communication Profile (revised)	Wirz *et al.* (1990)
Communicative Abilities in Daily Living (CADL)-Revised	Holland *et al.* (1998)

range of interactive contexts. Pragmatic assessments typically appraise the ability to use language within natural contexts, including knowledge of language structure and knowledge of the environment and social rules, as well as the ability to adapt to changing environmental demands (Penn, 1999). In contrast, functional communication assessments largely aim to evaluate the quality of communication attempts (Manochiopining *et al.*, 1992), or the impact of communication disorders on social and vocational roles, otherwise referred to as participation restrictions (Hinchliffe *et al.*, 2001b). Although a more in-depth discussion of these assessment tools is beyond the scope of this chapter, the incorporation of such measures is considered critical to any thorough clinical evaluation of language dysfunction resulting from subcortical lesions, as opposed to an exclusive impairment-driven approach. The reader is referred to Table 9.2 for some suggested functional and pragmatic assessments that may be applied in the management of subcortical language disorders.

Treatment of subcortical language disorders

Communication has been described as essential to all activities of daily living, and critical to maintaining psychosocial well-being and positive quality of life (Hinchliffe *et al.*, 2001b). Akin to any communication deficit, the efficacious treatment of language disorders resulting from subcortical lesions relies upon comprehensive assessment at impairment, activity and participation levels (Hinchliffe *et al.*, 2001b). On the basis of these findings, appropriate therapeutic goals and treatment programmes may then be developed.

A range of treatment approaches, largely adopted from the school of cognitive neuropsychology (Mazaux and Richer, 1998) may be applied to the rehabilitation of subcortical language disorders. Although previously discussed in the context of language deficits resulting from traumatic brain injury (Hinchliffe *et al.*, 2001b), restorative, compensatory and behavioural treatment principles are considered translatable to all language-disordered populations, including patients with subcortical language disorders.

Restorative treatment approaches

Restorative approaches operate on the premise that the repetitive undertaking of specific exercises, which train particular neuronal circuits, will improve functional abilities as a consequence of neuronal growth. In this manner, cognitive skills are re-established within the context of their premorbid status (Hinchliffe *et al.*, 2001b).

In applying this approach, specific linguistic deficits are determined by psychometric/impairment-based assessment and rehabilitation programmes implemented involving the repeated execution of structured tasks (Mateer *et al.*, 1990) which target areas of deficit. In relation to language rehabilitation, such tasks may involve lexical-semantic processing exercises (e.g. identifying synonyms and antonyms, defining words according to semantic criteria, categorization tasks), complex comprehension exercises (e.g. following instructions of increasing complexity, story retelling, defining multiple meaning words) or word-retrieval exercises (e.g. word-association tasks, synonym and antonym generation) (Hinchliffe *et al.*, 2001b).

Limitations of this approach do exist, however, and include a potential difficulty for some patients to generalize skills taught during structured clinical tasks to real-world situations, and may be related to an incomplete understanding of the relationship between the targeted deficit and the training task utilized (Snow and Ponsford, 1995). It has been suggested that the modification of such tasks to include functionally relevant stimuli on an individual basis may alleviate this downfall to some extent, as would combining this approach with the development of compensatory strategies (Hinchliffe *et al.*, 2001b).

Compensatory and behavioural treatment approaches

Compensatory approaches operate on the premise that function cannot be restored once lost. Alternatively, skills and strategies are developed to establish functional competence (Mazaux and Richer, 1998). Behavioural treatment approaches adopt behaviour-modification techniques which aim to reinforce desired behaviours and to extinguish undesirable behaviours, or to positively reinforce the learning of new skills. In applying compensatory approaches, patients are taught self-initiated methods by which to overcome language deficits, such as the use of aids (e.g. notebooks containing word cues in the case of word-finding difficulties) and external cues (e.g. requests for repetition of information in the case of comprehension deficits), with a view to automatization over time (Hinchliffe *et al.*, 2001b). Functional skills training may entail activity-based tasks within relevant communicative environments (e.g. telephone-answering routines, role playing, direct instructions and scripting, fading of cues) (Hinchliffe *et al.*, 2001b). Functional skills training may also extend to environmental manipulation techniques, whereby the patient's communicative environment is modified to maximize communicative success (e.g. providing communication strategies for potential communication partners such as allowing increased time for a response, or reducing environmental distractions to enhance comprehension) (Hinchliffe *et al.*, 2001b).

Summary

The present chapter aimed to provide a summary of linguistic assessments that have been identified as sensitive in detecting language deficits which may arise as a consequence of subcortical pathology. In particular, it was emphasized that traditional aphasia tests fail to adequately profile the nature of language disturbances associated with subcortical lesions. Attention was specifically directed to tests of complex, or higher-level, language function, of which component tasks demand frontal lobe support in their execution. Such assessments include TLC-E, TWT-R, WSTLC and semantic fluency. Limitations of these assessments were also discussed, including a foundation in paediatrics and a subsequent lack of normative data relevant to adults, as well as a deficiency in functional parameters with which to assess the impact of communication deficits upon quality of life. Potential treatment approaches were also described, including restorative and compensatory/behavioural methods.

References

Chenery, H.J., Murdoch, B.E. and Ingram, J.C.L. (1996). An investigation of confrontation naming performance in Alzheimer's disease as a function of disease severity. *Aphasiology* 10, 423–41.

Clark, L.W. and White, K. (1995). Nature and efficiency of communication management in Alzheimer's disease. In R. Lubinski (ed.), *Dementia and Communication* (pp. 238–56). San Diego, CA: Singular Publishing.

Copland, D.A., Chenery, H.J. and Murdoch, B.E. (2000). Persistent deficits in complex language function following dominant nonthalamic subcortical lesions. *Journal of Medical Speech Language Pathology* 8(1), 1–14.

Frattali, C.M., Thompson, D., Holland, A., Wohl, C. and Ferketic, M. (1995). *American Speech Language and Hearing Association Functional Assessment of Communication Skills for Adults*. Rockville, MD: ASHA.

Guilford, A.M. and Nawojczk, D.C. (1988). Standardisation of the Boston Naming Test at the kindergarten and elementary school levels. *Language, Speech and Hearing Services in Schools* 19, 395–400.

Hinchliffe, F.J., Murdoch, B.E. and Chenery, H.J. (1998). Towards a conceptualisation of language and cognitive impairment in closed head injury: use of clinical measures. *Brain Injury* 12, 109–32.

Hinchliffe, F.J., Murdoch, B.E. and Theodoros, D.G. (2001a). Linguistic deficits in adults subsequent to traumatic brain injury. In B.E. Murdoch and D.G. Theodoros (eds), *Traumatic Brain Injury: Associated Speech, Language and Swallowing Disorders* (pp. 199–222). San Diego, CA: Singular Publishing.

Hinchliffe, F.J., Murdoch, B.E. and Theodoros, D.G. (2001b). Treatment of cognitive-linguistic communication disorders following traumatic brain injury. In B.E. Murdoch and D.G. Theodoros (eds), *Traumatic Brain Injury: Associated Speech, Language and Swallowing Disorders* (pp. 273–309). San Diego, CA: Singular Publishing.

Holland, A., Frattali, C.M. and Fromm, B. (1998). *Communication Activities of Daily Living (CADL-2)*. Austin, TX: Pro-Ed.

Huisingh, R., Barrett, M., Zachman, L., Blagden, C. and Orman, J. (1990). *The Word Test-Revised: a Test of Expressive Vocabulary and Semantics*. East Moline, IL: Linguisystems.

Ilmberger, J., Rau, S., Noachtar, S., Arnold, S. and Winkler, P. (2002). Naming tools and animals: asymmetries observed during direct electrical cortical stimulation. *Neuropsychologia* 40, 695–700.

Kaplan, E., Goodglass, H. and Weintraub, S. (1983). *Boston Naming Test*. Philadelphia, PA: Lippincott Williams and Wilkins.

Kushner, M., Reivich, M., Fieschi, C., Silver, F., Chawluk, J. *et al.* (1987). Metabolic and clinical correlations of acute ischaemic infarction. *Neurology* 37, 1103–10.

LaBarge, E., Balota, D.A., Stordandt, M. and Smith, D.S. (1992). An analysis of confrontation naming errors in senile dementia of the Alzheimer's type. *Neuropsychology* 6, 77–95.

LeDorze, G. and Nespoulous, J.-L. (1989). Anomia in moderate aphasia: problems in accessing the lexical representation. *Brain and Language* 37, 381–400.

Lethlean, J.B. and Murdoch, B.E. (1997). Performance of subjects with multiple sclerosis on tests of high level language. *Aphasiology* 11, 39–57.

Lomas, J., Pickard, L., Betser, S., Elbard, H., Finlayson, A. and Zoghaib, C. (1989). The communicative effectiveness index: development and psychometric evaluation of a functional communication meaure for adult aphasia. *Journal of Speech and Hearing Disorders* 54, 113–224.

Manochiopining, S., Sheard, C. and Reed, V.A. (1992). Pragmatic assessment in adult aphasia: a clinical review. *Aphasiology* 6, 519–34.

Mateer, C.A., Sohlberg, M.M. and Youngman, P.K. (1990). The management of acquired attention and memory deficits. In R.L.I. Wood and I. Fussey (eds), *Cognitive Rehabilitation in Perspective* (pp. 68–95). London: Taylor and Francis.

Mazaux, C.A. and Richer, E. (1998). Rehabilitation after traumatic brain injury in adults. *Disability and Rehabilitation* 20, 435–47.

Murdoch, B. and Leathlean, J.B. (1996). Language dysfunction in subcortical arteriosclerotic encephalopathy. *Journal of Medical Speech Language Pathology* 4(4), 275–88.

Payne, J.C. (1994). *Communication Profile: a Functional Skills Survey*. Tucson, AZ: Communication Skill Builders.

Penn, C. (1985). The profile of communicative appropriateness: a clinical tool for the assessment of pragmatics. *The South African Journal Communication Disorders* 32, 18–23.

Penn, C. (1999). Pragmatic assessment and therapy for persons with brain damage: what have clinicians gleaned in two decades? *Brain and Language* 68, 535–52.

Sarno, M.T. (1975). *The Functional Communication Profile*. New York: NYU Medical Centre, Institute of Rehabilitation Medicine.

Smith, S.R., Murdoch, B.E. and Chenery, H.J. (1989). Semantic abilities in dementia of the Alzheimer's type. *Brain and Language* 36, 314–24.

Snow, P. and Ponsford, J. (1995). Assessing and managing changes in communication and interpersonal skills following TBI. In J. Ponsford, S. Sloan and P. Snow (eds), *Traumatic Brain Injury Rehabilitation for Everyday Adaptive Living* (pp. 137–64). Hillsdale, NJ: Lawrence Erlbaum Associates.

Spreen, O. and Benton, A.L. (1977). *Neurosensory Centre Comprehensive Examination for Aphasia*. Victoria: University of Victoria.

Tranel, D., Logan, C.G., Frank, R. and Damasio, A.R. (1997). Explaining category-related effects in the retrieval of conceptual and lexical knowledge for concrete entities: operationalisation and analysis of factors. *Neuropsychologia* 35(10), 1329–39.

Whelan, B.-M. and Murdoch, B.E. (2005). Unravelling subcortical linguistic substrates: comparison of thalamic versus cerebellar cognitive-linguistic regulation mechanisms. *Aphasiology* 19(12), 1097–1106.

Whelan, B.-M., Murdoch, B.E., Theodoros, D.G., Silburn, P. and Harding-Clark, J.A. (2000). Towards a better understanding of the role of subcortical nuclei participation in language: the study of a case following bilateral pallidotomy. *Asia Pacific Journal of Speech, Language and Hearing* 5, 93–112.

Whelan, B.-M., Murdoch, B.E., Theodoros, D.G., Silburn, P. and Hall, B. (2002). A role for the dominant thalamus in language? A linguistic comparison of two cases subsequent to unilateral thalamotomy procedures in the dominant and non-dominant hemispheres. *Aphasiology* 16(12), 1213–26.

Whelan, B.-M., Murdoch, B., Theodoros, D.G., Hall, B. and Silburn, P. (2003). Defining a role for the sub-thalamic nucleus (STN) within operative theoretical models of subcortical participation in language. *Journal of Neurology Neurosurgery and Psychiatry* 74, 1543–50.

Whelan, B.-M., Murdoch, B., Theodoros, D.G., Hall, B. and Silburn, P. (2004a). Re-appraising contemporary theories of subcortical participation in language: proposing an interhemispheric regulatory function for the subthalamic nucleus (STN) in the mediation of high-level linguistic processes. *Neurocase* 10(5), 345–52.

Whelan, B.-M., Murdoch, B., Theodoros, D.G., Silburn, P. and Hall, B. (2004b). Redefining functional models of basal ganglia organisation: a role for the posteroventral pallidum in linguistic processing. *Movement Disorders* 19(11), 1267–78.

Whelan, B.-M., Murdoch, B., Theodoros, D.G., Hall, B. and Silburn, P. (2005a). Beyond verbal fluency: investigating the long-term effects of bilateral subthalamic (STN) deep brain stimulation (DBS) on language function in 2 cases. *Neurocase* 11, 93–102.

Whelan, B.-M., Murdoch, B.E., Theodoros, D.G., Silburn, P. and Hall, B. (2005b). Borrowing from models of motor control to translate cognitive processes: evidence for hypokinetic-hyperkinetic linguistic homologues? *Journal of Neurolinguistics* 18, 361–81.

Wiig, E.H. and Secord, W. (1989). *Test of Language Competence-Expanded Edition*. New York: The Psychological Corporation.

Wiig, E.H. and Secord, W. (1992). *Test of Word Knowledge*. New York: The Psychological Corporation.

Wiig, E.H. and Semel, E. (1974). Development of comprehension of logical grammatical sentences by grade school children. *Perceptual and Motor Skills* 38, 171–6.

Wirz, S.L., Skinner, C. and Dean, E. (1990). *Revised Edinburgh Functional Communication Profile*. Tucson, AZ: Communication Skill Builders.

Worrall, L. (1999). *The Everyday Communication Needs Assessment (ECNA)*. London: Winslow Press.

Section C   Subcortical speech disorders

10 Role of the subcortical structures in speech motor control

Introduction

As outlined in Chapter 1, motor speech disorders frequently occur in neurological disorders (e.g. Parkinson's disease, Huntington's disease, dystonia, etc.) considered to be primarily attributable to lesions involving subcortical structures such as the basal ganglia and cerebellum (Darley *et al.*, 1975; Murdoch, 1998), implying that these subcortical brain structures have a role in the normal regulation of the motor functioning of the speech musculature. Unfortunately, the precise nature of this role remains elusive. In recent years, several models have been proposed in an attempt to further elucidate the possible contribution of subcortical structures to motor control and to explain the occurrence of movement disorders subsequent to basal ganglia and cerebellar lesions. These models, which are discussed more fully later in this chapter, have served a valuable role by providing testable hypotheses and in some cases have guided the development of new pharmacological and neurosurgical treatments for movement disorders of subcortical origin.

The basal ganglia and cerebellum are two groups of subcortical nuclei that classically have been regarded as motor structures. In addition to their role in motor functions, anatomical studies and clinical research conducted over the past 10–15 years have increasingly implicated the basal ganglia and cerebellum in a range of behavioural functions, including several different types of cognitive, language and limbic function (see Chapter 8). Although it is acknowledged that subcortical structures such as the basal ganglia and cerebellum may have functions extending beyond motor activities, the present chapter will focus on their possible role in motor control, with particular emphasis on speech motor control. Both the macrostructure of the basal ganglia and cerebellum, including their connections with other brain structures, and the microstructural aspects, including details of neurotransmitter types, will be summarized briefly as an essential precursor to discussion of the functional role of these structures. Contemporary models and theories of subcortical participation in motor control will be described and discussed with particular emphasis given to how these models may explain the occurrence of motor speech disorders such as hyperkinetic, hypokinetic and ataxic dysarthria subsequent to neuropathology involving the basal ganglia or cerebellum. In doing so, however, it is acknowledged that other subcortical pathologies, such as damage to the corticobulbar tracts as they course through the subcortical white matter, may also be associated with dysarthria.

Functional neuroanatomy of the basal ganglia and cerebellum

Damage to the basal ganglia and cerebellum produces well-described alterations in motor function such as tremor, rigidity, akinesia or dysmetria, which may affect the speech-production mechanism. It is thought that many of these symptoms may be due to disruption of basal ganglia or cerebellar outputs to areas of the cerebral cortex involved in the control of movement. Models of basal ganglia–thalamocortical and cerebello-cortical circuits have therefore become central to research and theoretical approaches aimed at understanding the role of the basal ganglia and cerebellum in speech motor functions. Consequently, central to any attempt to understand the role of these subcortical structures in speech motor control is a knowledge of their basic neuroanatomy. A detailed description of the neuroanatomy of the basal ganglia, cerebellum and associated nuclei is presented in Chapter 2. The following sections therefore provide a brief outline and update of the functional neuroanatomy of the basal ganglia and cerebellum necessary for understanding models of subcortical mechanisms in speech motor control.

Functional neuroanatomy of the basal ganglia

Although the connections of the basal ganglia are not yet fully understood, with new findings continuing to be made, the basic anatomy of the circuitry connecting these structures was clearly described by Alexander *et al.* (1986). Essentially, according to their description, information originating in the cerebral cortex passes through the basal ganglia and returns via the thalamus to specific areas of the frontal lobe; this feedback circuit is often referred to as the cortico-striato-pallido-thalamo-cortical loop.

The major components of the basal ganglia include the putamen and caudate nucleus (collectively known as the neostriatum), the globus pallidus, the substantia nigra pars compacta and substantia nigra pars reticulata (SNr), and the subthalamic nucleus (STN). In general, the basal ganglia can be considered to comprise a group of 'input' structures (the caudate nucleus, putamen and ventral striatum) that receive direct input essentially from areas of the cerebral cortex and 'output' structures (the internal segment of the globus pallidus (GPi), the SNr and the ventral pallidum) that project back to the cerebral cortex via the thalamus. Over the past two decades, notions of the organization of the basal ganglia, the thalamus and connections with various cortical regions have been revised. Originally, the neostriatum was considered to serve primarily to integrate diverse inputs from the entire cerebral cortex and to 'funnel' these influences via the ventrolateral thalamus to the primary motor cortex alone. Consistent with the view held at the time that they functioned primarily in the domain of motor control, the basal ganglia were thus seen as a mechanism for funnelling information into the motor system. Based on recent research, it is now clear that output from the basal ganglia terminates in thalamic regions that gain access to a wider region of the frontal lobe than just the primary motor cortex. Rather, these subcortical nuclei appear to project to many or most of the same cortical areas that send efferents to them. Consequently the original notion of the basal ganglia acting as a mechanism to funnel information to the motor cortex has been superseded by the view of the neostriatum as a 'multi-laned throughway' which forms part of a series of multi-segregated circuits connecting the cortex, the basal ganglia and the thalamus (Alexander *et al.*, 1986; Graybiel and Kimura, 1995; Middleton and Strick,

2000). Thus basal ganglia anatomy is characterized by their participation in multiple 'loops' with the cerebral cortex, each of which follows the basic route of cortex→ striatum→globus pallidus/substantia nigra→thalamus→cortex in a unidirectional fashion.

Alexander *et al.* (1986) identified at least five separate, parallel cortico-basal ganglia circuits according to the specific region of the frontal lobe that serves as a target for their thalamocortical projections. One of these cortico-basal ganglia circuits projected to the skeletomotor areas of the frontal cortex while another projected to the oculomotor areas. The three remaining circuits projected to non-motor areas of the frontal cortex, including the dorsolateral prefrontal area (Brodmann area 46), the lateral orbitofrontal cortex (Brodmann area 12) and the anterior cingulate/medial orbitofrontal cortices (Brodmann areas 24 and 13). Importantly, these circuits appear to be, to a large extent, functionally segregated (Alexander *et al.*, 1986), suggesting that structural convergence and functional integration occur within rather than between each of the identified circuits. Given the segregated nature of the cortico-basal ganglia circuits, collectively they may be viewed as having a unified role in modulating the operations of the entire frontal lobe, thereby influencing such diverse frontal lobe processes as motor activities, behavioural, cognitive, language and even limbic processes. This anatomical arrangement, whereby the output from the basal ganglia gains access to multiple areas of the frontal lobe, including non-motor areas, has profound consequences for the possible functional roles of the basal ganglia system and provides a basic neuroanatomical mechanism whereby these subcortical structures can influence aspects of behaviour, cognition and language as well as motor function.

The cortico-basal ganglia circuit that has received the greatest attention in the literature, and which is of greatest relevance to movement disorders associated with motor speech impairments, is the so-called skeletomotor circuit (see Figure 2.3). At the cortical level this circuit comprises the pre- and postcentral sensorimotor areas while at the subcortical level it comprises sensorimotor areas in the basal ganglia and the ventral anterior and ventrolateral thalamus. Cortical projections of the motor circuit terminate largely in the putamen. According to current models of the organization of the basal ganglia, putaminal output is directed over two separate projection systems, the so-called 'direct' and 'indirect' pathways. The direct pathway originates from striatal neurones that contain γ-aminobutyric acid (GABA) plus the peptide substance P and/or dynorphin and conveys activity from the neostriatum monosynaptically to the GPi and SNr. In contrast, the indirect pathway arises from striatal neurones that contain GABA and enkephalin and conveys activity to the GPi and SNr polysynaptically via a sequence of connections involving the external segment of the globus pallidus (GPe) and the STN. In both cases the returning thalamocortical connections seem to reach precisely the regions of the frontal cortex that contribute as inputs to the neostriatum (Strick *et al.*, 1995). A diagrammatic representation of the basic circuitry of the basal ganglia is presented in Figure 10.1.

Imbalance between the activity in the direct and indirect pathways and the resulting alterations in the activity of the GPi and SNr are thought to account for the hypo- and hyperkinetic features of basal ganglia disorders, including hypo- and hyperkinetic dysarthria. The possible roles of the direct and indirect pathways to the development of hypo- and hyperkinetic movement disorders are discussed further below. It is noteworthy, however, that based on the findings of single-axon training studies in primates, the simple dual (direct/indirect) division of basal ganglia circuitry has recently been challenged (Parent *et al.*, 2001). Using a single-cell labelling procedure, Parent *et al.* (2001) showed that striatal axons are highly collateralized, suggesting that

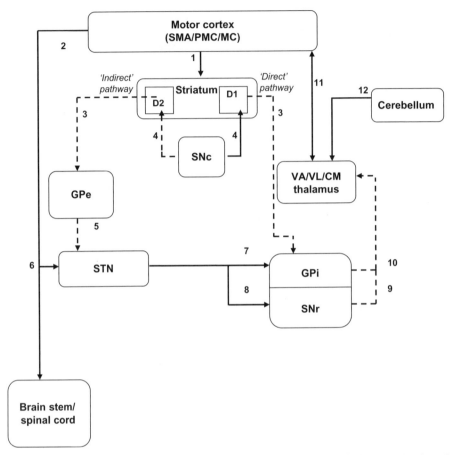

Figure 10.1 Modified schematic diagram of the basal ganglia–thalamocortical motor circuit under normal conditions based on DeLong (1990). SMA, supplementary motor area; PMC, pre-motor cortex; MC, motor cortex; D1, striatal output neurone receptor type D1; D2, striatal output receptor type D2; SNc, substantia nigra pars compacta; GPe, globus pallidus externus; STN, subthalamic nucleus; GPi, globus pallidus internus; SNr, substantia nigra pars reticulata; VA, ventral anterior nucleus of thalamus; VL, ventral lateral nucleus of thalamus; CM, centrum medianum; solid arrows, excitatory pathway; dashed arrows, inhibitory pathway. 1, Cortico-striatal pathway; 2, cortico-bulbar and cortico-spinal pathways; 3, striato-pallidal pathways; 4, nigro-striatal pathways; 5, pallido-subthalamic pathway, 6, cortico-subthalamic pathway; 7, subthalamo-pallidal pathway; 8, subthalamo-nigral pathway; 9, nigro-thalamic pathway; 10, pallido-thalamic pathway; 11, thalamo-cortical and cortico-thalamic pathways; 12, cerebello-thalamic pathway.

the basal ganglia should not be regarded as a simple dual (direct/indirect) neuronal system but rather should be viewed as a widely distributed network.

The nature of the neurotransmitters utilized by the neurones that comprise the cortico-basal ganglia circuits provides further insight as to the possible functional roles of these circuits. The cerebral cortex is connected to the neostriatum by way of excitatory neurones that use glutamate as a transmitter. In contrast, as noted above, the neurones connecting the neostriatum to globus pallidus use GABA, which exerts an inhibitory effect on targets in the medial and lateral globus pallidus and in the SNr, although these neurones also contain neuropeptides such as substance P and enkephalin. The globus pallidus neurones are themselves inhibitory and consequently there are two inhibitory synapses in series between the neostriatum and the thalamus. In effect these two inhibitory synapses in series act as an excitation. When the neostriatum is active the globus pallidus neurones disinhibit the thalamocortical projection via the direct pathway and thus presumably facilitate the initiation of movement (or some other frontal lobe activity). Briefly, the suggested mechanism for this initiation of movement is as follows: corticostriatal activation of the direct pathway produces a GABA-mediated inhibition of GPi-SNr neurones, leading in turn to disinhibition of their thalamic target, thereby facilitating the thalamic projection to the precentral motor fields. The overall effect of this sequence is positive feedback for cortically initiated movements. Suppression of unwanted movements (activities) probably ensues through inhibition of the thalamocortical projections via the indirect pathway (Wichmann *et al.*, 1994) because projections from the STN to the GPi are excitatory. Put simply, corticostriatal stimulation of the GABA/enkephalin neurones in the indirect pathway inhibits the GPi and secondarily facilitates the STN. The latter results in increased excitatory drive onto the GPi-SNr which respond by increasing their output, thereby further inhibiting their thalamic and brain stem targets. The overall effect of this sequence is to provide negative feedback for movement, thereby acting to inhibit undesired movements or to signal a halt to movements in progress.

Thus both excitatory and inhibitory influences converge on the globus pallidus and their balance probably determines the activity in the thalamocortical projections. The most important neuromodulator of the balance between the activity of the direct and indirect pathways at the level of the neostriatum is dopamine. The dopaminergic input to the neostriatum is provided by the nigrostriatal projections from the substantia nigra pars compacta. Release of dopamine from terminals of the nigrostriatal projections appears to facilitate transmission over the direct pathway and to inhibit transmission over the indirect pathway via dopamine subtype D1 and D2 receptors respectively (Gerfen, 1995) (see Figure 10.1). Consequently, reduced basal ganglia output from the GPi-SNr leading to increased activity of thalamocortical projection neurones is the outcome of striatal dopamine release. The role of abnormal striatal dopamine release in the occurrence of hypo- and hyperkinetic speech disorders is discussed below in the section dealing with subcortical models of hypo- and hyperkinetic dysarthria.

Functional neuroanatomy of the cerebellum

The cerebellum comprises two large cerebellar hemispheres which are connected by a mid-portion called the vermis. As in the case of the cerebral hemispheres, the cerebellar hemispheres are covered by a layer of grey matter of cortex. Unlike the cerebral cortex, however, the cerebellar cortex tends to be uniform in structure throughout its extent. The cerebellar cortex is highly folded into thin transverse folds or folia. A series of deep and definite fissures divides the cerebellum into a number of lobes. Although the lobe system of the cerebellum is classified differently by different authors, three lobes are commonly recognized: the anterior lobe, the posterior lobe and the flocculonodular lobe. The posterior lobe, also referred to as the neocerebellum, lies between the other two lobes and is the largest portion of the cerebellum. Phylogenetically it is the newest portion of the cerebellum and is most concerned with the regulation of voluntary movements. In particular it plays an essential role in the coordination of phasic movements and is the most important part of the cerebellum for the coordination of speech movements.

The central core of the cerebellum, like that of the cerebral hemispheres, is made up of white matter. Located within the white matter, on either side of the midline, are four grey masses called the cerebellar or deep nuclei. These are the dentate nucleus, the globose and emboliform nuclei (collectively referred to as the interpositus) and the fastigial nucleus. The majority of the Purkinje cell axons, which carry impulses away from the cerebellar cortex, terminate in these nuclei.

To be able to perform its primary function of synergistic coordination of muscular activity, the cerebellum requires extensive connections with other parts of the nervous system. Damage to the pathways making up these connections can cause cerebellar dysfunction and possibly ataxic dysarthria in the same way as damage to the cerebellum itself. Briefly, the cerebellum functions in part by comparing input from the motor cortex with information concerning the momentary status of muscle contraction, degree of tension of the muscle tendons, positions of parts of the body and forces acting on the surfaces of the body originating from muscle spindles, Golgi tendon organs, etc. and then sending appropriate messages back to the motor cortex to ensure smooth, coordinated muscle function. Consequently, the cerebellum requires input from the motor cortex, muscle and joint receptors, receptors in the internal ear detecting changes in the position and rate of rotation in the head, skin receptors, etc. Conversely, pathways carrying signals from the cerebellum back to the cortex are also required to complete the cerebrocerebellar loop.

The traditional view of cerebrocerebellar loops is that they receive information from widespread cortical areas in the frontal, parietal and temporal lobes with the major afferent pathway connecting the cerebral cortex and the cerebellum being the corticopontine-cerebellar pathway. This pathway originates primarily from the motor cortex and projects to the ipsilateral pontine nuclei, from where secondary fibres project mainly to the cortex of the neocerebellum. Other afferent pathways project to the cerebellum from structures in the brain stem such as the olive (olivo-cerebellar tracts), the red nucleus (rubro-cerebellar tracts), the reticular formation (reticulo-cerebellar tract), the midbrain (tectocerebellar tract) and the cuneate nucleus (cuneocerebellar tract) as well as from the spinal cord (spinocerebellar tracts).

Efferent pathways from the cerebellum originate almost entirely from the deep nuclei and project to many parts of the central nervous system, including the cerebral cortex (via the thalamus), basal ganglia, red nucleus, brain stem reticular formation and vestibular nuclei. Traditionally the output of cerebellar processing is thought to be directed at only a single cortical area, namely the primary motor cortex, consistent with the belief the corticocerebellar circuits function primarily in the domain of motor control. In recent years, however, this point of view has been challenged. For instance, anatomical evidence is now available that demonstrates that the site of termination of cerebellar efferents is not restricted to only the subdivisions of the ventrolateral thalamus that innervate the primary motor cortex. Rather, the regions of the thalamus that receive cerebellar input are now recognized as including those regions that project to many motor as well as non-motor areas of the cerebral cortex (Middleton and Strick, 1997, 2001). In support of the anatomical evidence, functional neuroimaging studies have demonstrated that, in addition to motor activities, the cerebellum is involved in functions that include higher cognitive functions such as language and attention (Schmahmann, 2001). As yet, clinical data on the cerebellar representations of speech motor control do not provide a coherent picture. Although some studies have emphasized the importance of medial cerebellar structures to speech, others suggest a predominant contribution from the lateral parts of the cerebellum (Acker-mann and Hertrich, 2000). Several investigations have linked ataxic dysarthria to bilateral damage to the cerebellum while others have reported dysarthria in associa-tion with unilateral lesions (Ackermann and Ziegler, 1992). Although Lechtenberg and Gilman (1978) observed a significantly higher prevalence of dysarthria in patients with a left cerebellar lesions, in a study of speech deficits associated with ischaemic cerebellar lesions Ackermann et al. (1992) reported that three of their four dysarthric subjects had unilateral right-sided ischaemia. The findings of these latter authors demonstrated that lesions of the cerebellar cortex without involvement of the dentate nucleus can cause dysarthria.

Subcortical speech disorders: hypokinetic, hyperkinetic and ataxic dysarthria

Research into the motor functions of the basal ganglia, thalamus and cerebellum has focused primarily on the role of these structures in regulating the activity of limb and trunk muscles. Very little attention has been paid to the possible role that these sub-cortical structures may play in regulating the functioning of craniofacial muscles, especially the muscles of the speech-production apparatus. The occurrence of motor speech disorders in association with neurological conditions caused by pathological changes in the basal ganglia (e.g. Parkinson's disease) and cerebellum has, however, been regarded as indicative of a role for these structures in the motor control of the speech-production mechanism. Three principal types of dysarthria are associated with lesions involving subcortical structures, including hypokinetic dysarthria, hyper-kinetic dysarthria and ataxic dysarthria. The major features of each of these dysarthria types are outlined below. (For a full description of hypo-/hyperkinetic and ataxic dysarthria see Chapter 11.)

Hypo- and hyperkinetic dysarthria

The speech characteristics associated with hypokinetic dysarthria follow largely from the generalized pattern of hypokinetic motor disorder which includes marked reduc-tion in the amplitude of voluntary movements, slowness of movement, initiation difficulties, muscular rigidity, loss of the automatic (associated) aspects of movement and tremor at rest. For example, a pervading feature of articulatory impairment in persons with Parkinson's disease includes a reduction in the amplitude of displace-ment of the articulators and a decrease in the velocity of movement (Forrest and Weismer, 1995). Hunker and Abbs (1984) suggested that tremor of the orofacial struc-tures in persons with Parkinson's disease may have a significant effect on their reac-tion times during speech, such that the patient may be unable to initiate a muscle contraction until it coincides with a tremor oscillation. Furthermore, Hunker and Abbs (1984) suggested that movement times of the articulators may be prolonged because of the superimposition of a number of tremor-related muscle inhibitions. The abnormal speech breathing characteristics of persons with Parkinson's disease have largely been attributed to rigidity of the respiratory muscles, which imposes limita-tions on the movements of the chest wall, resulting in reduced respiratory capacity and incoordination of the rib cage and abdomen during respiration (Murdoch et al., 1989; Solomon and Hixon, 1993).

Extensive perceptual, acoustic and physiological analyses of hypokinetic dysarthria have been conducted in an attempt to produce a definitive description of the speech disorder and provide a basis for treatment programming (for review see Theodoros and Murdoch 1998a). Although various studies have identified impairment in all aspects of speech production (respiration, phonation, resonance, articulation and prosody) involving the various subsystems of the speech production mechanism, the individual with Parkinson's disease is most likely to exhibit disturbances of prosody, phonation and articulation (Darley et al., 1975; Chenery et al., 1988; Zwirner and Barnes, 1992). The findings of these studies, however, have not always been consistent with respect to the type of disturbance, the frequency of occurrence and the degree of severity of the abnormal perceptual, acoustic and physiological speech features present in the speech of hypokinetic dysarthric speakers. These inconsistencies reflect the extensive variability in the presentation of the hypokinetic dysarthria associated with Parkinson's disease, which may in itself be related to the progressive nature of the disease and/or factors such as the individual responses to anti-Parkinsonian medication.

Hyperkinetic dysarthria is the name given to a diverse group of speech disorders characterized by excessive motor activity in the form of involuntary movements that disturb speech production. Darley et al. (1975) distinguished between two categories of hyperkinetic disorder: quick hyperkinesias and slow hyperkinesias. Quick hyper-kinesias include myoclonic jerks (e.g. palatopharyngolaryngeal myoclonus), tics, chorea and ballism and are characterized by rapid abnormal involuntary movements that are either unsustained or sustained only very briefly and are random in occur-rence with respect to the particular body part affected. In contrast, the abnormal involuntary movements seen in slow hyperkinesias build up to a peak slowly and are sustained for at least 1 s or longer. In some instances the abnormal muscle contrac-tions seen in association with slow hyperkinesias are sustained for many seconds or even minutes, with muscle tone waxing and waning to produce a variety of distorted postures. The three major conditions included in the category of slow hyperkinesias include athetosis, dyskinesia (lingual-facial-buccal dyskinesia) and dystonia.

The clinical characteristics of the speech disorder associated with these conditions have been reviewed by Theodoros and Murdoch (1998b); however, by way of example the clinical speech characteristics of one quick (chorea) and one slow (dystonia) hyperkinetic condition are presented briefly here. The most prevalent abnormalities reported in the speech of persons with chorea are prosodic disturbances which are thought to reflect the interruption of speech flow by the choreiform movements as well as the speaker's tendency to compensate for sudden, unpredictable arrests of respiratory, phonatory, resonatory or articulatory function. Specifically, the speech of persons with chorea is characterized by prosodic excess (prolonged intervals, inap-propriate silences, prolonged phonemes and excess and equal stress), prosodic insuf-ficiency (monopitch, monoloudness, reduced stress and short phrases) and variable rate (Murdoch, 1990; Theodoros and Murdoch, 1998b). Dystonias affecting the speech mechanism may result in motor speech deficits that predominantly involve articula-tion, phonation and prosody (Zraick et al., 1993) and to some extent respiration (La Blance and Rutherford, 1991). The main effects of dystonia on speech production include delays in the initiation of voluntary movements necessary for speech due to prolonged dystonic movements, and slowness and restricted range of voluntary speech movements once initiated (Murdoch 1990). Dystonias affecting the speech mechanism may result in respiratory irregularities and/or abnormal movement and bizarre posturing of the jaw (mouth opening and closing), lips (pursing and retraction), tongue (involuntary protrusion and rotation), face (facial spasm and grimacing) and neck (elevation of larynx, torsion of the neck and alteration of the vocal tract) (Theodoros and Murdoch, 1998b).

In describing hypo- and hyperkinetic speech disorders, it has generally been assumed that the speech musculature is affected by subcortical lesions in the same way as limb muscles, implying that the role of the basal ganglia in the motor control of limb and craniofacial muscles is the same. Recently, however, evidence arising from investigations into the effects of stereotactic neurosurgically induced lesions in the globus pallidus or thalamus on speech production has suggested that the role of the basal ganglia in controlling the speech-production muscles may not be the same as their role in regulating limb muscle function. Specifically some reports have suggested that, although surgically induced lesions of the globus pallidus may be effective in relieving symptoms such as akinesia in limb muscles, they do not produce a concomitant improvement in the functioning of the speech musculature; in some cases speech intelligibility actually declines following such surgery (Johannson *et al.*, 1997; Lang *et al.*, 1998; Samuels *et al.*, 1998, Theodoros and Murdoch, 1998a). Prior to examining this evidence further, however, there is a need to study models of the pathophysiological mechanisms that underlie such diverse symptomatology as the hypokinesia in Parkinson's disease and the involuntary movements associated with hyperkinetic disorders.

Subcortical models of motor control applicable to hypo- and hyperkinetic dysarthria

Hypo- and hyperkinetic movement disorders represent the extreme ends of the clinical spectrum of basal ganglia associated motor disturbances. Parkinsonism is characterized by a reduction in striatal dopaminergic transmission leading to increased basal ganglia output to the thalamus. In contrast, the major hyperkinetic syndromes such as chorea, athetosis, dystonia, etc. are all characterized by reduced basal ganglia output to the thalamus, leading to disinhibition of the thalamocortical neurones which in turn leads to the development of involuntary movements. DeLong (1990) suggested that hypo- and hyperkinetic movement disorders can be explained using a functional model of the basal ganglia–thalamocortical circuit derived from findings of experiments involving monitoring of the neuronal activity of various basal ganglia sites in primates treated with 1-methyl-4-phenyl-1,2,3,6-tetrahydropyridine (MPTP). In primates treated with MPTP, the dopaminergic cells in the substantia nigra pars compacta degenerate, and the animals subsequently develop a clinical syndrome that closely resembles human Parkinsonism (Miller and DeLong, 1987). What the findings of these studies suggest is that the hypokinetic movement disorders associated with Parkinson's disease may result from increased inhibition of the thalamocortical neurones that renders the cortical projection areas less responsive to other inputs normally involved in initiating movements. Briefly, according to the model of hypokinetic movement disorders proposed by DeLong (1990) (see Figure 10.2), loss of striatal dopamine leads to excessive inhibition of the GPe leading to disinhibition of the STN, which in turn provides excessive excitatory drive to the basal ganglia output nuclei (ie. the GPi and SNr) via the indirect pathway leading to thalamic inhibition. This effect is reinforced by reduced inhibitory input to the basal ganglia output nuclei through the direct pathway, also leading to inhibition of thalamocortical neurones. According to DeLong (1990), these effects are postulated to result in a reduction in the usual reinforcing influence of the subcortical motor circuit upon cortically

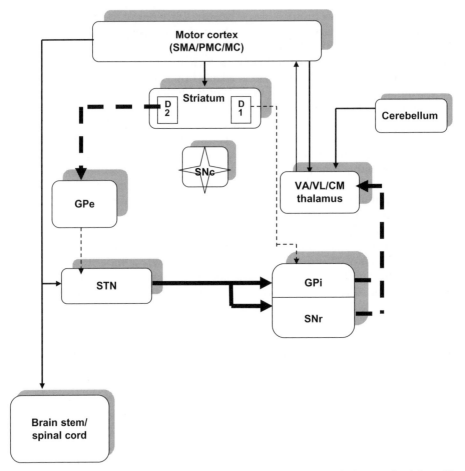

Figure 10.2 Modified schematic diagram of the basal ganglia–thalamocortical motor circuit in Parkinson's disease based on DeLong (1990). Abbreviations are as for Figure 10.1; solid arrows, excitatory pathway; dashed arrows, inhibitory pathway; star, lesion site.

initiated movements leading to symptoms such as akinesia and bradykinesia. The model proposed by DeLong (1990) is supported by data based on microelectrode recordings of basal ganglia neurone activity in MPTP-treated primates (Filion *et al.*, 1988; Filion and Tremblay, 1991) which have shown that neurones in the STN and GPi of these primates have higher discharge rates and show prominent changes in their discharge patterns, including a greater tendency to discharge in bursts. Further support has been derived from metabolic studies based on positron emission tomography (PET), which have demonstrated that the changes in basal ganglia discharge that results from dopamine depletion alter the neuronal activity in the thalamus and brain stem as well as cortical metabolic activity, consistent with the hypokinetic model (Brooks, 1991; Eidelberg, 1992; Calne and Snow, 1993; Leenders, 1997). Given that, according to the above hypokinetic model, motor disturbances in Parkinson's disease are postulated to result in large part from increased thalamic inhibition due to excess excitatory drive from the STN to the output nuclei of the basal ganglia, it has been speculated that induced lesions in the STN would ameliorate symptoms such as bradykinesia and akinesia (DeLong, 1990). Experiments involving selective lesioning of the STN with ibotenate (a fibre-sparing neurotoxin) in MPTP-treated monkeys have confirmed this hypothesis (DeLong, 1990).

In addition to the model of hypokinetic movement disorders, DeLong (1990) also proposed a functional model to explain hyperkinetic movement disorders. Evidence is available to suggest that a common mechanism underlies the various hyperkinetic movement disorders such as the choreiform movement in Huntington's disease and the dyskinetic movements seen in hemiballismus. In fact it has been suggested that these dyskinesias differ only by the intensity and amplitude of the movements. It is known that, early in the course of Huntington's disease, there is a selective loss of striatal GABA/enkephalin neurones that give rise to the indirect pathway. Experiments involving neurotoxin (ibotenate)-induced lesions in the STN of monkeys suggest ballismus is associated with disinhibition of the thalamus as a result of STN lesions. According to the model of hyperkinetic movement disorders proposed by DeLong (1990), reduced excitatory projections from the STN to the GPi due to either STN lesions (as in ballismus) or reduced striatopallidal inhibitory influences along the indirect pathway (as in Huntington's disease) (see Figure 10.3) lead to reduced inhibitory outflow from the GPi-SNr and excessive disinhibition of the thalamus. Dystonia has been likened to Parkinson's disease with evidence of excessive indirect pathway activity, yet differs in that direct pathway activity is also excessive, producing an overall reduction in GPi output (see Figure 10.4). In the case of levodopa-induced dyskinesias, disinhibition of the thalamus is thought to result from excessive dopaminergic stimulation of the striatal GABA/substance P neurones that send inhibitory projections to the output nuclei of the basal ganglia via the direct pathway (see Figure 10.5). The proposed overall effect is that of excessive positive feedback to the precentral motor fields engaged by the skeletomotor circuit resulting in hyperkinetic movements (DeLong, 1990).

Although the above models serve to explain the basic pathophysiological mechanisms underlying hypo- and hyperkinetic movement disorders, they do not account for a number of clinical and experimental observations. For example, the above models do not provide a satisfactory explanation for the lack of dyskinesias after pallidotomy, the lack of Parkinsonian signs after thalamotomy and the failure of experimental GPe lesions to abolish drug-induced dyskinesias. Although predicted by the model, according to Bathia and Marsden (1994), lesions of the thalamus are not associated with Parkinsonism even though such lesions could be expected to reduce or interrupt thalamocortical drive. Likewise, lesions of the GPi in normal monkeys or humans do not induce dyskinesias as would be predicted by the model (Baron *et al.*, 1997). Despite these limitations the primate-based models proposed by DeLong (1990) provide an ideal context for looking further at the role of the basal ganglia in speech motor control based on evidence provided by the study of patients with circumscribed, surgically induced lesions in specific nuclei of the basal ganglia system.

Ataxic dysarthria

Brain lesions involving the cerebellum or its connections are classically associated with a motor speech disorder called ataxic dysarthria. The clinical features of ataxic dysarthria follow on from the neuromotor abnormalities associated with damage to the cerebellum, in particular ataxia. The term 'ataxia' is used to define motor disturbances of cerebellar origin associated with a variety of clinical symptoms,

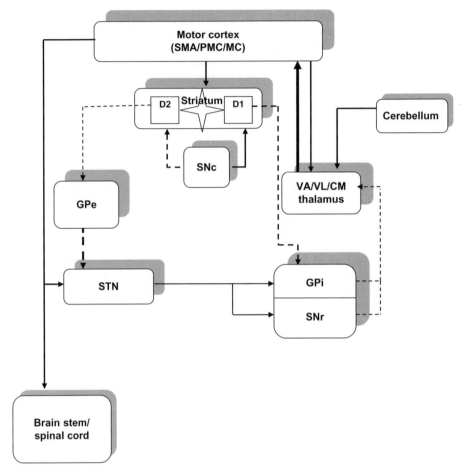

Figure 10.3 Modified schematic diagram of the basal ganglia–thalamocortical motor circuit in Huntington's disease based on DeLong (1990). Abbreviations are as for Figure 10.1; solid arrows, excitatory pathway; dashed arrows, inhibitory pathway; star, lesion site.

including dysmetria-hypermetria, asynergia, postural and gait instability, intention tremor and space-time motor incoordination. Dysmetria is a condition in which there is improper measuring of distance in muscular acts. The presence of dysmetria is shown by the patient's inability to stop a movement at the desired point. For example, when reaching for an object, the patient's hand may over-reach the intended point (hypermetria) or under-reach the intended point (hypometria). Dyssynergia represents a breakdown in the 'cooperative action of muscles' and is reflected in patients with cerebellar lesions in the separation of a series of voluntary movements that normally flow smoothly and in sequence into a succession of mechanical or puppet-like movements (decomposition of movement). It may also manifest as movement abnormalities such as delayed starting or stopping of movements. Disturbances of posture and gait may be very pronounced, the patient possibly being unable to maintain an upright posture or walking in a staggering fashion with a broad base of support. Tremor is another feature of cerebellar disease and refers to the presence of an involuntary, rhythmic oscillatory movement of a body part. The tremor of cerebel-

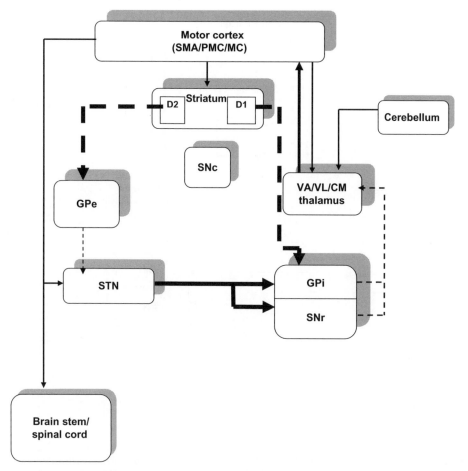

Figure 10.4 Schematic diagram of the basal ganglia–thalamocortical motor circuit in dystonia based on Starr *et al.* (2005). Abbreviations are as for Figure 10.1; solid arrows, excitatory pathway; dashed arrows, inhibitory pathway.

lar disease is typically exaggerated by goal-oriented movements (intention tremor) and is consequently seen during movement of a body part but is absent at rest. This is in contrast to the muscle tremor seen in Parkinson's disease, which is most obvious during rest and is reduced during movement.

The predominant features of ataxic dysarthria are a breakdown in the articulatory and prosodic aspects of speech. Unlike some forms of dysarthria (e.g. flaccid dysarthria), where the speech disorder can be linked to deficits in individual muscles, ataxic dysarthria is associated with decomposition of complex movements arising from a breakdown in the coordinated action of the muscles of the speech production apparatus to produce speech. Consequently, individual and repetitive movements of parts of the speech mechanism contain errors of force, range, timing and direction and tend to be slow, leading to irregularity of motor performance and to impaired coordination of simultaneous and sequenced movements. Increased variability in both limb and speech movement direction, force, velocity, amplitude, rate, movement onsets and terminations have been noted subsequent to cerebellar damage (Kent *et al.*, 1979;

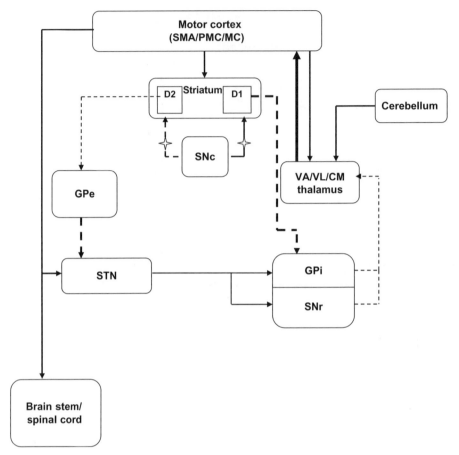

Figure 10.5 Modified schematic diagram of the basal ganglia–thalamocortical motor circuit subserving drug-induced dyskinesias based on DeLong (1990). Abbreviations are as for Figure 10.1; solid arrows, excitatory pathway; dashed arrows, inhibitory pathway; star, excessive dopaminergic stimulation of GABA/substance P neurones.

Schonle *et al.*, 1990; Hallett *et al.*, 1991; Ackermann and Hertrich, 1994; Ackermann and Hertrich, 2000). In particular, inaccuracy of movement, irregular rhythm of repetitive movement, discoordination, slowness of both individual and repetitive movements and hypotonia of affected muscles appear to be the principal neuromuscular deficits associated with cerebellar damage that underlie ataxic dysarthria.

As noted above, movement-timing disorders account for the majority of the reported movement disorders following cerebellar damage. The major speech-production timing deficit identified in cases of cerebellar disease has been increased durations for sentences, words, syllables and phonemes (Schonle *et al.*, 1990; Ackermann and Hertrich, 1994; Kent *et al.*, 1979, 1997). Other speech-timing deficits reported following cerebellar lesions include abnormal transitions from consonants to vowels, an inability to increase speech rate, reduced velocities and reduced speech movement acceleration (Kent and Netsell, 1975; Ackermann and Hertrich, 1995; Kent *et al.*, 1997). It would appear, however, that not all aspects of timing control are impaired in persons with cerebellar damage, with some individuals being able to preplan certain aspects of limb and utterance timing. For instance, some individuals with cerebellar damage have been observed to reduce initial limb movement and utterance segment duration as more segments are added to the movement in a manner similar to normal controls (Kent *et al.*, 1979; Bell-Barti and Chevrie-Muller, 1991). In addition, not all speech durations are abnormally long in these patients, with voice-onset time and tense vowel duration being reported to be less susceptible to lengthening (Kent and Netsell, 1975; Kent *et al.*, 1997). Further, recent evidence suggests that the timing dysregulation affects longer utterances in cerebellar pathology more than single-word productions (Kent *et al.*, 1997), suggesting that patients with cerebellar disorders are able to compensate for movement-timing disorders during production of single words.

In addition to its role in coordination of muscular activity, the cerebellum has also been shown to participate in motor learning (Sanes *et al.*, 1990; Topka *et al.*, 1993). The majority of evidence to support such a role in motor learning comes from simple motor learning paradigms such as reflex adaptation and classical conditioning (Lisberger, 1988) with both animals and humans with cerebellar lesions demonstrating deficits in the acquisition, learning and relearning of classically conditioned sensorimotor responses. A number of PET studies have also demonstrated cerebellar involvement during complex motor learning tasks, with normal controls demonstrating increased cerebellar metabolism during motor learning (Grafton *et al.*, 1992; Jenkins and Frackowiak, 1993). Interestingly, the cerebellum has also been shown to increase in activation during a verbal learning task (Raichle *et al.*, 1994).

In that stuttering has been characterized as a disorder of temporal coordination of the sensorimotor and/or cognitive-linguistic processes involved in speech, De Nil *et al.* (2001) have recently questioned the role of the cerebellum in the genesis of articulatory disruptions seen in stuttered speech. Based on the findings of a PET investigation of cerebellar activation during single-word reading and verb generation in stuttering and non-stuttering adults, De Nil *et al.* (2001) concluded that there is a need to consider cerebellar processes in investigations of the neural bases of stuttering.

Therefore, although the central contribution of the cerebellum to timing and coordination of sensorimotor actions is well established and the link between cerebellar damage and the occurrence of ataxic dysarthria well recognized, the exact contribution of the cerebellum to speech motor control is not fully understood. In particular the potential roles of the cerebellum in speech and oral learning and to the genesis of articulatory disturbances in stuttering has yet to be determined. As a further complication, based on the findings of a functional magnetic resonance imaging (fMRI) study, Wildgruber *et al.* (2001) confirmed a differential contribution of various cortical and subcortical structures, including the cerebellum and basal ganglia, to speech motor control depending on syllable production rate. In particular they found that cerebellar responses as determined by fMRI were primarily restricted to fast performance of silent repetitions. They suggested that in order to further characterize the specific role of the various cortical and subcortical areas involved in speech motor control, the production of different articulatory gestures at different frequencies and rhythm patterns must be evaluated via functional neuroimaging.

Subcortical structures in speech motor control: evidence from neurosurgical studies

The rationale behind neurosurgical procedures used in the treatment of motor disturbances associated with Parkinson's disease lies in the findings from studies on

primates using MPTP that increased basal ganglia output is a major pathophysiological step in the development of Parkinsonian motor signs. Neurosurgical procedures
such as pallidotomy, involving thermo-lesioning of the GPi, and thalamotomy, involving thermoablation of the ventral intermedius (Vim) of the ventrolateral thalamus,
therefore represent attempts to reduce basal ganglia output surgically. Although the
feasibility of this approach was first demonstrated with lesions involving the STN in
MPTP-treated primates (Wichmann et al., 1994), STN lesions in humans have been
considered potentially hazardous because of the risk of development of persistent
dyskinesias. Consequently, neurosurgical procedures for the treatment of Parkinson's
disease in humans have primarily involved pallidotomy and thalamotomy. More
recently, non-destructive neurosurgical procedures involving implantation of deep-
brain stimulators have been utilized to control basal ganglia output.

Thalamotomy, pallidotomy and deep-brain stimulation

Although relatively common in the 1960s (Svennilson et al. 1960; Allan et al., 1966),
thalamotomy and pallidotomy at that time were only supported by relatively primi-
tive neuroradiological procedures to confirm the precise location of the lesion. Not
unexpectedly, therefore, these techniques were associated with some complications.
Subsequently, the introduction of levodopa as an effective anti-kinetic treatment for
Parkinson's disease in 1967 led to a major reduction in the use of pallidotomy and
thalamotomy in the treatment of this condition. For a number of reasons, however,
recent years have witnessed a renaissance in the neurosurgical treatment of movement disorders associated with Parkinson's disease. These reasons include: enhanced
understanding of basal ganglia circuitry, function and pathophysiology based largely
on experiments conducted on the MPTP-treated primate model; advances in neuroimaging and neurosurgical techniques making lesion localization more accurate; a
degree of disillusionment with drug treatment for movement disorders, with a large
number of patients remaining disabled despite optimal medical therapy; and positive
reports of clinical studies suggesting that neurosurgical procedures are effective in
improving a number of movement disorders, including akinesia, dyskinesia, dystonia, tremor and rigidity (Iacono et al., 1995; Kelly, 1995).

Thalamotomy

For patients with Parkinson's disease in whom tremor is the dominant feature, the
Vim of the thalamus or its afferent projections is still the most commonly chosen surgical target (refer to Chapter 5 for more detailed account of surgical procedure).
Thalamotomies have been shown to be particularly effective in patients with significant tremor, rigidity or drug-induced dyskinesias, but they have not been shown to
be effective in patients with akinesia or bradykinesia (Selby, 1967). The rationale
underlying thalamotomy is that lesioning of the ventrolateral thalamus interrupts the
increased excitatory outflow from the thalamus, thus resulting in a reduction in
tremor. While the mechanisms of action of thalamotomy are largely uncharted,
researchers have hypothesized that the post-operative reduction in tremor may be
due to destruction of autonomous neural activity (i.e. synchronous bursts) that fires
at the same frequency as limb tremor.

Pallidotomy

Patients with tremor-dominant Parkinson's disease, however, constitute a small
minority. More common are patients with akinetic/rigid Parkinson's disease with

fluctuating on/off periods. For this latter group of patients, the GPi is considered to be a more appropriate surgical target (refer to Chapter 5 for more detailed account of surgical procedure). The rationale for pallidotomy is based on the theory that the major motor disturbances in Parkinson's disease are caused by overactivity of the GPi, which, in turn, is largely caused by excessive drive from the STN due to dopaminergic deficiency. Indeed, it is thought that the excessive inhibitory activity of the GPi inhibits the thalamic and cortical motor system, producing slowness, rigidity and poverty of movement. Therefore, lesioning the GPi results in a reduction in the GPi-mediated excess inhibition of brain stem and thalamocortical neurones. Pallidotomy has been shown to be effective against akinesia/bradykinesia, rigidity and tremor as well as dyskinesia/dystonia and motor fluctuations (Laitinen, 1995; Baron et al., 1997). Other symptoms such as postural disequilibrium, gait abnormalities and freezing episodes respond less well. Interestingly, the current models of Parkinson's disease pathophysiology do not predict that dyskinesia would improve following pallidotomy. Compelling clinical evidence that levodopa-induced dyskinesias improve following pallidotomy has led to serious reconsideration of the model. One possible explanation for the reduction in dyskinesia is that pallidotomy results in the elimination of the abnormal neuronal firing pattern in basal ganglia output neurones that communicate misinformation to cortical motor regions.

Deep-brain stimulation

In recent years, an increased understanding of the pathophysiology of Parkinson's disease has led to the development of new approaches to the treatment of motor disturbance associated with this condition. These approaches include non-destructive neurosurgical techniques that involve the implantation of chronic, high-frequency stimulation devices into various deep-brain structures (refer to Chapter 6 for more detailed account of surgical procedure). Chronic electrical stimulation was first developed as a treatment for tremor, using stimulation of the Vim nucleus of the thalamus; however, it has since been applied to other deep-brain structures, including the GPi and more recently the STN. Although the exact mechanism underlying the effects of deep-brain stimulation (DBS) is unknown, current researchers have postulated that DBS suppresses the neuronal firing pattern in the target via neural jamming or depolarization blockade, or by inducing the release of inhibitory transmitters.

High-frequency stimulation of the Vim has been observed to have the same effect in reducing Parkinsonian tremor as thermoablation of the Vim (Hirai et al., 1983) with some authors recommending the implantation of high-frequency thalamic stimulators as the surgical procedure of choice for the treatment of tremor disorders. Stated advantages of thalamic stimulation over thermo-lesioning of the thalamus include its reversibility and the ability to perform bilateral operations without causing permanent dysarthria (Koller and Hristova, 1996). Although the precise mechanism of action of implanted thalamic stimulators is unknown, neuronal jamming leading to deactivation of cyclic neuronal phenomena (Benabid et al., 1994) and decreased activity in the cerebellum (Dieber et al., 1993) have been proposed as possible mechanisms.

Stimulation of the GPi has been reported to reduce akinesia, rigidity, tremor and levodopa-induced dyskinesias (Gross et al., 1997) in a similar way to GPi ablation. Likewise preliminary studies suggest that STN stimulation improves all of the cardinal features of Parkinson's disease, with the further suggestion that these improvements are superior to those achieved with pallidal stimulation (Limousin *et al.*, 1997; Krack *et al.*, 1998). It is suggested that these positive effects are the outcome of the electrical stimulation of the STN counteracting the inhibitory effects on the thalamus arising from the globus pallidus, thereby increasing thalamocortical activation (Limousin *et al.*, 1995). The reduction in bradykinesia and tremor associated with stimulation of the GPi has been shown to be paralleled by increased activity (as measured by PET as increased regional blood flow) in the medial frontal cortex anterior to the supplementary motor area (Grafton and DeLong, 1997). These findings suggest that electrical stimulation alters inhibitory GPi output, resulting in increased activity in brain areas controlling movement, in a manner analogous to surgical ablation.

The DBS procedure has several advantages over ablative techniques including the fact that it is reversible and does not necessitate the creation of a destructive, permanent lesion. In addition, bilateral implantation can be performed during a single procedure with relative safety and stimulation settings can be adjusted at any time to optimize symptom relief and minimize adverse reactions. Finally, DBS does not preclude future treatments that require an intact basal ganglia system. Notwithstanding the advantages associated with DBS, there are also disadvantages associated with the procedure. In particular, DBS is an expensive procedure requiring a high degree of neurosurgical expertise and the adjustment of stimulation settings can be time consuming and inconvenient. Furthermore, the battery life of the DBS device is limited and there is a risk of complications associated with its implantation.

Effect of thalamotomy, pallidotomy and deep-brain stimulation on speech

Although the beneficial effects of thalamotomy, pallidotomy and DBS on general motor function in patients with Parkinson's disease have been well documented (Hirai *et al.*, 1983; Dieber *et al.*, 1993; Benabid *et al.*, 1994; Iacono *et al.*, 1995; Kelly, 1995; Limousin *et al.*, 1995), specific clinical evaluation of the effects of these surgical procedures on speech motor function has been limited. Of the studies that have reported the effects of pallidotomy, thalamotomy and DBS on speech, the majority of the data collected have been subjective, unsophisticated and perceptually based. Further, the results of those studies that have investigated the effects of these procedures on speech are equivocal, with some studies reporting improvements in speech and/or voice (Iacono *et al.*, 1995; Legg and Sonnenberg, 1998) and others reporting either no changes or a worsening of speech (Scott *et al.*, 1998; Schneider *et al.*, 1999) after procedures such as pallidotomy.

Iacono *et al.* (1995) investigated the effects of pallidotomy on speech production in a group of 62 patients with Parkinson's disease who underwent posteroventral pallidotomy. Based on one question taken from the Unified Parkinson's Disease Rating Scale (UPDRS) conducted pre- and post-surgery, they noted a decline in the severity of the speech impairment experienced by the patients post-surgery. However, although significant improvements in speech were reported in the total group performance, the subjects continued to exhibit residual speech deficits post-surgery. Although these findings suggest that pallidotomy has a positive effect on speech production in patients with Parkinson's disease, they provide very little information regarding the specific improvements observed post-surgery. Indeed, Iacono *et al.* (1995) did not evaluate the speech abilities of their subjects using a comprehensive perceptual and/ or physiological assessment battery and consequently were unable to provide specific information as to the characteristics of the speech disorder remaining post-operatively. In contrast to the findings of Iacono *et al.* (1995), a number of other studies have reported a lack of improvement in speech abilities post-pallidotomy, as measured by the UPDRS (Richards *et al.*, 1994; Johannson *et al.*, 1997; Barlow *et al.*, 1998). These equivocal findings may, at least in part, be due to poor inter-rater reliability of the UPDRS (Scott *et al.*, 1998).

Scott *et al.* (1998) used a more specific measure of speech function to investigate the effects of pallidotomy on the speech abilities of 20 post-pallidotomy patients with Parkinson's disease. Specifically, changes in the motor speech abilities were evaluated by the number of correct pronunciations of 'mama', 'papa', 'thanks', 'pitter-patter' and 'pataka' in 5 s, with eight subjects exhibiting reduced articulation rates following bilateral pallidotomy. Although unable to specify the quality or aetiology of these changes, the authors reinforced the need for more detailed and specialized investigation of the motor speech mechanism post-pallidotomy.

The Frenchay Dysarthria Assessment (FDA) was used by Legg and Sonnenburg (1998) to demonstrate improved speech abilities in a single case post-pallidotomy. In particular, the subject exhibited increased laryngeal modulation (evident in fewer audible pitch breaks), improved intonation, loudness and tongue function post-operatively. Involuntary movements and asymmetrical distortions of lips and jaw, however, remained unchanged and although overall speech was improved, the subject remained dysarthric. The speech changes observed in this case were attributed to relief of tremor in the thoracic regions of the body.

To date, only three studies reported in the literature, involving very small numbers of subjects, have used objective physiological or acoustic measures to evaluate the effects of neurosurgical treatment for Parkinson's disease on motor speech function (Barlow *et al.*, 1998; Schulz *et al.*, 1999; Theodoros *et al.*, 2000). Barlow *et al.* (1998) investigated perioral force and control and laryngeal aerodynamics immediately before and 48–144 h after pallidotomy in 11 subjects with Parkinson's disease. They reported a significant reduction in laryngeal airway resistance post-pallidotomy, while mean vocalic airflows were observed to increase to within normal limits. Other speech changes following pallidotomy included more consistent syllable-production rates, reduced voice-onset variability and improved force control of the perioral apparatus. A number of factors relating to the design of the study reported by Barlow *et al.* (1998), however, are the source of some concern. It is generally thought that assessment of motor function should occur when the neurological system is stable. Acutely, the lesion itself causes a core of neuronal death surrounded by an area of damaged cells (Samuels *et al.*, 1998). Additionally, perilesional oedema may become evident from 36 h onwards and may last up to 3–4 weeks post-operatively. The early effects of surgery observed by Barlow *et al.* (1998) may, therefore, be a result of sublethal neuronal perilesional damage and, due to the effects of oedema, an assessment carried out in the acute stage post-surgery may provide an inaccurate indication of the long-term effects of pallidotomy on speech production.

In a preliminary study involving a perceptual and physiological analysis of the effects of pallidotomy on motor speech function in persons with Parkinson's disease, a group of 12 subjects was found to have a significant reduction in speech intelligibility post-pallidotomy compared to pre-pallidotomy (Theodoros *et al.*, 2000). Physiological analysis of a subgroup of four subjects, using a range of assessment techniques covering respiratory, laryngeal, velopharyngeal and articulatory function, revealed that physiological changes in motor speech function following pallidotomy were either negative or non-existent in the majority of speech subsystems, with improvements in function noted in only few components of the speech-production mechanism

(Theodoros *et al.*, 2000). Intersubject variability was apparent across the four cases, even in those subjects who were closely matched for age, stage of disease and surgical procedure. Intrasubject variability was present in the form of differential subsystem impairment/improvement with respect to the specific subsystem affected and type of change that occurred. It was suggested that the observed negative effects of pallidotomy on motor speech function may be related to impaired muscle force generation (Barlow *et al.*, 1998) and movement preparation/motor set associated with lesioning of the motor circuit, the GPi (Alexander *et al.*, 1990) and/or to lesioning of specific neuronal fibres in the adjacent internal capsule. The positive effects demonstrated post-pallidotomy may be associated with improvements in general motor function resulting in more stable postural and speech musculature (Barlow *et al.*, 1998; Theodoros *et al.*, 2000).

Acoustic analysis of specific speech and voice parameters in six patients with Parkinson's disease following unilateral pallidotomy identified considerable variability among the subjects with respect to measures of phonation and articulation (Schulz *et al.*, 1999). Four of the six patients were reported to demonstrate positive changes post-pallidotomy in either phonatory or both phonatory and articulatory measures, with some subjects showing greater intensity, more syllables per second and longer extended vowel duration post-surgery (Schulz *et al.*, 1999).

As in the case of pallidotomy, few studies have documented the effects of thalamotomy on speech motor function. The few perceptual studies that have been reported suggest that in most instances thalamotomy has deleterious effects on speech. Tasker *et al.* (1983) reported that speech deteriorates post-operatively after Vim thalamotomy. In addition, operations involving the thalamus in the dominant hemisphere have been observed to be more likely to produce speech disturbances than equivalent neurosurgical procedures involving the non-dominant thalamus including dysarthria, monotonous voice, slow speech (Jenkins, 1968) and decreased loudness and articulation difficulties (Quaglieri and Celesia, 1977). Aspects of speech production including initiation of speech, maintenance and control of speech, fluency and vocal loudness have been reported to be disturbed in Vim thalamotomy involving either hemisphere (Petrovici, 1980). Diminished loudness, dysarthria and dysphasia have been observed subsequent to lesioning of the ventral lateral thalamus (Bell, 1968).

Although chronic high-frequency unilateral thalamic stimulation is effective in reducing both essential and Parkinsonian tremor (Koller and Hristova, 1996; Koller *et al.*, 1997), the effect of stimulation of the thalamus on speech remains uncertain. Stimulation of the thalamus has been reported to produce silencing and slowing of speech (Schaltenbrand, 1975), while stimulation of the left ventrolateral thalamus causes alterations in object naming in the form of agnosia, perseveration and anomia (Ojemann and Ward, 1971). Several studies have recently reported the effects of thalamic stimulation for essential tremor on speech (Carpenter *et al.*, 1998; Pahwa *et al.*, 1999; Taha *et al.*, 1999). Carpenter *et al.* (1998) reported that Vim stimulation that successfully controls hand tremor can also reduce the severity of vocal tremor, but with a less dramatic effect on the voice. Pahwa *et al.* (1999) noted that the speech deficits exhibited by some patients who become dysarthric following bilateral thalamic stimulation can often be ameliorated by adjusting stimulator settings, although this also frequently reduces the control of the tremor. In a study of 23 patients with thalamic stimulation, Taha *et al.* (1999) reported their perception that vocal tremor improved; however, no objective speech data were provided.

Although the effects of DBS on the motor disturbances associated with Parkinson's disease have been well documented, there is a relative paucity of evidence detailing the effects of DBS on speech function in individuals with Parkinson's disease. To date, research has generally comprised single case and small group studies involving GPi and STN stimulation and studies are equivocal as to the outcome for speech function. For example, a recent study found wide variation in the effects of GPi stimulation on the speech function of three Parkinson's disease participants with mild to moderate dysarthria (Solomon *et al.*, 2000). For example, GPi stimulation resulted in improved overall speech characteristics in one participant, whereas for another participant marked hypophonia became apparent.

Other studies have reported that speech function was relatively unaffected following STN DBS. In particular, a longitudinal study of 49 participants with advanced Parkinson's disease found that speech deficits appeared resistant to the effects of STN DBS (Krack *et al.*, 2003). Similarly, Bejjani *et al.* (2000) found that speech, swallowing and neck rigidity were less likely to improve from STN stimulation than other axial signs. Benabid *et al.* (2001) postulated that the lack of change in voice deficits following STN DBS was related to the location of stimulation targets. They speculated that stimulation targets made on the basis of limb symptoms may not be optimal for relieving orofacial deficits and that therefore the correct target for speech might be located in another area.

In contrast to findings of no change in speech function, other studies have documented significant improvements in parameters of oral control and voice in participants with Parkinson's disease following STN stimulation (Gentil *et al.*, 1999a, 1999b, 2000, 2003; Hoffman-Ruddy *et al.*, 2001). Interestingly, Gentil *et al.* (1999b) postulated that STN stimulation affected articulatory structures in an alternative manner to the dopaminergic pathways and hypothesized that articulatory system impairments may result mainly from non-dopaminergic lesions. Furthermore, Gentil *et al.* (2003) reported that bilateral STN stimulation produced improvements in maximal force and reaction time of articulators as well as sustained vowel duration and fundamental frequency stability in a group of 16 participants with moderate dysarthria.

Additional studies have documented that, although changes occurred in a few speech parameters following DBS of the STN, these changes did not represent functional changes in speech function. In particular, Dromey *et al.* (2000) examined the effects of bilateral STN stimulation in seven Parkinson's disease participants with mild to moderate dysarthria. Results revealed significant improvements in limb motor performance and small but significant increases in sound pressure level and fundamental frequency variability following bilateral STN stimulation. Overall, Dromey *et al.* (2000) concluded that speech measures did not change uniformly following DBS and that none of the speech changes was of a magnitude that would have a clinically relevant impact on functional communication.

Similarly, other studies have reported that bilateral STN DBS did not result in clinically relevant speech changes (Santens *et al.*, 2003). Specifically, Santens *et al.* (2003) investigated the effects of left, right and bilateral STN stimulation on perceptual ratings of prosody, articulation, speech intelligibility, voice quality, loudness and speech rate. Results revealed no significant differences in participants' perceptual speech characteristics between 'on' and 'off' bilateral STN stimulation conditions. Although there was no significant change in perceptual speech parameters following bilateral and right STN stimulation, left STN stimulation culminated in a significant deterioration in ratings of articulation, prosody and speech intelligibility. Tornqvist *et al.* (2005) investigated the effects of different stimulation parameter settings on the intelligibility of speech in 10 patients with bilateral STN DBS. Under DBS 'on' and 'off' conditions, five of the 10 patients did not exhibit a change in intelligibility between the two conditions, while four exhibited decreased intelligibility 'on' stimulation. Increases in the amplitude and frequency of stimulation were reported to cause significant impairments in intelligibility.

Based on the above reports, it is apparent that STN DBS can have a variable influence on speech function. Although the findings of a number of studies suggest that bilateral STN DBS may be associated with improvements in speech and non-speech oromotor measures, these benefits may not be clinically significant. Further, negative speech changes with STN DBS have also been reported. Given that negative side effects from STN DBS may be controlled through adjustment of the parameters of stimulation, it has been suggested that negative speech changes associated with STN DBS may be due to spread of electrical stimulation to the corticobulbar tracts in the internal capsule.

Summary of evidence from neurosurgical studies

In summary, although the beneficial effects of neurosurgical treatments for Parkinson's disease and other basal ganglia disorders on various aspects of general motor function are well documented, the effects of lesions induced by these procedures on the control of the speech musculature remains largely unknown. As a consequence, the potential of procedures such as pallidotomy, thalamotomy and DBS to yield new information regarding the role of specific subcortical structures in speech motor control has yet to be fully realized. Based on the preliminary evidence available to date, however, it would appear that procedures such as pallidotomy do not always have the positive effects on speech production as seen in the muscles in other parts of the body such as the limbs. To the contrary, in many instances speech intelligibility has been noted to decline post-pallidotomy. This difference may, at least in part, be an outcome of the segregated nature of the neuronal circuits that connect the cerebral cortex, basal ganglia and thalamus, with specific independent circuits subserving specific anatomical structures such as the orofacial structures versus the limb muscles (Alexander et al., 1990). Small inconsistencies in the site and volume of the lesions induced by stereotactic neurosurgery, therefore, could variably affect the functioning of the skeletal muscles in different regions of the body consistent with the case to case variability noted by several authors in their neurosurgical subjects. Another possible reason for the observed disparity between limb musculature and speech musculature is that subcortical modulation of the speech production muscles involves primarily non-dopaminergic subcortical pathways (Agid, 1998). Among these are neuronal systems originating in subcortical areas such as the cholinergic, serotoninergic and noradrenergic systems. This suggestion is based on the observation that although treatment of Parkinson's disease with levodopa results in improvements in symptoms such as bradykinesia, rigidity and tremor which arise from degeneration of the nigrostriatal system, other symptoms, such as abnormal gait/postural instability, dysarthria and cognitive impairment, considered to be produced by non-dopaminergic lesions do not (Agid, 1998). This hypothesis is supported by the knowledge that the effect of levodopa therapy on speech production is less effective than on limb function in patients with Parkinson's disease (Wolfe et al., 1975; Kompoliti et al., 2000). Kompoliti et al. (2000) examined the effect of central dopaminergic stimulation with apomorphine on speech in individuals with Parkinson's disease and reported that no index of laryngeal or articulatory function improved significantly after apomorphine stimulation. They concluded that laryngeal function and articulation are not under predominant dopaminergic control in Parkinson's disease leading them to suggest that treatment for dysarthria in Parkinson's disease should focus on non-dopaminergic pharmacology and other therapies. Bonnet *et al.* (1987) suggested that aggravation of Parkinson's disease following chronic levodopa therapy (e.g. increased involuntary abnormal movements, gait disorders and dysarthria) mainly results from increasing severity of cerebral non-dopaminergic lesions. Further research, involving the investigation of larger numbers of neurosurgical cases using a range of quantifiable physiological and acoustic assessments, is required if we are to achieve a greater understanding of the role of various subcortical structures in motor speech control.

Overall there are several conclusions that can be drawn regarding the effects of neurosurgical procedures on speech in Parkinson's disease. First, surgery to any of the commonly utilized sites (Vim, GPi, STN) has greater therapeutic effects on limb than on bulbar performance. Secondly, neurosurgical effects on speech are highly variable between patients. Thirdly, the effects of neurosurgery on speech may vary at the individual patient level, with some aspects of speech showing deterioration while others remain unchanged. Finally, the best neuroanatomical site for surgery to relieve the symptoms of Parkinson's disease with the best outcome for speech has yet to be determined, although STN is currently the preferred surgical target.

Summary

Although it has long been recognized that brain lesions involving subcortical structures may disrupt speech production, the precise role of subcortical structures such as the basal ganglia, thalamus and cerebellum in speech motor control remains elusive. To determine the basis of subcortical motor disorders, in recent years a number of theoretical models have been developed in an attempt to explain the roles of subcortical structures such as the basal ganglia, thalamus and cerebellum in speech motor control. Central to the development of these theoretical models has been experimentation based primarily on MPTP-treated primate models and functional neuroimaging studies which has led to a greater understanding of the basal ganglia-thalamocortical circuitry and cerebello-thalamocortical circuits, which are now recognized as comprising a series of parallel, multi-segregated circuits or 'loops'. Models developed that have incorporated this new knowledge of the neuroanatomy of the subcortical circuitry include those aimed at explaining the development of hypokinetic, hyperkinetic and ataxic movement disorders subsequent to basal ganglia pathology and cerebellar pathology. In recent years, renewed interest in the use of stereotactic neurosurgical procedures and DBS in the treatment of Parkinson's disease and other basal ganglia disorders has provided the opportunity for examining the effects of discrete circumscribed lesions in the globus pallidus and thalamus and electrical stimulation of the STN and thalamus on motor speech function. The preliminary data from this line of research suggest that the use of these techniques combined with functional neuroimaging based on PET and fMRI has the potential to further inform debate regarding the hypothesized roles of subcortical structures in speech motor control. In particular when combined with functional neuroimaging such as PET and fMRI, DBS has the potential to be a powerful technique for assessing the effect of discrete perturbations at different nodes of the basal ganglia–thalamocortical and cerebello-thalamocortical circuits (including the substantia nigra, globus pallidus, putamen, caudate nucleus, thalamus, STN and cerebellum). Utilization of such a combined approach would enable testing of contemporary models of subcortical functional organization through comparison of expected responses predicted by the models with specific changes in brain activity as identified by the functional neuroimaging. Such comparisons based on a range of task-specific speech-production activities would enable further determination of the differential contributions of various subcortical structures to speech motor control.

References

Ackermann, H. and Ziegler, W. (1992). Cerebellar dysarthria: a review. *Fortsch Neurology Psychiatry* 60, 28–40.

Ackermann, H. and Hertrich, I. (1995). Kinematic analysis of lower lip movements in ataxic dysathria. *Journal of Speech and Hearing Research* 38, 1252–9.

Ackermann, H. and Hertrich, I. (1994). Speech rate and rhythm in cerebellar dysarthria: an acoustic analysis of syllabic timing. *Folia Phoniatrica* 46, 70–8.

Ackermann, H. and Hertrich, I. (2000). The contribution of the cerebellum to speech processing. *Journal of Neurolinguistics* 13, 95–116.

Ackermann, H., Vogel, M., Petersen, D. and Poremba, M. (1992). Speech deficits in ischaemic cerebellar lesions. *Journal of Neurology* 239, 223–7.

Agid, Y. (1998). Levodopa: is toxicology a myth? *Neurology* 50, 858–63.

Alexander, G.E., DeLong, M.R. and Strick, P.L. (1986). Parallel organization of functionally segregated circuits linking basal ganglia and cortex. *Annual Review of Neuroscience* 9, 357–81.

Alexander, G.E., Crutcher, M.D. and DeLong, M.R. (1990). Basal ganglia-thalamocortical circuits: parallel substrates for motor, oculomotor, prefrontal and limbic functions. *Progress in Brain Research* 85, 119–46.

Allan, C.M., Turner, J.W. and Gadea-Ciria, M. (1966). Investigations into speech disturbance following stereotaxic surgery for Parkinsonism. *British Journal of Disorders of Communication* 1, 55–9.

Barlow, S.H., Iacono, R.P., Paseman, L.A., Biswas, A. and D'Antonio, L. (1998). The effects of posteroventral pallidotomy on force and speech aerodynamics in Parkinson's disease. In M.P. Cannito, C.M. Yorkston and D.R. Beukelman (eds), *Neuromotor Speech Disorders: Nature, Assessment and Management* (pp. 117–55). Baltimore, MD: Paul H. Brookes.

Baron, M.S., Jerrold, L., Vitek, J., Roy, A.E., Bakay, R. *et al.* (1997). Treatment of advanced Parkinson's disease by GPi pallidotomy: 1 year pilot study results. *Annals of Neurology* 40, 355–66.

Bathia, K.P. and Marsden, C.D. (1994). The behavioural and motor consequences of focal lesions of the basal ganglia in man. *Brain* 117, 859–76.

Bejjani, B.P., Gervais, D. and Arnulf, I. (2000). Axial parkinsonian symptoms can be improved: the role of levodopa and bilateral subthalamic stimulation. *Journal of Neurology, Neurosurgery and Psychiatry* 68, 595–600.

Bell, D.S. (1968). Speech functions of the thalamus inferred from the effects of thalamotomy. *Brain* 91, 619–38.

Bell-Barti, F. and Chevrie-Muller, C. (1991). Motor levels of speech timing: evidence from studies of ataxia. *Haskins Laboratories Status Report on Speech Research* SR-107/108, 87–92.

Benabid, A.L., Pollak, P. and Gross, C. (1994). Acute and long-term effects of subthalamic nucleus stimulation in Parkinson's disease. *Stereotactic Functional Neurosurgery* 62, 76–84.

Benabid, A.L., Ni, Z., Chabardes, S., Benazzouz, A. and Pollak, P. (2001). How are we inhibiting functional targets with high frequency stimulation? In K. Kultas-Ilinsky and I. Ilinsky (eds), *Basal Ganglia and Thalamus in Health and Movement* (pp. 309–15). New York: Kluwer Academic/Plenum Publishers.

Bonnet, A.M., Loria, Y., Saint-Hilaire, M.H., Lhermitte, F. and Agid, Y. (1987). Does long-term aggravation of Parkinson's disease result from non-dopaminergic lesions. *Neurology* 37, 1539–42.

Brooks, D.J. (1991). Detection of preclinical Parkinson's disease with PET. *Neurology* 41 (suppl. 2), 24.

Calne, D. and Snow, B.J. (1993). PET imaging in Parkinsonism. *Advances in Neurology* 60, 484.

Carpenter, M.A., Pahwa, R., Miyawaki, K.L., Wilkinson, S.B., Searl, J.P. *et al.* (1998). Reduction in voice tremor under thalamic stimulation. *Neurology* 50, 796–8.

Chenery, H.J., Murdoch, B.E. and Ingram, J.C.L. (1988). Studies in Parkinson's disease: 1. perceptual speech analysis. *Australian Journal of Human Communication Disorders* 16, 17–29.

Darley, F.L., Aronson, A.E. and Brown, J.R. (1975). Motor speech disorders. Philadelphia: W.B. Saunders.

DeLong, M.R. (1990). Primate models of movement disorders of basal ganglia origin. *Trends in Neurosciences* 13, 281–5.

De Nil, L.F., Kroll, R.M. and Houle, S. (2001). Functional neuroimaging of cerebellar activation during single word reading and verb generation in stuttering and nonstuttering adults. *Neuroscience Letters* 302, 77–80.

Dieber, M.P., Pollak, P. and Passingham, R. (1993). Thalamic stimulation and suppression of parkinsonian tremor: evidence of cerebellar deactivation using position emission tomography. *Brain* 116, 267–79.

Dromey, C., Kumar, R., Lang, A.E. and Lozano, A.M. (2000). An investigation of the effects of subthalamic nucleus stimulation on acoustic measures of voice. *Movement Disorders* 15, 1132–8.

Eidelberg, D. (1992). Positron emission tomography studies in Parkinsonism. *Neurology Clinics* 10, 421.

Filion, M. and Tremblay, L. (1991). Abnormal spontaneous activity of globus pallidus neurons in monkeys with MPTP-induced Parkinsonism. *Brain Research* 547, 142.

Filion, M., Tremblay, L. and Bedard, P.J. (1988). Abnormal influences of passive limb movement on the activity of globus pallidus neurons in Parkinsonian monkeys. *Brain Research* 444, 165.

Forrest, K. and Weismer, G. (1995). Dynamic aspects of lower lip movement in parkinsonian and neurologically normal geriatric speakers' production of stress. *Journal of Speech and Hearing Research* 38, 260–72.

Gentil, M., Garcia-Ruiz, P., Pollak, P. and Benabid, A.L. (1999a). Effects of stimulation of the subthalamic nucleus on oral control of patients with Parkinsonism. *Journal of Neurology, Neurosurgery and Psychiatry* 67, 329–33.

Gentil, M., Tournier, C.L., Pollak, P. and Benabid, A.L. (1999b). Effect of bilateral subthalamic nucleus stimulation and dopatherapy on oral control in Parkinson's disease. *European Neurology* 42, 136–40.

Gentil, M., Chauvin, P., Pinto, S., Pollak, P. and Benabid, A.L. (2000). Effect of bilateral stimulation of the subthalamic nucleus on Parkinsonian voice. *Brain and Language* 78, 233–40.

Gentil, M., Pinto, S., Pollak, P. and Benabid, A.L. (2003). Effect of bilateral stimulation of the subthalamic nucleus on Parkinsonian dysarthria. *Brain and Language* 85, 190–6.

Gerfen, C.R. (1995). Dopamine receptor function in the basal ganglia. *Clinical Neuropharmacology* 18, S162.

Grafton, S.T. and DeLong, M. (1997). Tracing the brain's circuitry with functional imaging. *Nature Medicine* 3, 602–3.

Grafton, S.T., Mazziotta, J.C., Presty, S., Friston, K.J., Frackowiak, R.S. *et al.* (1992). Functional anatomy of human procedural learning determined with regional cerebral blood flow and PET. *Journal of Neuroscience* 12, 2542–8.

Graybiel, A.M. and Kimura, M. (1995). Adaptive neural networks in the basal ganglia. In J.D. Houk, J.L. Davis and D.G. Beiser (eds), *Models of Information Processing in the Basal Ganglia* (pp. 103–16). Cambridge, MA: MIT Press.

Gross, C., Rougier, A., Guehl, D., Boraud, T., Julien, J. *et al.* (1997). High-frequency stimulation of the globus pallidus internalis in Parkinson's disease: a study of seven cases. *Journal of Neurosurgery* 87, 491–8.

Hallett, M., Berardelli, A., Matheson, J., Rothwell, J. and Marsden, C.D. (1991). Physiological analysis of simple rapid movements in patients with cerebellar deficits. *Journal of Neurology, Neurosurgery and Psychiatry* 53, 124–33.

Hirai, T., Miyazaki, M., Nakajima, H., Shibazaki, T. and Ohye, C. (1983). The correlation between tremor characteristics and the predicted volume of effective lesions in the stereotaxic nucleus ventralis intermedius thalamotomy. *Brain* 106, 1001–18.

Hoffman-Ruddy, B., Schulz, G., Vitek, J.L. and Evatt, M. (2001). A preliminary study of the effects of subthalamic nucleus (STN) deep brain stimulation (DBS) on voice and speech characteristics in Parkinson's disease. *Clinical Linguistics and Phonetics* 15, 97–101.

Hunker, C.J. and Abbs, J.H. (1984). Physiological analyses of parkinsonian tremors in the orofacial system. In M.R. McNeil, J.C. Rosenbek and A.E. Aronson (eds), *The Dysarthrias: Physiology, Acoustics, Perception, Management* (pp. 69–100). San Diego, CA: College-Hill Press.

Iacono, R.P., Shima, F., Lonser, R., Kuniyoshi, S., Maeda, G. *et al.* (1995). The results, indications and physiology of posteroventral pallidotomy for patients with Parkinson's disease. *Neurosurgery* 36, 1118–24.

Jenkins, A.C. (1968). Speech defects following stereotaxic operations for the relief of tremor and rigidity in Parkinsonism. *The Medical Journal of Australia* 7, 585–8.

Jenkins, I.H. and Frackowiak, R.S. (1993). Functional studies in human cerebellum with positron emission tomography. *Review Neurology Paris* 149, 647–53.

Johannson, F., Malm, J., Nordh, E. and Hariz, M. (1997). Usefulness of pallidotomy for advanced Parkinson's disease. *Journal of Neurology, Neurosurgery and Psychiatry* 62, 125–32.

Kelly, P. (1995). Pallidotomy in Parkinson's disease. *Neurosurgery* 36, 1154–7.

Kent, R.D. and Netsell, R. (1975). A case study of an ataxic dysarthric: cineradiographic and spectrographic observations. *Journal of Speech and Hearing Disorders* 40, 115–34.

Kent, R.D., Netsell, R. and Abbs, J. (1979). Acoustic characteristics of dysarthria associated with cerebellar disease. *Journal of Speech and Hearing Research* 22, 627–48.

Kent, R.D., Kent, J.F., Rosenbek, J.C., Vorperian, H.K. and Weismer, G. (1997). A speaking task analysis of the dysarthria in cerebellar disease. *Folia Phoniatrica and Logopedica* 49, 63–82.

Koller, W. and Hristova, A. (1996). Efficacy and safety of stereotaxic surgical treatment of tremor disorders. *European Journal of Neurology* 3, 507–14.

Koller, W., Pahwa, R., Busenbark, K., Hubble, S., Wilkinson, S.B. *et al.* (1997). High frequency unilateral thalamic stimulation in the treatment of essential and parkinsonian tremor. *Annals of Neurology* 42, 292–9.

Kompoliti, K., Wang, Q.E., Goetz, C.F., Leurgans, S. and Raman, W. (2000). Effects of central dopaminergic stimulation by apomorphine on speech in Parkinson's disease. *Neurology* 54, 458–62.

Krack, P., Pollak, P. and Limousin, P. (1998). Subthalamic nucleus or internal pallidal stimulation in young-onset Parkinson's disease. *Brain* 121, 451–7.

Krack, P., Batir, A., Van Blercom, N., Chabardes, S., Fraix, V. *et al.* (2003). Five-year follow-up of bilateral stimulation of the subthalamic nucleus in advanced Parkinson's disease. *New England Journal of Medicine* 349, 1925–34.

La Blance, G.R. and Rutherford, D.R. (1991). Respiratory dynamics and speech intelligibility in speakers with generalized dystonia. *Journal of Communication Disorders* 24, 141–56.

Laitinen, L.V. (1995). Pallidotomy for Parkinson's disease. *Neurosurgery Clinics North America* 6, 105.

Lang A.E., Lozano, A.M., Montgomery, E., Duffy, J., Tasker, R. *et al.* (1998). Posteroventral medial pallidotomy in advanced Parkinson's disease. *New England Journal of Medicine* 338, 262–3.

Lechtenberg, R. and Gilman, S. (1978). Speech disorders in cerebellar disease. *Annals of Neurology* 3, 285–90.

Leenders, K.L. (1997). Pathophysiology of movement disorders studied using PET. *Journal of Neural Transmission* 50, 39–46.

Legg, C.F. and Sonnenberg, B.R. (1998). Changes in aspects of speech and language functioning following unilateral pallidotomy. *Aphasiology* 12, 257–66.

Limousin, P., Pollack, P., Benazzouz, A., Hoffmann, D., Le Bas, J.F. *et al.* (1995). Effect of parkinsonian signs and symptoms of bilateral subthalamic nucleus stimulation. *Lancet* 345, 91–5.

Limousin, P., Greene, J., Pollak, P., Rothwell, J., Benabid, A.L. *et al.* (1997). Changes in cerebral activity pattern due to subthalamic nucleus or internal pallidum stimulation in Parkinson's disease. *Annals of Neurology* 42, 283–91.

Lisberger, S.G. (1988). The neural basis for learning of simple motor skills. *Science* 242, 728–35.

Middleton, F.A. and Strick, P.L. (1997). Dentate output channels: motor and cognitive components. *Progress in Brain Research* 114, 555–68.

Middleton, F.A. and Strick, P.L. (2000). Basal ganglia output and cognition: evidence from anatomical, behavioural and clinical studies. *Brain and Cognition* 42, 183–200.

Middleton, F.A. and Strick, P.L. (2001). Cerebellar projections to the prefrontal cortex of the primate. *Journal of Neuroscience* 21, 700–12.

Miller, W.C. and DeLong, M.R. (1987). Altered tonic activity of neurons in the globus pallidus and subthalamic nucleus in the primate MPTP model of parkinsonism. In M.B. Carpenter and A. Jayaraman (eds), *The Basal Ganglia II* (p. 415). New York: Plenum.

Murdoch, B.E. (1990). *Acquired Speech and Language Disorders: a Neuroanatomical and Functional Neurological Approach*. London: Chapman and Hall.

Murdoch, B.E. (1998). *Dysarthria: a Physiological Approach to Assessment and Treatment*. Cheltenham: Stanley Thornes.

Murdoch, B.E., Chenery, H.J., Bowler, S. and Ingram, J.C.L. (1989). Respiratory function in Parkinson's subjects exhibiting a perceptible speech deficit: a kinematic and spirometric analysis. *Journal of Speech and Hearing Disorders* 54, 610–26.

Ojemann, G.A. and Ward, A.A. (1971). Speech representation in ventrolateral thalamus. *Brain* 94, 669–80.

Pahwa, R., Lyons, K. and Wilkinson, S.B. (1999). Bilateral thalamic stimulation for the treatment of essential tremor. *Neurology* 53, 1447–50.

Parent, A., Lévesque, M. and Parent, M. (2001). A re-evaluation of the current model of the basal ganglia. *Parkinsonism and Related Disorders* 7, 193–8.

Petrovici, J.N. (1980). Speech disturbances following stereotaxic surgery in ventrolateral thalamus. *Neurosurgical Review* 3, 189–95.

Quaglieri, C.E. and Celesia, G.G. (1977). Effects of thalamotomy and levadopa therapy on the speech of Parkinson patients. *European Neurology* 15, 34–9.

Raichle, M.E., Fiez, J.A., Videen, T.O. *et al.* (1994). Practice-related changes in human brain functional anatomy during nonmotor learning. *Cerebral Cortex* 4, 8–26.

Richards, M., Marder, K., Cote, L. and Mayeux, R. (1994). Interrater reliability of the Unified Parkinson's Disease Rating Scale motor examination. *Movement Disorders* 9, 89–91.

Samuels, M., Caputo, E., Brooks, D.J., Schrag, A., Scaravilli, T. *et al.* (1998). A study of medial pallidotomy for Parkinson's disease: clinical outcome, MRI location and complications. *Brain* 121, 59–75.

Sanes, J.N., Dimitrov, B. and Hallett, M. (1990). Motor learning in patients with cerebellar dysfunction. *Brain* 113, 103–20.

Santens, P., De Letter, M., Van Borsel, J., DeReuck, J. and Caemaert, J. (2003). Lateralized effects of sub-thalamic nucleus stimulation on different aspects of speech in Parkinson's disease. *Brain and Language* 87, 243–58.

Schaltenbrand, G. (1975). The effects on speech and language of stereotactical stimulation in thalamus and corpus callosum. *Brain and Language* 2, 70–7.

Schmahmann, J.D. (2001). The cerebrocerebellar system: anatomic substrates of the cerebellar contribution to cognition and emotion. *International Review of Psychiatry* 13, 247–60.

Schneider, S.L., Duffy, J.R. and Uitti, R.J. (1999). *Motor speech changes following pallidotomy in patients with Parkinson's disease.* Paper presented at the American-Speech-Language-Hearing Association Annual Convention, San Francisco, CA.

Schonle, P.W., Dressler, D. and Conrad, B. (1990). Orofacial movement impairments in cerebellar dysarthria: a kinematic analysis with electromagnetic articulography. In A. Beradelli, R. Benecke, M. Manfredi and C.D. Marsden (eds), *Motor Disturbances II* (pp. 249–59). New York: Academic Press.

Schulz, G.M., Peterson, T., Sapienza, C.M., Greer, M. and Friedman, W. (1999). Voice and speech characteristics of persons with Parkinson's disease pre- and post-pallidotomy surgery: preliminary findings. *Journal of Speech, Language and Hearing Research* 42, 1176–94.

Scott, R.B., Gregory, R., Hines, N., Carroll, C., Hyman, N. *et al.* (1998). Neuropsychological, neurological and functional outcome following pallidotomy for Parkinson's disease: a consecutive series of eight simultaneous bilateral and twelve unilateral procedures. *Brain* 121, 659–75.

Selby, G. (1967). Stereotactic surgery for the relief of Parkinson's disease. I. A critical review. *Journal of Neurological Science* 15, 315.

Solomon, N.P. and Hixon, T.J. (1993). Speech breathing in Parkinson's disease. *Journal of Speech and Hearing Research* 36, 294–310.

Solomon, N.P., McKee, A.S., Larson, K.J., Nawrocki, M.D., Tuite, P.J. *et al.* (2000). Effects of pallidal stimulation on speech in three men with Parkinson's disease. *American Journal of Speech-Language Pathology* 9, 241–56.

Starr, P.A., Rau, S. and Davis, V. (2005). Spontaneous neuronal activity in human dystonia: comparison with Parkinson's disease and normal macaque. *Journal of Neurophysiology* 93, 3165–76.

Strick, P.L., Dunn, R.P. and Picard, N. (1995). Macro-organization of the circuits connecting the basal ganglia with the cortical motor areas. In J.C. Houk, J.L. Davis and D.G. Beiser (eds), *Models of Information Processing in the Basal Ganglia* (pp. 117–30). Cambridge, MA: MIT Press.

Svennilson, E., Torvik, A. and Lowe, R. (1960). Treatment of Parkinsonism by stereotactic thermolesions in the pallidal region. *Acta Psychiatry Neurology Scandinavia* 35, 358–77.

Taha, J.M., Janszen, M.A. and Favre, J. (1999). Thalamic deep brain stimulation for the treatment of head, voice and bilateral limb tremor. *Journal of Neurosurgery* 91, 68–72.

Tasker, R.R., Siqueira, J. and Hawrylyshyn, L.W.O. (1983). What happened to VIM thalamotomy for Parkinson's disease? *Applied Neurophysiology* 46, 68–83.

Theodoros, D.G. and Murdoch, B.E. (1998a). Hypokinetic dysarthria. In B.E. Murdoch (ed.), *Dysarthria: a Physiological Approach to Assessment and Treatment* (pp. 266–313). Cheltenham: Stanley Thornes.

Theodoros, D.G. and Murdoch, B.E. (1998b). Hyperkinetic dysarthria. In B.E. Murdoch (ed.), *Dysarthria: a Physiological Approach to Assessment and Treatment* (pp. 314–36). Cheltenham: Stanley Thornes.

Theodoros, D.G., Ward, E.C., Murdoch, B.E., Silburn, P. and Lethlean, J. (2000). Impact of pallidotomy on motor speech function in Parkinson's disease: preliminary perceptual and physiological findings. *Journal of Medical Speech-Language Pathology* 8, 315–22.

Topka, H., Valls-Sole, J., Massaquoi, S.G. and Hallett, M. (1993). Deficits in classical conditioning in patients with cerebellar degeneration. *Brain* 116, 961–9.

Tornqvist, A.L., Schalen, L. and Rehncrona, S. (2005). Effects of different electrical parameter settings on the intelligibility of speech in patients with Parkinson's disease treated with subthalamic deep brain stimulation. *Movement Disorders* 20, 416–23.

Wichmann, T., Bergman, H. and DeLong, M.R. (1994). The primate subthalamic nucleus. 1. Functional properties in intact animals. *Journal of Neurophysiology* 72, 494.

Wildgruber, D., Ackermann, H. and Grodd, W. (2001). Differential contributions of motor cortex, basal ganglia and cerebellum to speech motor control: effects of syllable repetition rate evaluated by fMRI. *Neuroimage* 13, 101–9.

Wolfe, V.I., Garvin, J.S., Bacon, M. and Waldrop, W. (1975). Speech changes in Parkinson's disease during treatment with L-dopa. *Journal of Communication Disorders* 8, 271–9.

Zraick, R.I., LaPointe, L.L., Case, J.L. and Duane, D.D. (1993). Acoustic correlates of vocal quality in individuals with spasmodic torticolis. *Journal of Medical Speech-Language Pathology* 1, 261–9.

Zwirner, P. and Barnes, G.J. (1992). Vocal tract steadiness: a measure of phonatory upper airway motor control during phonation in dysarthria. *Journal of Speech and Hearing Research* 35, 761–8.

11 Dysarthria associated with subcortical pathologies

Introduction

The occurrence of dysarthria in association with neurological conditions caused by pathological changes in the basal ganglia (e.g. Parkinson's disease, Huntington's disease) or cerebellum is well documented and is widely regarded as indicative of a role for subcortical structures in the motor control of the speech-production mechanism. Pathological changes involving the basal ganglia and cerebellum produce well-described alterations in motor function such as tremor, rigidity of the muscles, akinesia or dysmetria, which in turn may affect the normal functioning of the speech-production mechanism, leading to dysarthria. It is thought that many of these symptoms may be due to disruption of the basal ganglia or cerebellar outputs to areas of the cerebral cortex involved in the control of movement. In recent years, several models have been proposed in an attempt to further elucidate the possible contribution of subcortical structures to motor control and to explain the occurrence of movement disorders subsequent to basal ganglia and cerebellar lesions. These models are described and discussed fully in Chapter 10.

As in the case of movement disorders of basal ganglia origin affecting limb and trunk muscles, dysarthrias associated with lesions in the basal ganglia take the form of hypo- and hyperkinetic movement disorders. In general, hypokinetic disorders (e.g. Parkinson's disease) are associated with increased basal ganglia output, whereas hyperkinetic movement disorders (e.g. Huntington's disease) are associated with decreased output. Hypokinetic disorders are characterized by significant impairments in movement initiation (akinesia) and reduction in the velocity of voluntary movements (bradykinesia) and are usually accompanied by muscular rigidity and tremor at rest. By contrast, hyperkinetic disorders are characterized by excessive motor activity in the form of involuntary movements (dyskinesia) with varying degrees of hypotonia. With regard to their effect on the speech-production mechanism, these disorders manifest as hypokinetic dysarthria (classically associated with Parkinson's disease) and hyperkinetic dysarthria (seen in association with a range of hyperkinetic conditions such as Huntington's disease, dystonia, etc.).

Ataxic dysarthria is the motor speech disorder classically associated with brain lesions involving the cerebellum or its connections. As in the case of the basal ganglia dysarthrias mentioned above, the clinical features of ataxic dysarthria follow on from the neuromotor abnormalities associated with damage to the cerebellum, in particular ataxia. In contemporary neurological literature, the term ataxia is used to define motor disturbances of cerebellar origin associated with a variety of clinical symptoms including dysmetria-hypermetria, asynergia, postural and gait instability, intention tremor and space-time motor incoordination.

Dysarthrias associated with basal ganglia pathology: hypo- and hyperkinetic dysarthria

Hypokinetic dysarthria

Hypokinetic dysarthria is most commonly associated with Parkinson's disease. In fact, the term hypokinetic dysarthria was first used by Darley *et al.* (1969a, 1969b) to describe the resultant complex pattern of perceptual speech characteristics associated with Parkinsonism. More recently an acoustically similar form of dysarthria has also been observed in persons with progressive supranuclear palsy (Steele–Richardson–Olszewski syndrome) (Hanson and Metter, 1980; Metter and Hanson, 1986).

Parkinson's disease
Parkinson's disease is a progressive, degenerative, neurological disease associated with selective loss of dopaminergic neurones in the pars compacta of the substantia nigra (Uitti and Calne, 1993). The annual incidence of Parkinson's disease is estimated to be 20 per 100000. The cumulative lifetime risk for Parkinsonism is greater than 1 in 40, making it one of the more common neurological diseases. Onset is insidious and the course is that of slow progression of disability over many years. The degree and rate of progression, however, does vary from patient to patient. Parkinson's disease begins most commonly after age 40 with the mean age of onset between 58 and 62 years. The age-specific incidence of Parkinson's disease peaks in the age group 70–79 years (Martilla and Rinne, 1991). The cardinal signs of Parkinson's disease include akinesia/bradykinesia, rigidity, tremor at rest and postural reflex impairment. The degree to which each of these signs is present varies from patient to patient. Affected persons may complain of rigidity and tremor, immobility of facial expression, slowness of movements and diminished swinging of the arms and heaviness of the limbs when walking. Posture is often stooped forward, with the arms at the sides, elbows slightly flexed and fingers adducted. The patients often exhibit a characteristic gait, which involves short, slow, shuffling steps. Dementia occurs in approximately 41% of Parkinsonian cases. A speech disorder may in some cases be the first symptom to emerge (Hoehn and Yahr, 1967). Gracco *et al.* (1993) and Hanson (1991) found laryngeal dysfunction to be readily observable in subjects with early Parkinson's disease, and indicated that it may precede the appearance of symptoms elsewhere. It has been estimated that 60–80% of patients with Parkinson's disease exhibit a hypokinetic dysarthria with the prevalence increasing as the disease advances (Scott *et al.*, 1985; Johnson and Pring, 1990). For a full description of the neuropathology, clinical features and medical treatment of Parkinson's disease see Chapter 8.

Progressive supranuclear palsy
Progressive supranuclear palsy is conventionally taken to refer to the subcortical degenerative syndrome of unknown aetiology that produces an akinetic-rigid form of Parkinson's disease first described by Steele *et al.* (1964). Affected persons have an akinetic-rigid syndrome, pseudobulbar palsy and dementia of frontal type associated with lesions located in the basal ganglia (including the globus pallidus, caudate

nucleus and subthalamic nucleus), brain stem and cerebellar nuclei. Hypokinetic dysarthria is the prominent dysarthria type in progressive supranuclear palsy, but in the early stages of the disorder, the dysarthria is often mixed with hypokinetic, spastic and ataxic components (Kluin *et al.*, 1993). Onset of the disorder is usually in middle to later life and the condition is rapidly progressive, resulting in marked incapacity of the patient in 2–3 years.

Clinical characteristics of hypokinetic dysarthria
In contrast to other forms of dysarthria, the clinical characteristics of hypokinetic dysarthria were identified by a systematic analysis of patients with a specific disease, namely idiopathic Parkinson's disease. Overall, the speech characteristics associated with hypokinetic dysarthria follow largely from the generalized pattern of hypokinetic motor disorders which includes marked reductions in the amplitude of voluntary movement (akinesia), initiation difficulties, slowness of movement (bradykinesia), muscular rigidity, tremor at rest and postural reflex impairments. According to Darley *et al.* (1975), marked limitation of the range of movement of the muscles of the speech mechanism is the outstanding characteristic of hypokinesia as it affects speech. These authors stated that the reduced mobility, restricted range of movement and supranormal rate of the repetitive movements of the muscles involved in speech production lead to the various manifestations of hypokinetic dysarthria.

Although impairments in all aspects of speech production (i.e. respiration, phonation, resonance, articulation and prosody) involving the various subsystems of the speech-production mechanism have been identified in individuals with Parkinson's disease, these individuals are most likely to exhibit disturbances of prosody, phonation and articulation (Darley *et al.*, 1975; Chenery *et al.*, 1988; Zwirner and Barnes, 1992). The reported features of the speech disturbance in Parkinson's disease commonly include monotony of pitch and loudness, decreased use of all vocal parameters for effecting stress and emphasis, breathy and harsh voice quality, reduced vocal intensity, variable rate including short rushes of speech or accelerated speech, consonant imprecision, impaired breath support for speech, reduction in phonation time, difficulty in the initiation of speech activities and inappropriate silences (Darley *et al.*, 1969a, 1969b; Ludlow and Bassich, 1983, 1984; Scott *et al.*, 1985; Chenery *et al.*, 1988). Reduced pitch and loudness variation were among the most prominent speech deficits observed in patients with Parkinson's disease in the perceptual-based studies of Darley *et al.* (1969a, 1969b, 1975). Based on their average perceptual rating scores, the following hierarchy of deviant speech dimensions was observed in 32 patients with Parkinson's disease: (1) monopitch, (2) reduced stress, (3) monoloudness and (4) imprecise consonants.

The reported findings, however, have not always been consistent with respect to the type of disturbances, the frequency of occurrence, and the degree of severity of the abnormal perceptual, acoustic and physiological features present in the speech of persons with hypokinetic dysarthria. For example, Darley *et al.* (1975) reported that in 15 of their 32 patients with Parkinson's disease, the average perceived speech loudness levels were lower than those of other dysarthric groups, suggesting that reduced speech loudness is a distinctive feature of speech in Parkinson's disease and as such may have a useful role in the differential diagnosis of hypokinetic dysarthria. Nevertheless, reduced speech loudness does not appear to be present in all dysarthric patients with Parkinson's disease. Ludlow and Bassich (1984) reported that only 42% (5/12) of their dysarthric patients with Parkinson's disease were perceived to have reduced speech loudness. Similarly, in a more recent study Gamboa *et al.* (1997)

reported that only 49% of dysarthric patients with Parkinson's disease (20/41) self-reported they had developed hypophonia. It has been suggested that these values may underestimate the actual proportion of dysarthric patients with Parkinson's disease who are hypophonic, given that many of these people appear to be able to compensate for their hypophonia during formal speech testing. Further patients with Parkinson's disease may have perceptual deficits that make it difficult for them to accurately identify hypophonia in their own speech (Ho et al., 2000).

Respiratory function in hypokinetic dysarthria

A number of the perceptual features identified in hypokinetic dysarthria, such as reduction in overall loudness, decay of loudness, reduced phrase length, short rushes of speech and reduced phonation time, have been attributed to the impairment of respiration (Darley et al., 1975). In support of these assumptions, Chenery et al. (1988) identified a mild impairment of respiratory support for speech in the majority (89%) of their subjects with Parkinson's disease. In addition, more than half of their subjects demonstrated reductions in phrase lengths, short rushes of speech, reduced loudness and decay of loudness during speech. Similarly Ludlow and Bassich (1984) identified a reduction in overall loudness in 42% of their subjects, and the majority of the cases with Parkinson's disease demonstrated a variable rate of speech which could be partially attributed to respiratory insufficiency.

Patients with Parkinson's disease have been identified by several investigators to exhibit significant reductions in their vital capacity (Cramer, 1940; De La Torre et al., 1960). In particular, De La Torre et al. (1960) found that two-thirds of their subjects with Parkinson's disease recorded vital capacities 40% below the expected values. Laszewski (1956) reported that the majority of his subjects exhibited a marked reduction in vital capacity, with little measurable thoracic excursion during inhalation or exhalation. During a sustained phonation task, Mueller (1971) found that subjects with Parkinson's disease expended significantly smaller volumes of air than control subjects. Using spirographic analysis, Hovestadt et al. (1989) revealed that, on non-speech tasks, peak inspiratory and expiratory flow and maximum expiratory flow at a 50% level were significantly below normal for patients with relatively severe Parkinson's disease. In contrast, neither Murdoch et al. (1989) nor Solomon and Hixon (1993) identified significant overall reductions in vital capacity and lung volumes in their groups of subjects with Parkinson's disease.

Recent studies involving kinematic investigations of respiratory function in Parkinson's disease have also identified incoordinaton of the components of the chest wall during speech breathing. Murdoch et al. (1989) identified irregularities in chest-wall movement during the production of sustained vowels and syllable repetitions. These abnormal chest-wall movements took the form of abrupt changes in the relative contribution of the chest-wall components and featured both ribcage and abdominal paradoxical movements. In addition, Murdoch et al. (1989) found that the subjects with Parkinson's disease demonstrated a wide range of relative volume contributions of the ribcage and abdomen during speech breathing, with a predominance of ribcage involvement. However, Solomon and Hixon (1993), using different instrumentation, recorded smaller ribcage than abdominal contribution to lung volume change in speech breathing of patients with Parkinson's disease and found that ribcage and abdominal paradoxing were not specific to subjects with Parkinson's disease alone. Both studies, however, identified a significantly greater breathing rate and minute ventilation in subjects with Parkinson's disease compared with control subjects.

Speech and language disorders

Laryngeal function in hypokinetic dysarthria

Phonatory disturbance is often the initial symptom of the ensuing speech disorder associated with Parkinson's disease. In fact, Logemann *et al.* (1978) identified laryngeal problems as being the most prominent deviant features in their group of 200 subjects with Parkinson's disease, occurring in 89% of cases. Similarly, about half of the deviant speech dimensions identified by Darley *et al.* (1975) and Ludlow and Bassich (1983) as being the most distinguishing features of hypokinetic dysarthria related to phonatory disturbance. The deviant perceptual features associated with laryngeal dysfunction in Parkinson's disease include disorders of vocal quality and impairment of the overall levels and variability of pitch and loudness.

Descriptions of the vocal quality of the hypokinetic speaker have included a number of deviant vocal parameters including hoarseness, harshness, breathiness, vocal tremor and glottal fry. Inconsistencies in the frequency of occurrence of these deviant phonatory features are apparent across many of the reported perceptual studies. In relation to hoarseness and harshness, the perceptual findings would appear to be equivocal with respect to the prominence of either feature in the vocal output of persons with hypokinetic dysarthria. Hoarseness was perceived to be present in 45% of patients in Logemann *et al.*'s (1981) study, one-third of subjects examined by Ludlow and Bassich (1984), in each subject in the Chenery *et al.* (1988) study and in 84% of the subjects with Parkinson's disease assessed by Murdoch *et al.* (1995). Hoarseness, however, was not found to be a prominent deviant dimension in the study reported by Darley *et al.* (1975). Instead, harshness was listed among the 10 most deviant speech features identified by these latter authors. A harsh vocal quality has been perceived to be present in 77–84% of patients with hypokinetic dysarthria (Ludlow and Bassich, 1984; Chenery *et al.*, 1988; Zwirner and Barnes, 1992). Although there is some degree of inconsistency in the reported frequency of occurrence of breathiness in hypokinetic dysarthria, it would appear that a breathy vocal quality is also a relatively common characteristic of this type of dysarthria (Darley *et al.*, 1975). Breathiness has been reported to occur in approximately 50–95% of patients with hypokinetic dysarthria (Chenery *et al.*, 1988; Zwirner and Barnes, 1992; Murdoch *et al.*, 1995). Glottal fry has been identified in 60–85% of cases with hypokinetic dysarthria, whereas pitch unsteadiness or vocal tremor has been reported to be present in approximately 65% of subjects with Parkinson's disease (Chenery *et al.*, 1988; Murdoch *et al.*, 1995). The findings of acoustic studies suggest that the disorders of vocal quality perceived to be present in patients with Parkinson's disease result from phonatory inefficiency due to abnormal positioning of the vocal folds, irregular vocal-fold activity and problems with the synchronization of phonation and articulation.

In addition to deviations in vocal quality, the hypokinetic dysarthria associated with Parkinson's disease is characterized perceptually by the presence of monotony of pitch and loudness and a reduction in overall pitch and loudness levels. Both monotony of pitch and loudness have been identified as prominent features of verbal output of subjects with Parkinson's disease, being the first and third most deviant perceptual speech features of hypokinetic dysarthria documented by Darley *et al.* (1975), respectively. Later perceptual studies have confirmed the presence of monotony of pitch and loudness in the majority of subjects with Parkinson's disease (Ludlow and Bassich, 1984; Chenery *et al.*, 1988; Zwirner and Barnes, 1992). Similarly, acoustic findings have provided consistent evidence of a reduction in the variability of pitch and loudness in the speech output of these subjects (Metter and Hanson, 1986; Flint *et al.*, 1992; King *et al.*, 1994).

Unfortunately, few studies reported in the literature have been based on physiological investigation of laryngeal function in persons with Parkinson's disease. Collectively, those studies that have been reported have shown that individuals with Parkinson's disease demonstrate abnormal vocal-fold posturing and vibratory patterns and laryngeal aerodynamics (Hanson *et al.*, 1983; Hirose *et al.*, 1985; Gerratt *et al.*, 1987; Murdoch *et al.*, 1995). Physiological studies utilizing photoglottography (PGG) and electroglottography (EGG) have identified abnormal vocal-fold vibratory patterns in patients with Parkinson's disease (Hanson *et al.*, 1983; Gerratt *et al.*, 1987). Essentially these studies have demonstrated a proportionately greater amount of time spent in opening relative to closing duration with no well-defined closed period (Hanson *et al.*, 1983; Gerratt *et al.*, 1987). Hanson *et al.* (1983) noted that only 15% of the glottal cycle was spent in the 'closed period'. In addition these latter authors found that the waveform shape varied widely from cycle to cycle, suggesting variability in the control of vocal-fold posture. Abnormalities in the laryngeal aerodynamics of persons with Parkinson's disease as identified by instrumental studies are also generally consistent with impaired laryngeal function in this group. Murdoch *et al.* (1995) identified a hyperfunctional pattern of laryngeal activity in subjects with Parkinson's disease characterized by increased glottal resistance and reduced subglottal pressure, average phonatory sound pressure level and phonatory flow rate compared to matched control subjects. It was suggested by Murdoch *et al.* (1995) that the aerodynamic findings in their study reflected the presence of rigidity in the laryngeal musculature. In addition, their study indicated that dysarthric speakers with Parkinson's disease were not homogeneous, but rather exhibited differential impairment within the laryngeal subsystem. Overall, the laryngeal subsystem of the speech-production mechanism in subjects with Parkinson's disease would appear to demonstrate a greater degree of variability in perceptual, acoustic and physiological features than other subsystems of the speech-production apparatus.

Velopharyngeal function in hypokinetic dysarthria

Controversy surrounds the existence of a resonatory disturbance in persons with Parkinson's disease. Several authors have reported low incidences of perceived hypernasality in groups of subjects with Parkinson's disease (Darley *et al.*, 1975; Logemann *et al.*, 1978; Theodoros *et al.*, 1995). At the same time, hypernasality has been identified as one of the most useful perceptual features for differentiating between hypokinetic dysarthria and normal speech (Ludlow and Bassich, 1983). For some individuals with Parkinson's disease hypernasality has been found to be the most prominent deviant speech feature (Hoodin and Gilbert, 1989a, 1989b).

Physiological evaluation of velopharyngeal functioning using a variety of direct and indirect instrumental techniques has provided objective evidence of dysfunction of the velopharyngeal valve in subjects with Parkinson's disease. Hirose and colleagues (1981) conducted a study in which velar movements were directly observed by means of an X-ray microbeam system that tracked a lead pellet attached to the nasal side of the velum. During the rapid repetition of the monosyllable /ten/, Hirose *et al.* (1981) identified a gradual decrease in the degree of displacement of the velum. In effect, the lowering and elevation of the velum for the nasal and non-nasal consonants, respectively, were found to be incomplete towards the end of the speech task. At a rapid rate of repetition, the interval between each utterance was noted to be inconsistent and the displacement and rate of velar movements were found to be markedly reduced (Hirose *et al.*, 1981).

In a study involving the use of videofluoroscopy to examine velar movements during speech in patients with Parkinson's disease, Robbins *et al.* (1986) identified a significant reduction in velar elevation, which was considered to reflect a reduced range of velar movement. Nasal accelerometry has also revealed a significantly greater degree and increased frequency of hypernasality in the speech output of a group of hypokinetic speakers with Parkinson's disease (Theodoros *et al.*, 1995). Specifically, the individuals with Parkinson's disease, as a group, recorded significantly higher Horii Oral Nasal Coupling (HONC) indices compared with the controls. Of the 23 individuals with Parkinson's disease, 17 (74%) were identified by Theodoros *et al.* (1995) as exhibiting increased nasality.

Clinicians, therefore, should be alert to the existence of resonatory disturbance in Parkinson's disease and be aware that this abnormality may manifest itself, to varying degrees, in some individuals and not others. Further research, involving the simultaneous use of both direct and indirect instrumental measures together with perceptual evaluation, is required to determine the exact nature of velopharyngeal function in hypokinetic dysarthria.

Articulatory function in hypokinetic dysarthria

By far the majority of speakers with hypokinetic dysarthria exhibit disorders of articulation. Articulatory impairments such as consonant and vowel imprecision and prolongation of phonemes have been observed, with consonant imprecision identified as the most common articulatory disturbance (Darley *et al.*, 1975; Logemann *et al.*, 1978; Chenery *et al.*, 1988; Zwirner and Barnes, 1992). Consonant articulation has been found to be characterized by errors in the manner of production involving incomplete closure for stops and partial construction of the vocal tract for fricatives, resulting in the abnormal production of stop-plosives, affricates and fricatives (Canter, 1965; Logemann and Fisher, 1981).

In addition to abnormalities of articulation, disordered speech rate is also frequently observed in patients with Parkinson's disease. Perceptually, individuals with Parkinson's disease have been noted to demonstrate both a faster (Darley *et al.*, 1975; Enderby, 1986; Chenery *et al.*, 1988; Zwirner and Barnes, 1992) and a slower overall rate of speech than normal (Chenery *et al.*, 1988; Zwirner and Barnes, 1992), with most studies suggesting that the speech rate of these patients is generally variable (Ludlow and Bassich, 1983; Scott *et al.*, 1985; Hoodin and Gilbert, 1989a). In addition, subjects with Parkinson's disease have been noted to demonstrate short rushes of speech, or what is perceived as an 'accelerated' speech pattern (Darley *et al.*, 1975; Chenery *et al.*, 1988; Zwirner and Barnes, 1992). The production of short rushes of speech in the verbal output of speakers with Parkinson's disease was found by Darley *et al.* (1975) to be one of the most prominent features of hypokinetic dysarthria. Furthermore, this deviant speech dimension was identified in 84% of the subjects with Parkinson's disease assessed by Chenery *et al.* (1988). In some cases, a progressive acceleration of speech within a speech segment has also been perceived to be present (Scott *et al.*, 1985; Chenery *et al.*, 1988).

Acoustic analysis of the speech rate disturbance in Parkinson's disease has generally confirmed the perceptual impression of a variety of rate disturbances being evident in these subjects. Studies have demonstrated a normal rate of speech production (Ackermann and Ziegler, 1991; Flint *et al.*, 1992), a normal to increased rate (Kent and Rosenbek, 1982; Weismer, 1984), and an increased rate (Hammen *et al.*, 1989; Lethlean *et al.*, 1990), whereas some groups of subjects with Parkinson's disease have been found to exhibit rate disturbance on a continuum from slower to faster than normal (Metter and Hanson, 1986). Interestingly, however, while many individuals with Parkinson's disease demonstrate a faster than normal rate of speech, Ludlow and Bassich (1984) found that, when specifically required to increase their speech rate, the subjects were often unable to do so.

Physiological investigations of the articulatory function of patients with Parkinson's disease have identified the presence of abnormal patterns of muscle activity, reductions in the range and velocity of articulatory movement, impaired strength, endurance and fine force control of the articulators and tremor in the orofacial structure. These investigations have included a wide variety of instrumental techniques including direct recordings of muscle activity such as electromyography (Hunker *et al.*, 1982; Hirose, 1986; Moore and Scudder, 1989) and a range of kinematic procedures including strain-gauge transduction systems (Abbs *et al.*, 1983; Connor *et al.*, 1989), lead-pellet tracking (Hirose *et al.*, 1982), electromagnetic articulography (Ackermann *et al.*, 1993) and optoelectrics (Svensson *et al.*, 1993). Overall, the most common physiological findings relating to the articulatory subsystem of subjects with Parkinson's disease include a reduction in the amplitude of displacement of the articulators and a decrease in velocity of movement (Forrest and Weismer, 1995). The physiological findings of reduced amplitude and velocity of the articulatory movements provide support for the so-called articulatory undershoot hypothesis proposed to explain the articulatory imprecision evident in persons with Parkinson's disease (Hunker *et al.*, 1982).

In summary, the findings of the perceptual, acoustic and physiological studies relating to articulatory function in Parkinson's disease have generally been consistent in identifying articulatory deficits in this group. Further research, however, is needed to determine the specific relationships among the deviant perceptual, acoustic and physiological speech features to define the precise nature of articulatory dysfunction. Such an approach requires a comprehensive perceptual, acoustic and physiological assessment of the articulatory subsystem of individual speakers with hypokinetic dysarthria.

Prosodic function in hypokinetic dysarthria

According to Darley *et al.* (1975), prosodic disturbances constitute the most prominent features of hypokinetic dysarthria. Descriptions of the speech of persons with Parkinson's disease frequently refer to the dysprosodic aspects of speech production in relation to stress and intonation, fluency and rate. Impairment of stress patterning, variable rate, short rushes of speech or 'accelerated' speech, difficulty in the initiation of speech, phoneme repetition, palilalia, inappropriate silences and monotony of pitch and loudness have been identified in these individuals (Darley *et al.*, 1975; Ludlow and Bassich, 1983, 1984; Chenery *et al.*, 1988; Zwirner and Barnes, 1992).

For a detailed description of the assessment and treatment of hypokinetic dysarthria see Chapter 12.

Hyperkinetic dysarthria

Hyperkinetic dysarthria is a collective name for a diverse group of speech disorders in which the deviant speech characteristics are the product of abnormal involuntary movements that disturb the rhythm and rate of motor activities, including those involved in speech production. These involuntary movements, which may involve the limbs, trunk, neck, face, etc., may be rhythmic or irregular and unpredictable, rapid or slow. The abnormal involuntary movements involved vary considerably in their form and locus across the different diseases of the basal ganglia. Consequently, there is considerable heterogeneity in the deviant speech dimensions that manifest as the speech disorders termed hyperkinetic dysarthria. Any or all of the major subcomponents of the speech-production apparatus may be involved, including the respiratory system, phonatory valve, resonatory valve and articulatory valve. Disturbances in prosody are also present.

In that the various different types of hyperkinetic dysarthria are each associated with one of the hyperkinetic movement disorders (Freed, 2000), clinically the hyperkinetic dysarthrias are usually described in the context of the underlying movement disorders causing the speech disturbance. With this construct in mind, Darley *et al.* (1975) distinguished between two categories of hyperkinetic disorder: quick hyperkinesias and slow hyperkinesias. Quick hyperkinesias include myoclonic jerks (e.g. palatopharyngolaryngeal myoclonus), tics, chorea and ballism, and are characterized by rapid, abnormal, involuntary movements that are either unsustained or sustained only very briefly, and are random in occurrence with respect to the particular body part affected. In contrast, the abnormal involuntary movements seen in slow hyperkinesias build up to a peak slowly and are sustained for at least one second or longer. In some instances the abnormal muscle contractions seen in association with slow hyperkinesias are sustained for many seconds or even minutes, with muscle tone waxing and waning to produce a variety of distorted postures. The three major conditions included in the category of slow hyperkinesias are athetosis, dyskinesia (lingual-facial-buccal dyskinesia) and dystonia. The major types of hyperkinetic disorder are outlined in Table 11.1.

Quick hyperkinesias: myoclonic jerks

Myoclonic jerks are abrupt, sudden, unsustained muscle contractions, which occur irregularly. These involuntary muscle contractions may occur as single jerks of a body part or may be repetitive, with the muscles of the limbs, face, oral cavity, soft palate, larynx and diaphragm being affected, among others. In those instances where the involuntary movements are repetitive, they can be either rhythmic or non-rhythmic in nature. According to Simon *et al.* (1999), myoclonic jerks are classified according to their distribution, relationship to precipitating stimuli or aetiology. Although myoclonic jerks are sometimes focal, involving only isolated muscles (focal myoclonus), they may also be multifocal, occurring simultaneously in larger groups of muscles (generalized myoclonus).

Myclonic jerks may occur as a normal phenomenon in healthy persons as an isolated abnormality, or in association with lesions located in a variety of different sites in the central nervous system, ranging from the cerebral cortex (e.g. cortical reflex myoclonus) to the spinal cord (e.g. spinal myoclonus). Myoclonus may also occur as part of a convulsive disorder (epilepsy) or in association with diffuse metabolic, infectious or toxic disturbances of the nervous system such as diffuse encephalitis and toxic encephalopathies. Although often occurring spontaneously, myoclonic jerks may also be induced by various sensory stimuli (e.g. visual, auditory or tactile stimuli) or in some instances by voluntary muscle activity (action myoclonus).

The muscles of the speech mechanism may be affected by myoclonic jerks in the same way as the muscles of the limbs. Myoclonic jerks may involve the muscles of the soft palate, larynx and diaphragm either individually or in combination. In those rare cases where it occurs in isolation, palatal myoclonus usually involves the rhythmical contraction of the soft palate which may result in temporary hypernasality and

Disorder	Symptoms	Effect on speech
Myoclonic jerks	Characterized by abrupt, sudden, unsustained muscle contractions which occur irregularly. Involuntary contractions may occur as single jerks of the body or may be repetitive. Two forms may affect speech – palatal myoclonus and action myoclonus.	Speech disorder in palatal myoclonus is usually characterized by phonatory, resonatory and prosodic abnormalities; for example, vocal tremor, rhythmic phonatory arrests, intermittent hypernasality, prolonged intervals and inappropriate silences. Action myoclonus: speech disrupted as a result of fine, arrhythmic, erratic muscle jerks, triggered by activity of the speech musculature.
Tics	Gilles de la Tourette's syndrome characterized by development of motor and vocal tics plus behavioural disorders. Vocal tics include simple vocal tics (for example, grunting, coughing, barking, hissing, etc.) and complex vocal tics (for example, stuttering-like repetitions, palilalia, echolalia and copralalia).Brief, unsustained, recurrent, compulsive movements. Usually involve a small part of the body, for example, facial grimace.	
Chorea	A choreic movement consists of a single, involuntary, unsustained, isolated muscle action producing a short, rapid, uncoordinated jerk of the trunk, limb, face, tongue, diaphragm, etc. Contractions are random in distribution and timing is irregular. Two major forms: Sydenham's chorea and Huntington's disease.	A perceptual study of 30 patients with chorea demonstrated deficits in all aspects of speech production (Darley et al., 1969a).
Ballism	Rare hyperkinetic disorder characterized by involuntary, wide-amplitude, vigorous, flailing movements of the limbs. Facial muscles may also be affected.	Least important hyperkinetic disorders with regard to occurrence of hyperkinetic dysarthria.
Athetosis	Slow hyperkinetic disorder characterized by continuous, arrhythmic, purposeless, slow, writhing-type movements that tend to flow one into another. Muscles of the face, neck and tongue are involved, leading to facial grimacing, protrusion and writhing of the tongue and problems with speaking and swallowing.	Descriptions of the speech disturbance in athetosis are largely related to athetoid cerebral palsy rather than hyperkinetic dysarthria in adults.
Dyskinesia	Two dyskinetic disorders are included under this heading: tardive dyskinesia and levodopa-induced dyskinesia. The basic pattern of abnormal involuntary movement in both of these conditions is one of slow, repetitive, writhing, twisting, flexing and extending movements often with a mixture of tremor. Muscles of the tongue, face and oral cavity are most often affected.	Accurate placement of the articulators of speech may be severely hampered by the presence of choreoathetoid movements of the tongue, lip pursing and smacking, tongue protrusion and sucking and chewing behaviours.
Dystonia	Characterized by abnormal involuntary movements that are slow and sustained for prolonged periods of time. Involuntary movements tend to have an undulant, sinuous character that may produce grotesque posturing and bizarre writhing, twisting movements.	Dystonias affecting the speech mechanisms may result in respiratory irregularities and/or abnormal movement and bizarre posturing of the jaw, lips, tongue, face and neck. In particular, focal cranial/orolingual-mandibular dystonia and spasmodic torticollis have the most direct effect on speech function.

articulatory imprecision. Laryngeal myoclonus most frequently occurs in combination with palatal myoclonus (Drysdale *et al.*, 1993), where it can have the additional effect of temporarily interrupting phonation. Diaphragmatic myoclonus can cause slight interruptions to airflow and is usually most easily detected in sustained phonation tasks.

In particular, two forms of myoclonus have a marked effect on speech: palatopharyngolaryngeal myoclonus (sometimes simply referred to as palatal myoclonus) and action myoclonus. Palatopharyngolaryngeal myoclonus is characterized by continuous synchronous jerks of the soft palate at the rate of 1–4 Hz with other brain stem-innervated muscles – particularly the larynx and pharynx – usually involved. The condition can be either symptomatic or idiopathic (essential rhythmical palatal myoclonus), with the symptomatic condition most often the result of cerebrovascular lesions involving the brain stem or cerebellum (Deuschl *et al.*, 1990). However, a variety of other conditions, including tumours, multiple sclerosis, encephalitis and degenerative diseases can also lead to palatal myoclonus. Hyperkinetic dysarthria due to palatopharyngolaryngeal myoclonus rarely exists as an isolated speech disturbance, but more frequently occurs in conjunction with another type of dysarthria. Although palatopharyngolaryngeal myoclonus has direct effects on the speech musculature, speech deficits may not be readily perceived during conversational speech because of the low amplitude and brevity of the myoclonic movements (Duffy, 1995). Where a speech disturbance is apparent, it is usually characterized by phonatory, resonatory and prosodic abnormalities such as vocal tremor, momentary rhythmic phonatory arrests, intermittent hypernasality, prolonged intervals and inappropriate silences (Darley *et al.*, 1975; Aronson, 1990).

Action myoclonus is differentiated from other myoclonic conditions such as palatopharyngolaryngeal myoclonus by the fact that it is triggered by muscle activity. In this condition speech function is disrupted as a result of fine, arrhythmic, erratic muscle jerks that are triggered by muscle activity associated with a conscious attempt at a task requiring precision of movement (e.g. speech production) (Lance and Adams, 1963). The muscle jerks may present one at a time or in a series and are usually less than 200 ms in duration (Lance and Adams, 1963). Documentation of the speech impairment associated with action myoclonus is restricted to one unpublished report. Aronson *et al.* (1984; cited in Duffy, 1995) identified articulatory and phonatory impairments in a study of four cases. Despite demonstrating normal orofacial features at rest, myoclonic spasms of the lips were evident when speech was attempted, resulting in a reduced speech rate. Phonatory disturbances observed in these four cases included repetitive fluctuations in phonation and adductor vocal arrests that were synchronized with the myoclonic jerks of the lip muscles.

Quick hyperkinesias: tics
Tics are brief, unsustained, recurrent, compulsive movements that involve a relatively small part of the body and occur out of a background of normal motor activity. They usually occur spontaneously without provocation by any particular stimulus and are generally considered as involuntary movements. Although tics may be briefly controlled voluntarily, such periods of suppression are often followed by a period of more intensive involuntary contraction.

Tics can be classified into four groups depending on whether they are simple or multiple and transient or chronic. Transient simple tics are very common in children, usually terminating spontaneously within 1 year, and generally requiring no treatment. Chronic simple tics can develop at any age but often begin in childhood, and treatment is not necessary in most cases. The syndrome of multiple motor and vocal tics is generally referred to as Gilles de la Tourette's syndrome. First described by Frenchman Gilles de la Tourette in 1885, the first signs of Tourette's consist of motor tics in 80% of cases and vocal tics in 20% (Simon *et al.*, 1999; Alsobrook and Pauls, 2002). The condition primarily affects boys (4:1 ratio) and development of motor and vocal tics is accompanied by a variety of behavioural disorders, including obsessive compulsive disorder, attention-deficit hyperactivity disorder and other forms of general behavioural disturbances such as conduct disorder, panic attacks, multiple phobias, mania, etc. In those cases where the initial sign is a motor tic, it most commonly involves the face, taking the form of sniffing, barking, blinking or forced eye closure. The motor tics progressively involve the face, neck, upper limbs and eventually the entire body. Vocal tics include both simple and complex vocal tics. Simple vocal tics include grunting, coughing, barking, throat clearing, hissing and snorting (Serra-Mestres *et al.*, 1998). This may occur as isolated events or be embedded with involuntary verbal utterances. In addition, complex vocal tics such as stuttering-like repetitions, unintelligible sounds, palilalia (repetition of self-generated words or phrases) and echolalia have also been reported. Copralalia (involuntary, compulsive swearing) although not universal, is another characteristic complex vocal tic observed in Gilles de la Tourette's syndrome. Soft neurological signs, such as mild incoordination in motor skills and slight asymmetry of motor function, including deep tendon reflexes, are also occasionally evident on examination of the child. The incidence of Tourette's syndrome is less than 1 in 100 000 (Friedhoff, 1982) and drug therapy utilizing antidopaminergic agents has been shown to be effective in some cases.

Quick hyperkinesias: chorea

The term chorea is derived from the Greek word for dance and was originally applied to the dance-like gait and continual limb movements seen in acute infectious chorea. A choreic (or choreiform) movement consists of a single, unsustained, isolated muscle action producing a short, rapid, uncoordinated jerk of the trunk, limb, face, tongue, diaphragm, etc. They are random in their distribution and their timing is irregular and unpredictable. Choreiform movements range in severity from gross displacements of body parts to subtle abnormal involuntary movements. Choreiform contractions are slower than myoclonic jerks, each lasting from 0.1 to 1 s and can occur at rest or during sustained postures, or may be superimposed on voluntary movements. When superimposed on normal movements, the abnormal involuntary movements can cause characteristic symptoms such as dance-like gait. When superimposed on the normal movements of the speech mechanism during speech production, choreic movements can cause momentary disturbances in the course of contextual speech.

A variety of different conditions may be associated with the occurrence of chorea, including metabolic and toxic conditions (e.g. hepatic encephalopathy, Wilson's disease, hyperthyroidism and dopaminergic medications), inflammatory/infectious disorders (e.g. Sydenham's chorea, encephalitis), vascular lesions involving the basal ganglia or thalamus and degenerative conditions (e.g. Huntington's disease). Pregnant women can also on occasion manifest choreiform movements. Chorea can also occur as an idiopathic disorder. Two of the most common choreiform disorders are Sydenham's chorea and Huntington's disease. Sydenham's chorea occurs principally in children and adolescents, and Huntington's disease occurs principally in adults. Both disorders are characterized by hyperkinesia, as well as speech, language, cognitive and psychiatric disorders. (For a description of the language disorders associated with Huntington's disease, see Chapter 8.)

Sydenham's chorea

First described by Thomas Sydenham in 1686 as St Vitus' dance, Sydenham's chorea is a movement disorder occurring primarily in association with β-haemolytic strep-tococcal throat infections or with rheumatic heart disease (Goldenberg *et al.*, 1992; Simon *et al.*, 1999). The symptom complex of the condition includes involuntary, purposeless, rapid movements which are often associated with incoordination, muscle weakness and/or behavioural abnormalities. These spontaneous movements may involve any portion of the body and occur at rest but disappear during sleep. The condition usually occurs in childhood or adolescence, with onset usually being noted between the ages of 5 and 10 years. Females are affected more than males and the onset of choreic involuntary movements may be either acute or insidious. The prog-nosis for Sydenham's chorea is good and recovery is the general rule with symptoms usually subsiding within 4–6 months (Simon *et al.*, 1999). The course of the condition, however, is extremely variable, with some cases recovering in a few weeks and others showing persistence of the abnormal involuntary movements over a period of years. Frequent relapses occur in some patients with Sydenham's chorea. Pathological changes in Sydenham's chorea have been reported in the cerebral cortex, cerebellum, thalamus, caudate nucleus, putamen and midbrain. These changes consist of wide-spread neuronal degeneration, vascular changes and, rarely, focal brain lesions from embolization resulting from endocarditis. Neuropathological and radiological find-ings in the acute stage are rare and no consistent neuropathological lesions have been identified in Sydenham's chorea.

Hyperkinetic dysarthria associated with Sydenham's chorea has received little attention in the research literature. Further, the few studies reported have largely only documented the presence of dysarthria in persons with Sydenham's chorea rather than providing specific details as to the clinical features of the condition. Nausieda *et al.* (1980) reported the findings of a retrospective study of 240 individuals with Syden-ham's chorea noting that 39% had dysarthria. Swedo *et al.* (1993) examined 11 mod-erately affected children reporting that all exhibited a dysarthria which manifested as 'slurred or incoherent speech . . . with two children rendered mute' (p. 707). In all but two of the children, the dysarthria subsided within months of initiation of medical treatment and was noted not be present at an 18 month follow-up assessment. Further studies reporting the presence of dysarthria in Sydenham's chorea were conducted by Goldenberg *et al.* (1992) who examined 187 children in Brazil and Kulkarni and Anees (1996) who examined 60 children in India.

Huntington's disease

Huntington's disease is a chronic degenerative neurological disorder that is mani-fested by progressive chorea or, at times, other extrapyramidal symptoms as well as progressive intellectual deterioration. The condition is inherited as an autosomal dominant trait, with onset of symptoms typically occurring in the fifth decade of life. As the condition is a progressive disorder, the degree of choreiform movements gradually becomes greater and greater as the condition advances and is usually fatal within 10–15 years post-onset. Pathologically, Huntington's disease is marked by a loss of neurones in the caudate nucleus and putamen and these structures are grossly shrunken and atrophic. The globus pallidus is usually well preserved, as is the sub-stantia nigra. Although major pathological changes are seen in the striatum and cerebral cortex, some changes have also been noted in the cerebral white matter, the thalamus and the hypothalamus. (For a description of the changes in the basal ganglia circuitry in Huntington's disease, see Chapter 10.)

The clinical picture in the advanced stages of Huntington's disease includes facial grimacing (involving the lips, tongue and cheeks), jerks of the head, weaving movements of the arms and shoulders, twists and jerks of the body, as well as superimposed voluntary movements (e.g. an involuntary upward jerk of the arm may be fused into a scratching of the head). The patient's gait at this stage is often markedly involved, consisting of jerky lurching steps that represent a combination of voluntary and involuntary movements. Muscular strength, however, is unimpaired. Unlike Parkinson's disease, the ability to initiate voluntary movements is intact. However, the conduct of a continuous movement (e.g. walking or speech production) is frequently impeded by superimposed muscle jerks.

The pervasive choreiform movements evident in patients with Huntington's disease and other forms of chorea have a profound effect on the individual's attempts at speech production because of the sudden, rapid and unpredictable nature of the involuntary movements which interfere with respiratory, laryngeal, velopharyngeal and articulatory speech activity. The laboured and effortful speech is presumed to be a manifestation of inaccuracy in the direction of movement, irregularity in rhythm, range, force and muscle tone, and a reduced rate of individual and repetitive movements of the muscles of the speech mechanism (Darley et al., 1969b). Hyperkinetic dysarthria associated with chorea is distinguished from other types of dysarthria by the sporadic and transient nature of the abnormal speech features. Individuals with chorea may, in fact, demonstrate normal speech intelligibility, punctuated by distorted speech production during the periods of hyperkinesias.

To date, relatively few studies based on perceptual, acoustic and/or physiological assessments have documented the clinical features of hyperkinetic dysarthria associated with Huntington's disease. The most comprehensive perceptual study to have been reported was performed by Darley et al. (1969a). They reported that all basic motor-speech processes were disturbed. The 10 most deviant speech dimensions observed in patients with chorea by Darley et al. (1969a) were, in rank order, (1) imprecise consonants, (2) prolonged intervals, (3) variable speaking rate, (4) monopitch, (5) harsh voice quality, (6) inappropriate silences, (7) distorted vowels, (8) excess loudness variation, (9) prolonged phonemes and (10) monoloudness. In particular, they reported that choreic patients were most distinctive from other patients with dysarthria in the area of prosodic alterations, being more deviant than any other neurological group on the speech dimensions of excess loudness variation, variable rate and prolonged intervals. According to Darley et al. (1975), the prosodic changes appear to represent an attempt by the choreic speaker to avoid articulatory and phonatory interruptions by variably altering their rate of speech, prolonging their phonemes and prolonging the intervals between words, equalizing the stress on syllables and introducing inappropriate silences.

Hartelius et al. (2003) also examined the speech of speakers with mild and moderate Huntington's disease and, consistent with Darley et al. (1969a, 1969b), observed significant speech deviations in all areas of speech production tested. The most severe speech deviations observed by this group were in phonation, oral motor performance including oral diadochokinesis, and prosody. Although no correlation was found between age or gender and severity of dysarthria, a significant difference in the severity of dysarthria was found between the group with mild Huntington's disease and the group with moderate Huntington's disease. The most frequently occurring perceptual deviations found in continuous speech were mainly related to speech timing and phonation and were hypothesized to reflect the underlying excessive and involuntary movement pattern.

Imprecise consonant and distorted vowel production and irregular articulatory breakdowns have been reported to characterize the articulation of patients with chorea (Darley *et al.*, 1975) and are consistent with the expected adverse effects of choreiform movements on lip, tongue and jaw function. Support for this conclusion has been provided by several acoustic studies of the speech output of patients with Huntington's disease. Zwirner and Barnes (1992) identified greater than normal variability in the first and second formants of a sustained vowel, reflecting abnormal jaw movements (first formant) and aberrations of tongue position and shape (second formant). In addition, Ackermann *et al.* (1995) found that, on an oral diadochokinetic task, their patients with Huntington's disease exhibited increased syllable durational variability and, in some cases, incomplete articulatory gestures which could be attributed to the effects of choreic activity.

The excessive loudness variation exhibited by patients with Huntington's disease was considered to be a characteristic of this form of hyperkinetic dysarthria by Darley *et al.* (1969a, 1969b). In some cases, voice stoppages or arrests were observed in these patients. Objective acoustic assessments of voice in patients with Huntington's disease have identified high phonatory instability (increased variability in fundamental frequency and sudden reductions in frequency of approximately one octave) consistent with involuntary laryngeal movements (Ramig, 1986; Ramig *et al.*, 1988; Zwirner *et al.*, 1991; Zwirner and Barnes, 1992).

Hypernasality when present in patients with Huntington's disease is usually only mild and intermittent, reflecting the variable nature of the choreiform movements affecting soft-palate function. Darley *et al.* (1969a) reported that only approximately 40% of their patients with Huntington's disease exhibited hypernasality. Likewise, these researchers only observed abnormal respiratory patterns in six of their 30 patients with chorea, the abnormal respiratory pattern taking the form of sudden, forced and involuntary inspiration and/or expiration. However, Darley *et al.* (1969a) found this abnormal respiratory pattern to be unique to this form of hyperkinetic dysarthria.

Quick hyperkinesias: ballism (hemiballismus)
Hemiballismus is a rare hyperkinetic movement disorder characterized by involuntary, wide-amplitude, vigorous, flailing movement of the limbs, particularly the arm, on one side of the body. Facial muscles may also be affected. The most consistent neuropathological finding associated with hemiballismus is vascular damage to the subthalamic nucleus or its immediate connections on the side contralateral to the involuntary movement disorder. Ballism can also be caused by other conditions including infections, drugs, autoimmune disorders, primary brain tumours and acquired immunodeficiency syndrome (AIDS). Ballism is the least important of all the quick hyperkinesias in relation to the occurrence of hyperkinetic dysarthria.

Slow hyperkinesias: athetosis
Athetosis is a slow hyperkinesia characterized by continuous, arrhythmic, purposeless, slow, writhing-type movements that tend to flow one into the other. The abnormal movements cease only during sleep and the affected muscles are always hypertonic and may show transient stages of spasms. Athetoid movements particularly involve the distal musculature of the limbs. The muscles of the face, neck and tongue, however, may also be affected, leading to facial grimacing, protrusion and writhing of the tongue, and problems with speaking and swallowing.

Athetosis occurs most often as part of a congenital complex of neurological signs that results from disordered development of the brain, birth injury or other aetiological factors and represents a subcategory of cerebral palsy (Morris *et al.*, 2002). The term, therefore, is rarely used to describe movement disorders acquired in adulthood with many neurologists regarding athetosis as synonymous with dystonia when referring to the acquired condition. Consequently, the majority of reports in the literature relating to the occurrence and nature of speech disorders associated with athetosis are largely based on studies of children or adults with cerebral palsy. Intelligibility of connected speech has been reported to be markedly decreased though phonemic competence is intact, suggesting that athetoid individuals lack the neuromuscular control for articulatory precision (Platt *et al.*, 1980). The articulatory abnormalities noted in individuals with athetosis include wide-ranging jaw movements, inappropriate tongue placement, intermittent velopharyngeal closure, retrusion of lower lip and prolonged transition time for articulatory movements (Kent and Netsell, 1978).

Slow hyperkinesias: dyskinesia (lingual-facial-buccal dyskinesia)
The term dyskinesia is often used in a general way to refer to abnormal, involuntary, hyperkinetic movements without regard to aetiology (Miller and Jankovic, 1990). Although when used in this way all involuntary movements could be described as dyskinetic, only two dyskinetic disorders are usually considered under this heading: tardive dyskinesia and levodopa-induced dyskinesia. As both of these conditions may be limited to the bulbar musculature, they are sometimes referred to as focal dyskinesias. Further, because the muscles of the tongue, face and oral cavity are most often affected, these two disorders are also termed lingual-facial-buccal dyskinesias. The basic pattern of abnormal involuntary movement in both of these conditions is one of slow, repetitive, writhing, twisting, flexing and extending movements, often with a mixture of tremor.

Tardive dyskinesia
Tardive dyskinesia is a late-onset, acquired movement disorder resulting from long-term neuroleptic treatment (treatment with a pharmacological agent having antipsychotic action) (Jeste and Wyatt, 1982). Although neuroleptic drugs have been prescribed for psychiatric disorders since the 1930s, the condition was first described by Schonecker (1957), when the term tardive dyskinesia was coined. Also sometimes referred to as Meige syndrome, tardive dyskinesia is regarded by some neurologists as a form of focal dystonia involving the cranial-cervical region (Ferguson, 1992). The syndrome occurs relatively late in the course of neuroleptic therapy.

The abnormal involuntary movements seen in tardive dyskinesia are usually of the choreoathetoid type, are sometimes stereotyped and principally affect the tongue, lips and jaw and, to a lesser degree, the larynx and respiratory musculature (Feve *et al.*, 1995). The limbs and trunk are also occasionally involved. A combination of tongue twisting and protrusion, lip smacking and puckering and chewing movement in a repetitive and stereotypic fashion is often observed (Jankovic, 1995). In addition, the soft palate may also elevate and lower involuntarily. When asked to do so, patients with tardive dyskinesia may be able to suppress the involuntary mouth movements. These movements may also be suppressed by voluntary actions such as putting food in the mouth or talking.

Speech production is often markedly affected in tardive dyskinesia due to the abnormal involuntary, rhythmic movements of the orofacial, lingual and mandibular structures. The accurate placement of the articulators of speech may be severely hampered by the presence of choreoathetoid movements of the tongue, lip pursing and smacking, tongue protrusion and sucking and chewing behaviours (Matthews and Glaser, 1984; Vernon, 1991). According to Darley *et al.* (1969a, 1969b) articulatory deviations were the most prominent features of the hyperkinetic dysarthria exhibited by their patients with tardive dyskinesia. Other perceptually based studies have also identified prosodic, phonatory and respiratory impairments, in addition to articulatory disorders, in small groups of subjects with tardive dyskinesia (Gerratt, 1983; Gerratt *et al.*, 1984). In a perceptual study of 12 patients with tardive dyskinesia, Gerratt *et al.* (1984) reported that these patients exhibited marked disturbances in the temporal organization of speech (prosodic impairment) and phonation, while articulatory deficits (irregular articulatory breakdowns and imprecise consonants) were perceived to be less severely impaired. Respiratory dysfunction, involving respiratory dysrhythmia, involuntary grunts and gasping sounds, have also been reported in patients with tardive dyskinesia (Weiner *et al.*, 1978; Faheem *et al.*, 1982).

The most comprehensive perceptual study of the hyperkinetic dysarthria associated with tardive dyskinesia was conducted by Khan *et al.* (1994). They reported that the 17 male psychiatric patients with tardive dyskinesia examined in their study demonstrated significantly reduced phonation times, levels of speech intelligibility and speech rate compared to 10 neuroleptically treated patients without tardive dyskinesia. La Porta *et al.* (1990) phonetically analysed the speech of two subjects with tardive dyskinesia during reading, sentence repetition and spontaneous conversation tasks. Both cases were found to produce high frequencies of abnormal consonants, compared to a single control subject who had received long-term neuroleptic treatment but did not exhibit tardive dyskinesia. Specifically the two patients with tardive dyskinesia made the most number of errors on alveolar, alveo-dental and palatal phonemes, consistent with abnormal movements of the tongue in tardive dyskinesia. Interestingly, La Porta *et al.* (1990) found that vowel production was unimpaired in these two subjects.

Support for the above perceptual findings in relation to articulation and phonation has come from acoustic investigations of the dysarthria associated with tardive dyskinesia. For example, Gerratt (1983) investigated motor steadiness of the vocal tract musculature superior to the glottis during vowel production in five subjects with tardive dyskinesia using a measure of formant frequency fluctuation as an indicator of changes in vocal-tract configuration. Consistent with the articulatory and phonatory deficits identified perceptually by La Porta *et al.* (1990) and Khan *et al.* (1994), their results indicated that formant frequency fluctuations were markedly higher for four of the five subjects compared to normal controls, reflecting a reduction in motor steadiness supraglottally.

Physiological investigations of the speech mechanism in patients with tardive dyskinesia have involved objective analyses of buccolingual, tongue and respiratory function using a variety of instrumental techniques. Caligiuri *et al.* (1988), using a head-mounted transduction system and a pursuit tracking paradigm, evaluated the fine motor control of lip, jaw and tongue movements in 11 patients with tardive dyskinesia. Greater tracking errors were demonstrated by the patients with tardive dyskinesia for the lip (31%), tongue (36%) and jaw (31%) compared with non-tardive dyskinetic patients (lip 12%, tongue 12%, jaw 13%). Using position transducers, Caligiuri *et al.* (1989) identified greater motor instability in the tongue in 13 patients with tardive dyskinesia compared to control subjects and non-tardive dyskinesia patients. Physiological assessment of respiratory function in patients with tardive dyskinesia, using respiratory inductance plethysmography, has confirmed perceptual observations of respiratory impairments in these patients. Wilcox *et al.* (1994) found that patients with tardive dyskinesia demonstrated rapid, shallow breathing characterized by irregular tidal breathing patterns, with greater variability in both tidal volume and time of the total respiratory cycle than control subjects.

As indicated above, tardive dyskinesia occurs later in the course of neuroleptic therapy, often after a decrease in the drug dosage or discontinuation of the drug therapy. The involuntary lingual-facial-buccal movements often persist for months or years after the neuroleptic therapy has been discontinued. If recognized early, however, the symptoms of tardive dyskinesia (including the associated hyperkinestic dysarthria) may recede with the discontinuation of neuroleptic treatment (Drummond and Fitzpatrick, 2004).

Levodopa-induced dyskinesia

Combined lingual-facial-buccal dyskinesia is not unique to tardive dyskinesia but may also be seen as part of the hyperkinesia of Huntington's disease and following high-dose levodopa therapy in Parkinson's disease. As in tardive dyskinesia, the abnormal involuntary movements seen in the latter condition are also typically choreic and also characteristically involve the muscles of the tongue, face and mouth. The tongue may demonstrate 'fly-catcher' movements in which it involuntarily moves in and out of the mouth repeatedly. Simultaneously, the lips may pucker and retract while the jaw may open and close or move from side to side spontaneously. The induction of lingual-facial-buccal dyskinesia by levodopa therapy is consistent with the proposal of Ludlow and Bassich (1984) that patients with Parkinson's disease treated with levodopa have a speech disorder resembling a hyperkinetic rather than a hypokinetic dysarthria.

Slow hyperkinesias: dystonia

Dystonia is a collective term for a variety of neurogenic movement and posture disorders characterized by abnormal, involuntary muscle contractions which may be accompanied by irregular repetitive movements. Dystonic movements are abnormal, involuntary movements which are slow and sustained for prolonged periods of time. Affected muscles are hypertonic and the involuntary movements tend to have an undulant, sinuous character which may produce grotesque posturing and bizarre writhing movements. Dystonia tends to involve large parts of the body, particularly the muscles of the trunk, neck and proximal parts of the limbs. However, the muscles of the speech mechanism may also be involved, in which case the patient may exhibit spasms of the face, producing facial grimacing, forceful spasmodic eye closing (blepharospasm), pursing of the lips, jaw spasm, involuntary twisting and protrusion of the tongue, and respiratory irregularities. The most distinguishing feature of dystonia involves the maintenance of an abnormal or altered posture, on some occasions involving only a single focal part of the body while on others involving a diffuse region of the body. The abnormal involuntary contractions usually build up slowly, produce a prolonged distorted posture such as twisting of the trunk about the long axis (torsion spasm) and then gradually recede. Occasionally, dystonic movements begin with a jerk and then build up to a peak before subsiding.

A variety of conditions may lead to dystonia, including encephalitis, head trauma, vascular diseases and drug toxicity. In addition, various progressive degenerative diseases of the central nervous system such as Wilson's disease and Huntington's disease often manifest dystonic features at some time in their course. One type of dystonia, dystonia musculorum deformans, is an inherited disease. In many cases, however, the cause of dystonia is unknown. Although it is often reported that dystonia is a disorder of the basal ganglia, lesions in the corpus striatum and globus pallidus having been described, no consistent and specific pathophysiology or pathomorphologic alteration in the brain has been identified.

Depending on the distribution of the abnormal involuntary movements dystonia can be classified into several subtypes including:

■ focal dystonia (involving only a single segment or part of the body),
■ segmental dystonia (involving two or more contiguous body segments),
■ multifocal dystonia (involving two non-contiguous body parts),
■ generalized dystonia (involving one or both legs plus another area of the body).

Focal dystonias that may affect speech and voice include orolingual-mandibular dystonia, laryngeal dystonia and cervical dystonia (also known as spasmodic torticollis). Patients with orolingual-mandibular dystonia have abnormal movements of the vocal tract, including sustained tongue movements, clenched jaw or forced jaw opening (Yoshida et al., 2002; Yoshida and Iizuki, 2003). These signs often occur with blepharospasm, and this complex has been referred to as focal cranial dystonia or Meige syndrome (Jankovic, 1988). According to Darley et al. (1975), articulation, phonation and prosody may all be significantly disturbed in patients with dystonia. In a study of 30 dystonia cases, Darley et al. (1969a) found that the deviant speech dimensions of imprecise consonants, disturbed vowels, harsh voice quality, irregular articulatory breakdown, strained-strangled voice quality, monopitch, monoloudness, inappropriate silence, short phrases and prolonged intervals to be the 10 major features of the hyperkinetic dysarthria seen in dystonia. Notably, three of the four most prominent deviant characteristics were related to articulatory disturbance. Resonatory disturbances have not been found to be characteristic features of dysarthria associated with dystonia. Approximately 30% of cases have been found to demonstrate hypernasality, with the majority of subjects exhibiting this abnormality to a mild degree (Darley et al., 1969a, 1969b; Golper et al., 1983). Likewise, except for two patients in Golper et al.'s (1983) study who were perceived to exhibit respiratory muscle spasms, studies of the speech output of patients with dystonia have generally failed to identify specific impairments of respiration. A number of perceptual features identified in this population, such as excessive loudness variations, short phrases and alternating loudness could, however, reflect the contribution of respiratory impairment in this population.

As a reflection of the phenomenon of laryngospasm during phonation, laryngeal dystonia is referred to as spasmodic dysphonia. Three subtypes of spasmodic dysphonia are recognized based on the specific aspect of vocal-fold movement impaired. These subtypes include adductor, abductor and mixed spasmodic dysphonia of which adductor is by far the most common (Blitzer and Brin, 1992). Three syllable-level adductor spasmodic dysphonia signs have been identified by various researchers as being key to the classification of the adductor spasmodic dysphonia voice: pitch shift (Sapienza et al., 1999, 2000), phonatory break (Langeveld et al., 2000) and aperiodicity (Sapienza et al., 1999, 2000).

Spasmodic torticollis, a condition in which tonic or clonic spasm in the neck muscles (especially the sternocleidomastoid and trapezius muscles) cause the head to be deviated to the right or left, or sometimes forward (antecollis) and backward (retrocollis), has also been reported to disrupt speech production (Case et al., 1990; La Pointe et al., 1993; Zraick et al., 1993). Acoustic speech/voice characteristics of the hyperkinetic dysarthria associated with spasmodic torticollis include reduced maximum phonation duration, slower sequential articulatory movement rates, slower alternate articulatory movement rates, longer phonatory reaction time, slower reading rate (in words per minute), lower overall intelligibility rating, increased jitter, increased shimmer, increased harmonic-to-noise ratio (females), lower habitual fundamental frequency (females), lower ceiling fundamental frequency (females) and restricted frequency range (females).

Essential voice tremor

Tremors are involuntary movements resulting from the contraction of opposing muscle groups, which produces rhythmic or alternating movement of a joint or group of joints. A number of different types of tremor are recognized, which include:

■ physiological tremor (e.g. tremor associated with cold or nervousness),
■ essential tremor (e.g. familial, action and senile),
■ toxic tremor (e.g. tremor in thyrotoxicosis and alcoholism),
■ pathological tremor (e.g. intention tremor in cerebellar disorders and rest tremor in Parkinson's disease).

Essential tremor is a hyperkinetic movement disorder that most often affects the head, arms or hands. It is the most common of the movement disorders, with approximately 50% of cases being familial and the bulk of the rest being idiopathic (Duffy, 1995). The condition is usually regarded as an exaggeration of normal physiological tremors. Although often referred to as a benign disorder, the symptoms of essential tremor are typically progressive and potentially disabling and may force affected persons to change jobs or seek early retirement. This type of tremor is absent at rest and appears when the patient acts to move or support a body part (hence the name, action tremor). Essential tremor is not associated with other evidence of neurological disease.

Essential or organic voice tremor is a focal presentation of essential tremor (Murdoch, 1990). The typical form of essential voice tremor occurs when the alternating contractions of the adductors and abductors of the vocal folds are of equal strength, in contrast to other presentations such as adductor and abductor spasmodic dysphonia where either the adductor or abductor movements of the vocal folds are disproportionately stronger. During contextual speech, essential voice tremor may not be apparent, especially when the tremor is mild. Vowel prolongation is typically the best task for eliciting voice-tremor (Aronson, 1990), which can be perceived as rhythmical frequency modulations of 4–7 Hz, sometimes accompanied by fluctuations in loudness. Although essential voice tremor may occur in isolation, it is usually accompanied by head or extremity tremor.

Dysarthria associated with cerebellar pathology

Damage to the cerebellum or its connections leads to a condition called ataxia, in which movements become uncoordinated. If the ataxia affects the muscles of the speech mechanism, the production of speech may become abnormal, leading to a cluster of deviant speech dimensions collectively referred to as ataxic dysarthria.

Although even simple movements are affected by cerebellar damage, the movements most disrupted by cerebellar disorders are the more complex, multicomponent sequential movements. Following damage to the cerebellum, complex movements tend to be broken down or decomposed into their individual sequential components, each of which may be executed with errors of force, amplitude and timing, leading to uncoordinated movements. As speech production requires the coordinated and simultaneous contraction of a large number of muscle groups, it is easy to understand how cerebellar disorders could disrupt speech production and cause ataxic dysarthria.

Ataxic dysarthria

As indicated above, ataxic dysarthria is associated with decomposition of complex movements arising from a breakdown in the coordinated action of the muscles of the speech-production mechanism. In particular, inaccuracy of movement, irregular rhythm of repetitive movement, uncoordiantion, slowness of both individual and repetitive movements and hypotonia of affected muscles seem to be the principal neuromuscular deficits associated with cerebellar damage that underlie ataxic dysarthria. To fully understand the pathophysiological basis of ataxic dysarthria, however, requires an understanding of the basic neuroanatomy and functional neurology of the cerebellum.

Neurological framework of ataxic dysarthria

The neuroanatomy and functional role of the cerebellum in motor function are described in detail in Chapter 2. Consequently, only the major features of cerebellar coordination of voluntary motor functions will be summarized here to explain the pathophysiological basis of the clinical features of ataxic dysarthria.

Although the cerebellum does not initiate any muscle contractions itself, it monitors those areas of the brain that do in order to coordinate the actions of muscle groups and time their contractions so that movements involving the skeletal muscles are performed smoothly and accurately. It is thought that the cerebellum achieves this coordination by translating the motor intent of the individual into response parameters that then control the action of the peripheral muscles. In order to be able to perform its primary function of synergistic coordination of muscular activity, the cerebellum requires extensive connections with other parts of the nervous system. Damage to the pathways comprising these connections can cause cerebellar dysfunction and possibly ataxic dysarthria, the same as damage to the cerebellum itself. Briefly, the cerebellum functions in part by comparing input from the motor cortex with information concerning the momentary status of muscle contraction, degree of tension of the muscle tendons, position of parts of the body and forces acting on the surfaces of the body originating from muscle spindles, Golgi tendon organs and so on, and then sending appropriate messages back to the motor cortex to ensure smooth, coordinated muscle function. Consequently, the cerebellum requires input from the motor cortex, from muscle and joint receptors, receptors in the internal ear detecting changes in the position and rate of rotation of the head, skin receptors and so on. Conversely, pathways carrying signals from the cerebellum back to the cortex are also required.

Connections with other parts of the brain are provided on either side by three bundles of nerve fibres called the cerebellar peduncles. These include the inferior peducle (restiform body), the middle peduncle (the brachium pontis) and the superior peduncle (brachium conjunctivum). The major afferent pathway connecting the cerebral cortex and the cerebellum is the cortico-pontine-cerebellar pathway. This pathway originates primarily from the motor cortex and projects to the ipsilateral pontine nuclei from where secondary fibres project mainly to the cortex of the neocerebellum. Other afferent pathways project to the cerebellum from structures in the brain stem such as the olive (olivo-cerebellar tract), the red nucleus (rubro-cerebellar tract), the reticular formation (reticulo-cerebellar tract), the midbrain (tecto-cerebellar tract) and the cuneate nucleus (cuneo-cerebellar tract) as well as from the spinal cord (spino-cerebellar tracts).

Efferent pathways from the cerebellum originate almost entirely from the deep nuclei and project to many parts of the central nervous system, including the motor cortex (via the thalamus), the basal ganglia, red nucleus, brain stem, reticular formation and the vestibular nuclei. The feedback loop provided by the extensive afferent and efferent connections of the cerebellum give it the means to both monitor and modify motor activities taking place in various parts of the body to produce a smooth, coordinated motor action.

Diseases of the cerebellum linked to ataxic dysarthria

The major diseases of the cerebellum are listed in Table 11.2. The signs and symptoms of cerebellar dysfunction are generally the same, regardless of aetiology. In those disorders where the lesion is slowly progressive (for example, cerebellar tumour), however, symptoms of cerebellar disease tend to be much less severe than in conditions where the lesion develops acutely (for example, traumatic brain injury, cerebrovascular accidents, etc.). In addition, considerable recovery from the effects of an acute lesion can usually be expected.

Clinical characteristics of ataxic dysarthria

The disrupted speech output exhibited by individuals with cerebellar lesions has often been termed scanning speech, a term probably first used by Charcot (1877). According to Charcot (1877), 'the words are as if measured or scanned: there is a pause after every syllable, and the syllables themselves are pronounced slowly' (p. 192). The most predominant features of ataxic dysarthria include a breakdown in the articulatory and prosodic aspects of speech. According to Brown et al. (1970), the 10 deviant speech dimensions most characteristic of ataxic dysarthria can be divided into three clusters: articulatory inaccuracy, characterized by imprecision of consonant production, irregular articulatory breakdowns and distorted vowels; prosodic excess, characterized by excess and equal stress, prolonged phonemes, prolonged intervals and slow rate; and phonatory-prosodic insufficiency, characterized by harshness, monopitch and monoloudness. Brown et al. (1970) believed that the articulatory problems were the product of ataxia of the respiratory and oral-buccal-lingual musculature, and prosodic excess was thought by these authors to result from slow movements. The occurrence of phonatory-prosodic insufficiencies was attributed to the presence of hypotonia.

Respiratory function in ataxic dysarthria

Perceptual correlates of respiratory inadequacy have been noted in a number of perceptual studies of ataxic dysarthria (Kluin et al., 1988; Chenery et al., 1991). In a study of 16 subjects with ataxic dysarthria, Chenery et al. (1991) reported the presence of significantly reduced ratings of respiratory support for speech as well as a respiratory pattern characterized by sudden forced inspiratory and expiratory sighs. Kluin et al. (1988) documented subjective reports of audible inspiration in ataxic dysarthric speakers investigated in their laboratory.

Table 11.2 Diseases of the cerebellum

Diseases	Example	General features
Chromosomal disorders	Trisomy	Diffuse hypotrophy of the cerebellum may be present, and can be associated with either no clinical symptoms of cerebellar dysfunction or some dysfunction through to marked limb ataxia.
Congenital anomalies	Cerebellar agenesis	Partial to almost total non-development of the cerebellum. May in some cases not be associated with any clinical evidence of cerebellar dysfunction. In other cases, however, a gait disturbance may be evident in addition to limb ataxia (especially involving the lower limbs) and dysarthria.
Demyelinating disorders	Multiple sclerosis	Usually associated with demyelination in a number of regions of the central nervous system including the cerebellum. Consequently, the dysarthria, if present, usually takes the form of a mixed dysarthria rather than purely an ataxic dysarthria. Paroxysmal ataxic dysarthria may occur as an early sign of multiple sclerosis.
Hereditary ataxias	Friedreich's ataxia	The most commonly encountered spinal form of hereditary ataxia. Pathological degeneration primarily involves the spinal cord with degeneration of neurones occurring in the spino-cerebellar tracts. Some degeneration of neurones in the dentate nucleus and brachium conjunctivum may also occur. The first clinical sign of the disease is usually clumsiness of gait. Later limb ataxia (especially involving the lower extremities) also occurs. A large percentage of cases also exhibit dysarthria and nystagmus and cognitive deficits.
Infections	Cerebellar abscess	Most frequently caused by purulent bacteria but can also occur with fungi. Cerebellar abscesses most frequently arise by direct extension from adjacent infected areas such as the mastoid process or from otologic disease.
Toxic metabolic and endocrine disorders	Exogenous toxins; for example, industrial solvents, heavy metals, carbon tetrachloride, etc.	Signs of cerebellar involvement usually associated with symptoms of diffuse involvements of the central nervous system following these intoxications rather than appearing in isolation to other neurological deficits.
	Enzyme deficiencies for example, pyruvate dehydrogenase deficiency	Ataxia most marked in lower limbs.
	Hypothyroidism	Individuals with cretinism show poor development of the cerebellum. Ataxia present in 20–30% of myxoedema cases.
Trauma	Penetrating head wounds	May be associated with either mild slowly developing cerebellar dysfunction or rapid, severe cerebellar dysfunction.
Tumours	Medulloblastomas, astrocytomas and ependymomas	Primary tumours of the cerebellum occur more frequently in children than in adults. Medulloblastomas occur most commonly in the midline of the cerebellum in children and usually have a rapid course with a poor prognosis. Astrocytomas are more benign than medulloblastomas and generally occur in children of an older age group than medulloblastomas. Ependymomas are relatively slow growing and again are more common in children than adults.

Evidence is also available from physiological studies to suggest that speech breathing is disturbed in ataxic dysarthria. Murdoch *et al.* (1991) employed both spirometric and kinematic techniques to investigate the respiratory function of a group of 12 subjects with ataxic dysarthria associated with cerebellar disease. Their results showed that almost one-half of the ataxic cases had vital capacities below the normal limits of variation. In addition, the ataxic dysarthric speakers also demonstrated unusual patterns of chest-wall two-part contribution to lung volume change, including the presence of abdominal and ribcage paradoxing, abrupt changes in movements of the ribcage and abdomen and a tendency to initiate utterances at lower than normal lung volume levels. Murdoch *et al.* (1991) suggested that these findings were an outcome of impaired coordination of the chest wall and speculated that such respiratory anomalies had the potential to underlie some of the prosodic abnormalities observed in ataxic dysarthria.

Laryngeal function in ataxic dysarthria
Phonatory disturbances are frequently listed among the most deviant or most frequently occurring perceptually deviant speech dimensions in ataxic dysarthria (Brown *et al.*, 1970; Darley *et al.*, 1975; Enderby, 1986; Chenery *et al.*, 1991). The perceptual features listed that can be attributed to laryngeal dysfunction in ataxic dysarthria include disorders of vocal quality (for example, a harsh voice, strained-strangled phonation, pitch breaks and vocal tremor), impairment of pitch level (for example, elevated or lower pitch), and deficits in variability of pitch and loudness (for example, monopitch, monoloudness and excess loudness variation). It should be noted that, as indicated by Darley *et al.* (1975), although attributed to phonatory dysfunction, many of the above speech deviations could also result, at least partly, from dysfunction at other levels of the speech-production mechanism (for example, the respiratory system).

Unfortunately, only one study reported to date has used physiological instrumentation to investigate laryngeal activity in ataxic dysarthria. Grémy *et al.* (1967) used electroglottography to identify increased variability of vocal-fold vibrations in ataxic subjects.

Velopharyngeal function in ataxic dysarthria
The presence of hypernasal speech and nasal emission is not a commonly reported feature of ataxic dysarthria, suggesting that functioning of the velopharyngeal port may be normal in patients with cerebellar lesions. Duffy (1995) did report, however, that in some rare cases ataxic subjects may exhibit mild hyponasality, possibly as a consequence of improper timing of velar and articulatory gestures for nasal consonants. Oral examination of patients with cerebellar disorders most often reveals that elevation of the soft palate during phonation is normal.

Articulatory and prosodic function in ataxic dysarthria
The most prominent features of ataxic dysarthria involve a breakdown in articulatory and prosodic aspects of speech. The imprecise articulation leads to improper formation and separation of individual syllables leading to a reduction in intelligibility while the disturbance in prosody is associated with loss of texture, tone, stress and rhythm of individual syllables.

As indicated earlier, Brown *et al.* (1970) concluded that the 10 deviant speech dimensions perceived to be the most characteristic of ataxic dysarthria fell into three clusters: articulatory inaccuracy, prosodic excess and phonatory-prosodic insufficiency. Based on the performance of ataxic speakers on the Frenchay Dysarthria Assessment, Enderby (1986) also observed perceptual correlates of articulatory and prosodic inadequacy to be prominent among the 10 features she believed to be the most characteristic of ataxic dysarthria, including poor intonation, poor tongue movement in speech, poor alternating movement of the tongue in speech, reduced rate of speech, reduced lateral movement of the tongue, reduced elevation of the tongue, poor alternating movement of the lips and poor lip movements in speech.

In addition to the perceptual studies of ataxic dysarthria mentioned above, a number of researchers have used either acoustic and/or physiological procedures to study the articulatory and prosodic aspects of ataxic dysarthria. Kent *et al.* (1979) examined the acoustic features of five patients with ataxic dysarthria. They reported that the most marked and consistent abnormalities observed in the spectrograms of these speakers were alterations in the normal timing patterns and a tendency towards equalized syllable durations. These authors concluded that general timing is a major problem in ataxic dysarthria. Further, they speculated that ataxic speakers fail to decrease syllable duration when appropriate because such reductions require flexibility in sequencing complex motor instructions. The lack of flexibility may lead to a syllable-by-syllable motor control strategy with subsequent abnormal stress patterns.

Only a few studies reported to date have used physiological instrumentation to investigate the functioning of the articulators in ataxic dysarthria. In support of the concept that ataxic speakers are impaired in motor control, McClean *et al.* (1987) reported the case of an ataxic speaker who performed poorly on a non-speech visuomotor tracking task involving the lower lip and jaw. Kent and Netsell (1978) and Netsell and Kent (1976) analysed articulatory position and movements in ataxic speakers using cineradiography. They observed a number of abnormal articulatory movements including abnormally small adjustments of anterior-posterior tongue movements during vowel production, which they thought may form the basis of the perception of vowel distortions. Although movements of the lips, tongue and jaw were generally coordinated, these authors reported that individual movements of these structures were often slow. In addition, they noted that articulatory contacts for consonant production were occasionally incomplete.

Hirose *et al.* (1978) used an X-ray microbeam technique and electromyography to investigate articulatory dynamics in two dysarthric patients, one of whom had cerebellar degeneration. In particular they examined the movement patterns in the jaw and lower lip. Their results showed that the ataxic speaker demonstrated inconsistency in articulatory movements, being characterized by inconsistency in both range and velocity of movement. Further, Hirose *et al.* (1978) found that electromyography showed a breakdown of rhythmic patterns in articulatory muscles during syllable repetition. Overall, the findings of Hirose *et al.* (1978) are consistent with the perception that ataxic speech contains irregular articulatory breakdowns.

In an examination of four ataxic speakers, McNeil *et al.* (1990) investigated isometric force and static position control of the upper and lower lip, tongue and jaw during non-speech tasks. They reported that the ataxic speakers had greater force and position instability than normal speakers, although impairment on one task did not necessarily predict impairment on other tasks.

Summary

Neurological disorders associated with lesions in the basal ganglia or cerebellum have been documented to cause a range of motor speech disorders the symptoms of which reflect the effects of the lesion on the functioning of the muscles of the speech-production mechanism. Specifically, lesions involving the basal ganglia system are associated with two major forms of dysarthria, namely hypokinetic and hyperkinetic dysarthria. Hypokinetic dysarthria is seen almost exclusively in cases of Parkinson's disease but has also been reported as a feature of progressive supranuclear palsy. Hyperkinetic dysarthria, in contrast, is a collective name applied to a range of hyper-kinetic movement disorders all of which are characterized by the presence of abnormal, involuntary movements that may disrupt the normal functioning of the muscles of the speech-production mechanism. These latter disorders are further subdivided into quick and slow hyperkinetic disorders on the basis of the speed and duration of the abnormal involuntary movements associated with each condition. Quick hyper-kinesias include myoclonus, tics, chorea and ballism, whereas slow hyperkinesias include athetosis, dyskinesia and dystonia. Damage to the cerebellum is associated with ataxic dysarthria, a condition caused by the decomposition of complex movements arising from a breakdown in the coordinated action of the muscles of the speech-production mechanism to produce speech. Ataxic dysarthria is predominantly characterized by a breakdown in the articulatory and prosodic aspects of speech. Collectively these motor speech impairments associated with either basal ganglia or cerebellar lesions are indicative of a role for subcortical brain structures in the motor control of speech production.

References

Abbs, J.H., Hunker, C.J. and Barlow, S.H. (1983). Differential speech motor subsystem impairment with supranuclear lesions: neurophysiological framework and supporting data. In W.R. Berry (ed.), *Clinical Dysarthria* (pp. 21–56). San Diego, CA: College-Hill Press.

Ackermann, H. and Ziegler, W. (1991). Articulatory deficits in Parkinson's dysarthria: an acoustic analysis. *Journal of Neurology, Neurosurgery and Psychiatry* 54, 1093–8.

Ackermann, H., Grone, B.F., Hoch, G. and Schonle, P.W. (1993). Speech freezing in Parkinson's disease: a kinematic analysis of orofacial movements by means of electromagnetic articulography. *Folia Phoniatrica et Logopaedica* 45, 84–9.

Ackermann, H., Hertrich, I. and Hehr, T. (1995). Oral diadochokinesis in neurological dysarthrias. *Folia Phoniatrica et Logopaedica* 47, 15–23.

Alsobrook, J.P. and Pauls, D.L. (2002). A factor analysis of tic symptoms in Gilles de la Tourette's syndrome. *American Journal of Psychiatry* 159, 291–6.

Aronson, A.E. (1990). *Clinical Voice Disorders.* New York: Georg Thieme.

Aronson, A.E., O'Neill, B.P. and Kelly, J.J. (1984). *The dysarthria of action myoclonus: a new clinical entity.* Paper presented at the Clinical Dysarthria Conference, February.

Blitzer, A. and Brin, M.F. (1992. The dystonic larynx. *Journal of Voice* 6, 294–7.

Brown, J.R., Darley, F.L. and Aronson, A.E. (1970). Ataxic dysarthria. *International Journal of Neurology* 7, 302–18.

Caligiuri, M.P., Harris, M.J. and Jeste, D.V. (1988). Quantitative analyses of voluntary orofacial motor control in schizophrenia and tardive dyskinesia. *Biological Psychiatry* 24, 787–800.

Caligiuri, M.P., Jeste, D.V. and Harris, M.J. (1989). Instrumental assessment of lingual motor instability in tardive dyskinesia. *Neuropsychopharmacology* 2, 309–12.

Canter, G. (1965). Speech characteristics of patients with Parkinson's disease. II. Physiological support for speech. *Journal of Speech and Hearing Disorders* 30, 44–9.

Case, J., La Pointe, L. and Duane, D. (1990). *Speech and voice characteristics in spasmodic torticollis.* Paper presented at the International Congress of Movement Disorders, Washington DC.

Charcot, J.M. (1877). *Lectures on the Diseases of the Nervous System.* London: New Sydenham Society.

Chenery, H.J., Murdoch, B.E. and Ingram, J.C.L. (1988). Studies in Parkinson's disease. I. Perceptual speech analysis. *Australian Journal of Human Communication Disorders* 16, 17–29.

Chenery, H.J., Ingram, J.C.L. and Murdoch, B.E. (1991). Perceptual analysis of speech in ataxic dysarthria. *Australian Journal of Human Communication Disorders* 18, 19–28.

Connor, N.P., Ludlow, C.L. and Schulz, G.M. (1989). Stop consonant production in isolated and repeated syllables in Parkinson's disease. *Neuropsychologia* 27, 829–38.

Cramer, W. (1940). De spraak bij patienten met Parkinsonisme. *Logopaedie en Phoniatrie* 22, 17–23.

Darley, F.L., Aronson, A.E. and Brown, J.R. (1969a). Differential diagnostic patterns of dysarthria. *Journal of Speech and Hearing Research* 12, 246–69.

Darley, F.L., Aronson, A.E. and Brown, J.R. (1969b). Clusters of deviant speech dimensions in the dysarthrias. *Journal of Speech and Hearing Research* 12, 462–96.

Darley, F.L., Aronson, A.E. and Brown, J.R. (1975). *Motor Speech Disorders.* Philadelphia, PA: WB Saunders.

De La Torre, R., Mier, M. and Boshes, B. (1960). Studies in Parkinsonism: IX. Evaluation of respiratory function – preliminary observations. *Quarterly Bulletin of the Northwestern University Medical School* 34, 232–6.

Deuschl, G., Mischke, G. and Schenck, E. (1990). Symptomatic and essential rhythmic palatal myoclonus. *Brain* 113, 1645–72.

Drummond, S. and Fitzpatrick, A. (2004). Speech and swallowing performances in tardive dyskinesia: a case study. *Journal of Medical Speech Language Pathology* 12, 9–19.

Drysdale, A.J., Ansell, J. and Adeley, J. (1993). Palato-pharyngo-laryngeal myoclonus: an unusual cause of dysphagia and dysarthria. *Journal of Laryngology and Otology* 107, 746–7.

Duffy, J. (1995). *Motor Speech Disorders: Substrates, Diagnosis and Management.* St Louis, MO: Mosby.

Enderby, P. (1986). Relationships between dysarthric groups. *British Journal of Disorders of Communication* 21, 180–97.

Faheem, A.D., Brightwell, D.R., Burton, G.C. and Struss, A. (1982). Respiratory dyskinesia and dysarthria from prolonged neuroleptic use: tardive dyskinesia? *American Journal of Psychiatry* 139, 517–18.

Ferguson, A. (1992). Speech control in persistent tardive dyskinesia: a case study. *European Journal of Disorders of Communication* 27, 89–93.

Feve, A., Angelard, B. and Lacau St Guily, J. (1995). Laryngeal tardive dyskinesia. *Journal of Neurology* 242, 455–99.

Flint, A.J., Black, S.E. and Campbell-Taylor, I. (1992). Acoustic analysis in the differentiation of Parkinson's disease and major depression. *Journal of Psycholinguistic Research* 21, 383–99.

Forrest, K. and Weismer, G. (1995). Dynamic aspects of lower lip movement in Parkinsonian and neurologically normal geriatric speakers' production of stress. *Journal of Speech and Hearing Research* 38, 260–72.

Freed, D. (2000). *Motor Speech Disorders: Diagnosis and Treatment.* San Diego, CA: Singular-Thompson Learning.

Friedhoff, A. (1982). Gilles de la Tourette syndrome. *Advances in Neurology* 35, 335–9.

Gamboa, J., Jimenez-Jimenez, F.L., Nieto, A., Montojo, J., Orti-Pareja, M. *et al.* (1997). Acoustic voice analysis in patients with Parkinson's disease treated with dopaminergic drugs. *Journal of Voice* 11, 314–20.

Gerratt, B.R. (1983). Formant frequency fluctuation as an index of motor steadiness in the vocal tract. *Journal of Speech and Hearing Research* 26, 297–304.

Gerratt, B.R., Goetz, C.G. and Fisher, H.B. (1984). Speech abnormalities in tardive dyskinesia. *Archives of Neurology* 41, 273–6.

Gerratt, B.R., Hanson, D.G. and Berke, G.S. (1987). Glottographic measures of laryngeal function in individuals with abnormal motor control. In T. Baer, C. Sasaki and K. Harris (eds), *Laryngeal Function in Phonation and Respiration* (pp. 521–31). Boston, MA: College-Hill Press.

Goldenberg, J., Ferraz, M.B., Fonseca, A., Hilario, M.O., Bastos, W. *et al.* (1992). Sydenham chorea: clinical and laboratory findings. Analysis of 187 cases. *Revista Paulista de Medicina* 110, 152–7.

Golper, L., Nutt, J., Rau, M. and Coleman, R. (1983). Focal cranial dystonia. *Journal of Speech and Hearing Disorders* 48, 128–34.

Gracco, L.C., Marek, K.L. and Gracco, V.L. (1993). Laryngeal manifestations of early Parkinson's disease: imaging and acoustic data. *Neurology* 43 (suppl. 2), A285.

Grémy, F., Chevrie-Muller, C. and Garde, E. (1967). Etude phoniatrique clinique et instrumentale des dysarthries. *Review Neurologique* 116, 401–26.

Hammen, V.L., Yorkston, K.M. and Beukelman, D.R. (1989). Pausal and speech duration characteristics as a function of speaking rate in normal and Parkinsonian dysarthric individuals. In K.M. Yorkston and D.R. Beukelman (eds), *Recent Advances in Clinical Dysarthria* (pp. 213–23). Boston, MA: College-Hill Press.

Hanson, D.G. (1991). Neuromuscular disorders of the larynx. *Otolaryngologic Clinics of North America* 24, 1035–51.

Hanson, D.G., Gerratt, B.R. and Ward, P.H. (1983). Glottographic measurement of vocal dysfunction: a preliminary report. *Annals of Otology, Rhinology and Laryngology* 92, 413–20.

Hanson, W.R. and Metter, E.J. (1980). DAF as instrumental treatment for dysarthria in progressive supranuclear palsy: a case report. *Journal of Speech and Hearing Disorders* 45, 268–75.

Hartelius, L., Carlstedt, A., Ytterberg, M., Lillvik, M. and Laakso, K. (2003). Speech disorders in mild and moderate Huntington disease: results of dysarthria assessment of 19 individuals. *Journal of Medical Speech Language Pathology* 11, 1–14.

Hirose, H. (1986). Pathophysiology of motor speech disorders (dysarthria). *Folia Phoniatrica et Logopaedica* 38, 61–88.

Hirose, H., Kiritani, S., Ushijima, T. and Sawashima, M. (1978). Analysis of abnormal articulatory dynamics in two dysarthric patients. *Journal of Speech and Hearing Disorders* 4, 46–105.

Hirose, H., Kiritani, S., Ushijima, Y., Yoshioka, H. and Sawashima, M. (1981). Patterns of dysarthric movements in patients with Parkinsonism. *Folia Phoniatrica et Logopaedica* 33, 204–15.

Hirose, H., Kiritani, S. and Sawashima, M. (1982). Patterns of dysarthric movement in patients with amyotrophic lateral sclerosis and pseudobulbar palsy. *Folia Phoniatrica et Logopaedica* 34, 106–12.

Hirose, H., Sawashima, M. and Niimi, S. (1985). *Laryngeal dynamics in dysarthric speech.* Paper presented at the Thirteenth World Congress of Otorhinolaryngology, Miami Beach.

Ho, A.K., Bradshaw, J.L. and Iansek, R. (2000). Volume perception in Parkinsonian speech. *Movement Disorders* 15, 1125–31.

Hoehn, M.M. and Yahr, M.D. (1967). Parkinsonism: onset, progression, and mortality. *Neurology* 17, 427–42.

Hoodin, R.B. and Gilbert, H.R. (1989a). Nasal airflows in Parkinsonian speakers. *Journal of Communication Disorders* 22, 169–80.

Hoodin, R.B. and Gilbert, H.R. (1989b). Parkinsonian dysarthria: an aerodynamic and perceptual description of velopharyngeal closure for speech. *Folia Phoniatrica et Logopaedica* 41, 249–58.

Hovestadt, A., Bogaard, J.D., Meerwaldt, J.D., van der Meche, F.G.A. and Stigt, J. (1989). Pulmonary function in Parkinson's disease. *Journal of Neurology, Neurosurgery and Psychiatry* 42, 329–33.

Hunker, C., Abbs, J.H. and Barlow, S. (1982). The relationship between Parkinsonian rigidity and hypo-kinesia in the orofacial system: a quantitative analysis. *Neurology* 32, 755–61.

Jankovic, J. (1988). Cranial-cervical dysarthrias: an overview. In J. Jankovic and E. Tolosa (eds), *Advances in Neurology: Facial Dyskinesias*, vol. 49 (pp. 289–306). New York: Raven Press.

Jankovic, J. (1995). Tardive syndromes and other drug-induced movement disorders. *Clinical Neurophar-macology* 18, 197–214.

Jeste, D.V. and Wyatt, R.J. (1982). *Understanding and Treating Tardive Dyskinesia*. New York: Guildford Press.

Johnson, J.A. and Pring, T.R. (1990). Speech therapy in Parkinson's disease: a review and further data. *British Journal of Disorders of Communication* 25, 183–94.

Kent, R.D. and Netsell, R. (1978). Articulatory abnormalities in the athetoid cerebral palsy. *Journal of Speech and Hearing Disorders* 43, 353–73.

Kent, R.D. and Rosenbek, J.C. (1982). Prosodic disturbance and neurological lesion. *Brain and Language* 15, 259–91.

Kent, R.D., Netsell, R. and Abbs, J.H. (1979). Acoustic characteristics of dysarthria associated with cerebel-lar disease. *Journal of Speech and Hearing Disorders* 22, 613–26.

Khan, R., Jampala, V.C., Dong, K. and Vedak, C.S. (1994). Speech abnormalities in tardive dyskinesia. *American Journal of Psychiatry* 151, 760–2.

King, J.B., Ramig, L.O., Lemke, J.H. and Harii, Y. (1994). Parkinson's disease: longitudinal changes in acoustic parameters of phonation. *Journal of Medical Speech Language Pathology* 2, 29–42.

Kluin, K.J., Gilman, S., Markel, D.S., Koeppe, R.A., Rosenthal, G. *et al.* (1988). Speech disorders in olivo-pontocerebellar atrophy correlate with positron emission tomography findings. *Annals of Neurology* 23, 547–54.

Kluin, K.J., Gilman, S., Berent, S. and Gilman, S. (1993). Perceptual analysis of speech disorders in pro-gressive supranuclear palsy. *Neurology* 43, 563–6.

Kulkarni, M. and Anees, S. (1996). Sydenham's chorea. *Indian Pediatrics* 33, 112–15.

Lance, J.W. and Adams, R.D. (1963). The syndrome of intention or action myoclonus as a sequel to anoxic encephalopathy. *Brain* 87, 111–33.

Langeveld, T.P.M., Drost, H.A., Frijns, J.H.M., Zwinderman, A. and Baatenburg de Jong, R.J. (2000). Per-ceptual characteristics of adductor spasmodic dysphonia. *Annals of Otology, Rhinology and Laryngology* 109, 741–8.

La Pointe, L., Case, J. and Duane, D. (1993). Perceptual-acoustic speech and voice characteristics of sub-jects with spastic torticollis. In J. Till, K. Yorkston and D. Beukelman (eds), *Motor Speech Disorders: Assessment and Treatment* (pp. 40–5). Baltimore, MD: Paul H. Brookes.

La Porta, M., Archambault, D., Ross-Chouinard, A. and Chouinard, G. (1990). Articulatory impairment associated with tardive dyskinesia. *Journal of Nervous and Mental Disease* 178, 660–2.

Laszewski, Z. (1956). Role of the Department of Rehabilitation in preoperative evaluation of Parkinsonian patients. *Journal of the American Geriatric Society* 4, 1280–4.

Lethlean, J.B., Chenery, H.J. and Murdoch, B.E. (1990). Disturbed respiratory and prosodic function in Parkinson's disease: a perceptual and instrumental analysis. *Australian Journal of Human Communica-tion Disorders* 18, 83–98.

Logemann, J.A. and Fisher, H.B. (1981). Vocal tract control in Parkinson's disease: phonetic feature analysis of misarticulations. *Journal of Speech and Hearing Disorders* 46, 348–52.

Logemann, J.A., Fisher, H.B., Boshes, B. and Blonsky, E.R. (1978). Frequency co-occurrence of vocal tract dysfunctions in the speech of a large sample of Parkinson's patients. *Journal of Speech and Hearing Disorders* 43, 47–57.

Ludlow, C.L. and Bassich, C.J. (1983). The results of acoustic and perceptual assessment of two types of dysarthria. In W.R. Berry (ed.), *Clinical Dysarthria* (pp. 121–47). San Diego, CA: College-Hill Press.

Ludlow, C.L. and Bassich, C.J. (1984). Relationship between perceptual ratings and acoustic measures of hypokinetic speech. In M.R. McNeil, J.C. Rosenbek and A.E. Aronson (eds), *The Dysarthrias: Physiology, Acoustics, Perception, Management* (pp. 163–95). San Diego, CA: College-Hill Press.

Martilla, J.R. and Rinne, U.K. (1991). Progression and survival in Parkinson's disease. *Acta Neurologica Scandinavia* 84 (suppl. 136), 24–8.

Matthews, W.B. and Glaser, G.H. (1984). *Recent Advances in Clinical Neurology*. Edinburgh: Churchill Livingstone.

McClean, M.D., Beukelman, D.R. and Yorkston, K.M. (1987). Speech-muscle visuomotor tracking in dysarthric and nonimpaired speakers. *Journal of Speech and Hearing Research* 30, 276–82.

McNeil, M.R., Weismer, G., Adams, S. and Mulligan, M. (1990). Oral structure nonspeech motor control in normal, dysarthric, aphasic, and apraxic speakers: isometric force and static position. *Journal of Speech and Hearing Research* 33, 255–68.

Metter, E.J. and Hanson, W.R. (1986). Clinical and acoustical variability in hypokinetic dysarthria. *Journal of Communication Disorders* 19, 347–66.

Miller, L.G. and Jankovic, J. (1990). Drug-induced dyskinesias. In S.H. Appel (ed.), *Current Neurology 10* (pp. 127–36). Chicago, IL: Mosby-Yearbook.

Moore, C.A. and Scudder, R.H. (1989). Co-ordination of jaw muscle activity in Parkinsonian movement: description and response to traditional treatment. In K.M. Yorkston and D.R. Beukelman (eds), *Recent Advances in Clinical Dysarthria* (pp. 147–63). Boston, MA: College-Hill Press.

Morris, J.G., Grattan-Smith, P., Jankelowitz, S.K., Fung, V.S., Clouston, P.D. *et al.* (2002). Athetosis II: the syndrome of mild athetoid cerebral palsy. *Movement Disorders* 17, 1281–7.

Mueller, P.B. (1971). Parkinson's disease: motor speech behaviour in a selected group of patients. *Folia Phoniatrica et Logopaedica* 23, 333–46.

Murdoch, B.E. (1990). *Acquired Speech and Language Disorders: a Neuroanatomical and Functional Neurological Approach*. London: Chapman and Hall.

Murdoch, B.E., Chenery, H.J., Bowler, S. and Ingram, J.C.L. (1989). Respiratory function in Parkinson's subjects exhibiting a perceptible speech deficit: a kinematic and spirometric analysis. *Journal of Speech and Hearing Disorders* 54, 610–26.

Murdoch, B.E., Chenery, H.J., Stokes, P.D. and Hardcastle, W.J. (1991). Respiratory kinematics in speakers with cerebellar disease. *Journal of Speech and Hearing Research* 34, 768–80.

Murdoch, B.E., Manning, C.Y., Theodoros, D.G. and Thompson, E.C. (1995). *Laryngeal function in hypokinetic dysarthria*. Paper presented at the 23rd World Congress of the International Association of Logopedics and Phoniatrics, Cairo.

Nausieda, P., Grossman, B., Koller, W., Weiner, W. and Klawans, H. (1980). Sydenham chorea: an update. *Neurology* 30, 331–4.

Netsell, R. and Kent, R. (1976). Paroxysmal ataxic dysarthria. *Journal of Speech and Hearing Disorders* 41, 93–109.

Platt, L., Andrews, G. and Howie, P. (1980). Dysarthria of adult cerebral palsy II. Phonemic analyses of articulation errors. *Journal of Speech and Hearing Research* 23, 41–5.

Ramig, L.A. (1986). Acoustic analyses of phonation in patients with Huntington's disease. *Annals of Otology, Rhinology and Laryngology* 95, 288–93.

Ramig, L.A., Scherer, R.C., Titze, I.R. and Ringel, S.P. (1988). Acoustic analysis of voices of patients with neurologic disease: rationale and preliminary data. *Annals of Otology, Rhinology and Laryngology* 97, 164–72.

Robbins, J.A., Logemann, J.A., Kirshner, H.S. (1986). Swallowing and speech production in Parkinson's disease. *Annals of Neurology* 19, 283–7.

Sapienza, C.M., Walton, S. and Murry, T. (1999). Acoustic variations in adductor spasmodic dysphonia as a function of speech task. *Journal of Speech, Language and Hearing Research* 42, 127–40.

Sapienza, C.M., Walton, S. and Murry, T. (2000). Adductor spasmodic dysphonia and muscle tension dysphonia: acoustic analysis of sustained phonation and reading. *Journal of Voice* 14, 502–20.

Schonecker, M. (1957). Ein eigentümliche syndrome im oralen Bereich bei megaphenapplikation. *Nervenarzt* 28, 35.

Scott, S., Caird, F.I. and Williams, G.O. (1985). *Communication in Parkinson's Disease.* London: Croom Helm.

Serra-Mestres, J., Robertson, M.M. and Shetty, T. (1998). Palicoprolalia: an unusual variant of pallilalia in Gilles de la Tourette's syndrome. *Journal of Neuropsychiatry and Clinical Neuroscience* 10, 117–18.

Simon, R., Arminoff, M. and Greenberg, D. (1999). *Clinical Neurology*, 4th edn. Stamford, CA: Appleton and Lange.

Solomon, N.P. and Hixon, T.J. (1993). Speech breathing in Parkinson's disease. *Journal of Speech and Hearing Research* 36, 294–310.

Steele, J.C., Richardson, J.C. and Olszewski, J. (1964). Progressive supra-nuclear palsy. *Archives of Neurology* 10, 333.

Svensson, P., Henningson, C. and Karlsson, S. (1993). Speech motor control in Parkinson's disease: a comparison between a clinical assessment protocol and a quantitative analysis of mandibular movements. *Folia Phoniatrica et Logopaaedica* 45, 157–64.

Swedo, S., Leonard, H., Schapiro, M., Casey, B., Mannheim, G. *et al.* (1993). Sydenham's chorea: physical and psychological symptoms of St Vitus dance. *Pediatrics* 91, 706–13.

Theodoros, D.G., Murdoch, B.E. and Thompson, E.C. (1995). Hypernasality in Parkinson's disease: a perceptual and physiological analysis. *Journal of Medical Speech Language Pathology* 3, 73–84.

Uitti, R.J. and Calne, D.B. (1993). Pathogenesis of idiopathic Parkinsonism. *European Neurology* 33 (suppl. 1), 6–23.

Vernon, G.M. (1991). Drug-induced and tardive movement disorders. *Journal of Neuroscience Nursing* 23, 183–7.

Weiner, W.J., Goetz, C.G., Nausieda, P. and Klawans, H.L. (1978). Respiratory dyskinesias: extrapyramidal dysfunction and dyspnea. *Annals of Internal Medicine* 88, 327–31.

Weismer, G. (1984). Acoustic descriptions of dysarthric speech: perceptual correlates and physiological inferences. *Seminars in Speech and Language* 5, 293–313.

Wilcox, P.G., Bassett, A., Jones, B. and Fleetham, J.A. (1994). Respiratory dysrhythmias in patients with tardive dyskinesia. *Chest* 105, 203–7.

Yoshida, K., Kaji, R., Shibasaki, H. and Iizuka, T. (2002). Factors influencing the therapeutic effect of muscle afferent block for oromandibular dystonia and dyskinesia and implications for their distinct pathophysiology. *International Journal of Oral and Maxillofacial Surgery* 31, 499–505.

Yoshida, K. and Iizuki, T. (2003). Jaw deviation dystonia evaluated by movement-related cortical potentials and treated with muscle afferent block. *Cranio – The Journal of Craniomandibular Practice* 21, 295–300.

Zraick, R., La Pointe, L., Case, J. and Duane, D. (1993). Acoustic correlates of vocal quality in spasmodic torticollis. *Journal of Medical Speech Language Pathology* 1, 261–9.

Zwirner, P. and Barnes, G.J. (1992). Vocal tract steadiness: a measure of phonatory and upper airway motor control during phonation in dysarthria. *Journal of Speech and Hearing Research* 35, 761–8.

Zwirner, P., Murry, T. and Woodson, G. (1991). Phonatory function of neurologically impaired patients. *Journal of Communication Disorders* 24, 287–300.

12 Subcortical dysarthrias: assessment and treatment

Introduction

Subcortical dysarthrias represent motor speech disorders typically resulting from damage to or diseases of subcortical structures. Akin to movement disorders of the limbs and trunk, subcortical dysarthrias are commonly grouped into hyper- and hypokinetic, as well as ataxic subtypes, which usually result from pathology of the basal ganglia or cerebellum (or related brain regions), respectively. The clinical symptoms and associated syndromes of each of the above dysarthrias were discussed in Chapter 11. The current chapter will focus on current speech-pathology management strategies relative to the assessment and treatment of these disorders.

Assessment strategies

The motor speech examination typically comprises four essential components, namely (1) history taking, (2) examination of motor speech apparatus structure and musculature during non-speech tasks, (3) perceptual evaluation of speech and (4) assessment of speech intelligibility (Duffy, 2005). Subcortical dysarthrias are no exception to this rule. The above assessment principles will be described in brief in the ensuing section; however, the reader is referred to Duffy (2005) for a more detailed account of these evaluation methods.

Case history

In general, case-history taking involves the compilation of information pertaining to the onset and course of the particular motor speech deficit, the patient's perception of the disorder and the way in which the speech deficit impacts upon the patient's functional abilities and quality of life.

Non-speech examination of motor speech apparatus

Non-speech examination of the motor speech apparatus aims to provide information regarding the speed, strength, range, tone, accuracy, symmetry, size and steadiness of orofacial muscle movements, particularly in reference to the lips, tongue, jaw and palate. Examination of these motor speech subsystems is typically conducted at rest, during the production of sustained postures, and during movement. Reflexes such as the gag and jaw jerk reflexes are also evaluated.

Perceptual speech evaluation

According to Duffy (2005), the perceptual evaluation of speech aims to elicit behaviours which allow the identification of deviant speech dimensions, leading to the diagnosis and appropriate management of the relevant motor speech disorder. The classification of distinctive deviant speech characteristics relevant to dysarthric subtypes, including clusters of deviant speech dimensions within specific subtypes, was initiated by the seminal work of Darley *et al.* (1975). In more detail, 38 speech dimensions pertaining to respiratory, prosodic, pitch, loudness, phonatory, and articulatory characteristics, as well as descriptions of speech intelligibility and bizarreness, have been described across six dysarthric subtypes (i.e. flaccid, spastic, ataxic, hypokinetic, hyperkinetic and mixed). On the basis of these descriptions, perceptual rating scales may then be applied to individual patients, which classify the presence of relevant speech dimensions on an abnormality spectrum. Darley *et al.* (1975) utilized a seven-point abnormality scale; however, more concise scales have also been developed since this time (e.g. four-point scale: normal-mild-moderate-marked-severe ratings) (Duffy, 2005). When conducting a perceptual evaluation, the clinician typically identifies and documents deviant speech dimensions for a particular patient and then matches those features with the dysarthric subtype common to those perceptual features.

Tasks useful for eliciting speech for perceptual evaluation include vowel prolongation (i.e. provides information relative to pitch, loudness and vocal quality), alternating motion/diadochokinetic rates (i.e. provides information pertaining to speed and consistency of rapid and repetitive muscle movements (e.g. puh-puh-puh-puh) in relation to articulatory precision, efficiency of velopharyngeal closure, phonatory and respiratory support), sequential motion rates (i.e. involves rapid and sequential movements from one articulatory posture to another (e.g. puh-tuh-kuh)) and contextual speech (i.e. provision of a conversational, narrative or reading sample).

There is only one published diagnostic dysarthria test, the Frenchay Dysarthria Assessment (FDA) (Enderby, 1983). It consists of a rating scale which is applicable to information provided by the patient pertaining to their speech disorder, the clinician's perception of specific speech features, observations of non-speech structure and function, intelligibility, speaking rate, and status of hearing, vision, dentition, language, mood, posture and sensation. It encompasses assessment tasks which require speech and non-speech activities relevant to each motor speech subsystem (i.e. respiration, lips, tongue, jaw, velopharynx and larynx), as well as an evaluation of intelligibility. On the basis of assessment results, each patient's profile may be classified according to dysarthria subtype (e.g. flaccid, spastic, ataxic, hypokinetic, mixed, etc.).

Evaluation of speech intelligibility

The assessment of speech intelligibility (i.e. ease with which the acoustic signal may be understood) provides information regarding the impact of a motor speech disorder on a patient's general ability to communicate. The focus of this section will be on methods of evaluating speech intelligibility, as published measures of speech intelligibility are widely available and clinically applied. It has been suggested, however, that less widely utilized measures of comprehensibility (i.e. how understandable the acoustic signal is in addition to other cues which may influence comprehension such as knowledge of topic, gestures, etc.) and efficiency (i.e. the rate at which comprehensible or intelligible information is communicated) may also be helpful in establishing the functional limitations of a motor speech disorder (Duffy, 2005).

The most basic method of evaluating speech intelligibility may involve the clinician estimating a percentage of intelligibility on the basis of clinical observations. Published assessments, however, include the Assessment of Intelligibility of Dysarthric Speech (ASSIDS) (Yorkston and Beukelman, 1981a), which has been described as the most widely applied measure of speech intelligibility in dysarthric populations (Duffy, 2005), the Sentence Intelligibility Test (Yorkston and Beukelman, 1996), Word Intelligibility Test (Kent, 1989) and the intelligibility subtests of the Frenchay Dysarthria Assessment (Enderby, 1983).

The ASSIDS enables the quantification of single word and sentence intelligibility via the calculation of intelligibility scores (i.e. percentage of correctly identified words), as well as a communicative efficiency ratio in relation to normal speakers. The Sentence Intelligibility Test is a revised version of the sentence intelligibility component of the ASSIDS. Although it requires clinicians to transcribe sentences produced by patients, computerized software generates intelligibility scores. The Word Intelligibility Test involves single words that are composed of phonetic stimuli deemed to be potentially vulnerable in dysarthric populations. Patients are required to read phonetically contrasting words which are transcribed by the examiner, and an intelligibility score is then calculated on the basis of percentage of intelligible words generated.

Treatment approaches

Subsequent to motor speech evaluation and differential diagnosis, appropriate treatment strategies may be implemented. As mentioned previously, subcortical dysarthrias are typically classified as hypokinetic, hyperkinetic or ataxic. The following section summarizes the relevant treatment approaches (i.e. behavioural, biofeedback, prosthetic) commonly used to remediate these motor speech disorders, typically within the context of affected motor speech subsystems. Surgical and pharmacological management strategies have also been discussed, where relevant.

Hypokinetic/Parkinsonian dysarthria

Hypokinetic dysarthria is typically characterized by phonatory, articulatory and prosodic impairments; however, it may involve all motor speech subsystems (i.e. also encompass resonatory and respiratory disturbances as well) (Darley et al., 1975; Chenery et al., 1988), as a potential consequence of variability in disease state and progression (Theodoros and Murdoch, 1998b). Treatment strategies have primarily focused upon behavioural and instrumental techniques specially designed for this population, or have evolved from more traditional dysarthria therapy techniques (Theodoros and Murdoch, 1998b). Alternative techniques which may also have some bearing on speech function include surgical procedures and drug regimens.

Treatment of phonatory dysfunction in hypokinetic dysarthria
The treatment of phonatory dysfunction represents the mainstay of speech pathology intervention in Parkinson's disease populations, and has typically incorporated behavioural, prosthetic and biofeedback techniques (Theodoros and Murdoch, 1998b). Behavioural strategies have largely focused on improving breathy vocal quality, reduced vocal intensity, monopitch and monoloudness (Ramig *et al.*, 1994).

The Lee Silverman Voice Treatment programme (LSVT) represents a contemporary and efficacious behavioural therapeutic approach aimed at recalibrating the amplitude of motor output in patients with Parkinsonian dysarthria (Ramig *et al.*, 2001a, 2001b) via the production of intensive, repetitive and high-effort motor behaviour (Fox *et al.*, 2002). The programme was developed around the central hypothesis that reduced phonatory and respiratory drive underlie the perceptual manifestations of reduced volume and prosodically flat speech perceived in the speech of Parkinson's disease patients (Duffy, 2005). The programme focuses on increasing vocal effort via intensive (i.e. 16 sessions per month) and repeated maximum phonation drills which subsequently retrain respiratory and phonatory patterns (Ramig *et al.*, 1994; Kleinow *et al.*, 2001), ranging from vowel to conversation-level production (Duffy, 2005). Prolonged improvements in vocal loudness have been demonstrated for up to 24 months following treatment with this technique (Ramig *et al.*, 2001a), and generalization of increased function across motor speech subsystems has also been reported, including improvements in pitch, rate, facial expression, swallowing and speech intelligibility (Dromey *et al.*, 1995; Smith *et al.*, 1995).

In cases where behavioural therapy fails to facilitate improvements in phonatory function, prosthetic devices such as vocal amplifiers are recommended (Theodoros and Murdoch, 1998b). Biofeedback instruments have also been demonstrated as effective in the treatment of phonatory dysfunction associated with hyperkinetic dysarthria, including visual feedback devices pertaining to vocal intensity levels (e.g. the Vocalite, a voice-operated light source) (Scott and Caird, 1983), vocal loudness (e.g. Jedcom vocal loudness indicator) (Johnson and Pring, 1990) and pitch (e.g. sound level meter known as Visispeech) (Johnson and Pring, 1990); as well as oscillographic displays of vocal intensity and pitch levels, such as the VisiPitch and Laryngograph (Theodoros and Murdoch, 1998b); and portable devices which provide auditory feedback regarding insufficient vocal intensity levels (Rubow and Swift, 1985). Delayed auditory feedback techniques have also been applied within this population which aim to increase vocal intensity to compensate for increased background noise (Adams and Lang, 1992).

Treatment of articulatory dysfunction in hypokinetic dysarthria
Articulatory dysfunction observed in Parkinson's disease patients has been attributed to reductions in fine-force control, rate, range and strength of lip, tongue and jaw musculature (Theodoros and Murdoch, 1998b), also referred to as articulatory undershoot (Kent and Rosenbek, 1982). Behavioural techniques aimed at remediating the articulatory deficits associated with hypokinetic dysarthria principally include articulation drills which focus on the production of frequently occurring articulation errors (Logemann and Fisher, 1981), as well as non-speech tasks which concentrate on improving the strength, rate and range of lip, tongue and jaw movements (Theodoros and Murdoch, 1998b).

Biofeedback tools have also been applied to the treatment of articulatory dysfunction in hypokinetic dysarthria. Electromyographic feedback from the lip muscles has been shown to be effective in normalizing labial muscle activity in patients with Parkinson's disease (Hand *et al.*, 1979; Netsell and Cleeland, 1973). In addition, electropalatography (i.e. using a device which provides information regarding the timing and location of tongue-to-palate contact during speech) (Hardcastle *et al.*, 1991) may also be modified for articulatory biofeedback purposes in Parkinson's disease patients.

Treatment of prosodic dysfunction in hypokinetic dysarthria

Increased speech rate is a common feature of hypokinetic dysarthric speech and a range of behavioural and prosthetic approaches have been applied in treating this characteristic (Theodoros and Murdoch, 1998b). Pacing techniques involving hand tapping, metronomes, pacing boards and computerized pacing software have been successful in altering pause and articulation timing in patients with Parkinson's disease. Other strategies such as the utilization of short phrase lengths and breath group patterning have also been effective in reducing the speech rate of these patients (Robertson and Thomson, 1984), as has the application of delayed auditory feedback techniques (Theodoros and Murdoch, 1998b). Speech dysfluency in Parkinsonian speech such as phoneme repetition, initiation problems and palilalia may also be remediated via the rate-control techniques mentioned above (Theodoros and Murdoch, 1998b).

Impaired stress patterning and intonational contours are also commonly reported features of hypokinetic dysarthric speech. Therapeutic techniques aimed at improving stress patterning include contrastive stress drills, where sentence meanings are altered by producing alternative stress patterns (Fairbanks, 1960). The manipulation of vocal intensity and pitch using conventional techniques such as reading aloud items marked for pause time and intonation patterns (Moncur and Brackett, 1974), as well as biofeedback tools such as VisiPitch and Vocalite (Johnson and Pring, 1990), have also been effective in altering intonational contours within hypokinetic dysarthric speech.

Treatment of resonatory dysfunction in hypokinetic dysarthria

Velopharyngeal dysfunction and associated nasality impairments in Parkinson's disease patients are rare, with the majority of disturbances in this speech feature reported as mild (Theodoros and Murdoch, 1998b). In cases of overt velopharyngeal dysfunction, however, a range of behavioural therapeutic techniques which aim to improve velopharyngeal valving may be applied, including (1) oral-opening and tongue-movement exercises which improve the oral cavity's resonatory capacity (Moncur and Brackett, 1974), (2) speech rate reduction facilitating more effective velopharyngeal closure (Yorkston *et al.*, 1988) and (3) contrastive nasal and non-nasal articulation drills (Rosenbek and La Pointe, 1978). Biofeedback instruments which provide visual cues as to the effectiveness of velopharyngeal valving, such as the Nasometer (Kay Elemetrics) and accelerometry, may also be useful in remediating nasality disturbances in hypokinetic dysarthric speech (Theodoros and Murdoch, 1998b).

Treatment of respiratory dysfunction in hypokinetic dysarthria

Respiratory dysfunction in Parkinson's disease commonly involves the following: impaired breath support for speech, reduced vital capacity, short speech rushes, reduced overall volume and loudness decay, irregular breathing, shortened phonation time and phrase length, and incoordination of chest-wall movements (Theodoros and

Murdoch, 1998b). Behavioural techniques utilized in the treatment of these impairments have typically included exercises to improve breath control (e.g. progressive counting) and increase loudness, relaxing diaphragmatic breathing patterns and establishing appropriate phrasing and breath grouping for speech (Theodoros and Murdoch, 1998b). Most recently, the LSVT programme has also been shown to be effective in increasing respiratory support for speech (Ramig *et al.*, 1994). The accent method (Shimizu *et al.*, 1982) and inspiratory checking (Netsell and Hixon, 1992) techniques may be also be applied in cases where incoordinated speech breathing is a concern (Theodoros and Murdoch, 1998b). The accent method trains patients to establish an abdominal pattern of speech breathing, whereas inspiratory checking involves establishing maximal respiratory volume and air flow for speech.

Biofeedback methods which provide information about subglottal air pressure/respiratory volume during speech may also be useful in remediating respiratory dysfunction in dysarthric Parkinson's disease populations (Theodoros and Murdoch, 1998b). Most recently, kinematic instrumentation which provides feedback pertaining to chest-wall movements during speech (i.e. ribcage versus abdomen) has been recommended for use in populations with speech breathing disorders, including those with hypokinetic dysarthria (Theodoros and Murdoch, 1998b).

Surgical and pharmacological approaches to the treatment of hypokinetic dysarthria

Although the greatest effects of dopamine agonists such as levodopa, selegiline (Deprenyl) and carbidopalevodopa (Sinemet) have been largely observed relative to non-speech function in Parkinson's disease patients, some limited benefits have also been reported in motor speech abilities (Duffy, 2005). Of particular note for the clinician are evident variations in motor performance following the administration of dopamine agonists, which are thought to be drug-cycle dependent. Furthermore, clonazepam has also been reported as effective in treating increased speech rate and consonant imprecision in hypokinetic dysarthric speakers (Biary *et al.*, 1988).

As summarized in Chapters 5 and 6, neurosurgical techniques including thalamotomy, pallidotomy and deep-brain stimulation are now commonly applied in the modern-day management of movement disorders such as Parkinson's disease. Although not originally attempted with the aim of remediating speech deficits, some interesting effects from these procedures have been observed relative to the motor speech apparatus, including both improvements and decrements in function (see Chapter 10 for a detailed discussion of effects). For example, unilateral pallidotomy has been reported to effect improvements in phonation and articulation in some Parkinson's disease patients (Schulz *et al.*, 1999), whereas other studies have reported declines in speech intelligibility as a consequence of this procedure (Theodoros *et al.*, 2000; Uitti *et al.*, 2000). Bilateral pallidotomy has been associated with improvements in force control of oral structures as well as enhanced post-operative lip movement, more relaxed facial musculature and improved eating and drinking abilities (Barlow, 1998). Reports of significant worsening of dysarthria, saliva control difficulties, dysphagia and hypophonia have also been documented (Scott *et al.*, 1998). Thalamotomy has been consistently associated with post-operative development or worsening of dysarthria, particularly in the case of bilaterally placed lesions (Kelly *et al.*, 1987; Shannon, 2000). Residual dysarthria is a commonly reported side effect of deep-brain stimulation of the subthalamic nucleus (Limousin *et al.*, 1998; Rousseaux *et al.*, 2004), despite reports of both improvements and decrements in speech intelligibility following this procedure (Rousseaux *et al.*, 2004), as well as improvements in phonatory and articulatory speech subcomponents (McFarlane *et al.*, 1991; Maruska *et al.*, 2000). General consensus, however, dictates that the above surgical procedures are more commonly harmful than beneficial to hypokinetic dysarthric symptoms, and that more significant improvements in limb function as opposed to motor speech function may be typically elicited by these techniques (Pinto *et al.*, 2004).

Hyperkinetic dysarthria

Hyperkinetic dysarthria has been defined as a diverse group of speech disorders involving abnormal involuntary movements of the limbs, trunk, neck or face, which disturb the rate and rhythm of speech production (Theodoros and Murdoch, 1998a). Given the considerable heterogeneity of hyperkinetic symptoms (i.e. relative to type and locality of abnormal movements produced), each of the motor speech subsystems may be affected in hyperkinetic dysarthria. Indeed, specific speech symptoms associated with dystonia, chorea, myoclonus, tics, dyskinesia, tremor and athetosis are documented (Zraick and La Pointe, 2008).

Pharmacological intervention has provided the primary conventional treatment modality for the management of hyperkinetic dysarthria, with improvements in speech function associated with improvements in the movement disorder (Beukelman, 1983). More recently, surgical procedures (e.g. thalamotomy, pallidotomy and deep-brain stimulation) used to treat tremor, dystonia and dyskinesia have also produced some benefit in the alleviation of hyperkinetic dysarthric symptoms (Duffy, 2005).

At a subsystem level, phonatory and respiratory dysfunction have received significant attention in the treatment of hyperkinetic dysarthria; however, the mainstay of evaluated speech therapy techniques involves the application of behavioural, biofeedback and prosthetic methods of increasing postural and/or articulatory stability, and hence speech intelligibility, as well as techniques which promote the monitoring and control of excessive movements. As such, the ensuing discussion on hyperkinetic dysarthria focuses upon individual treatment strategies versus levels of subsystem dysfunction (in contrast to the sections on hypokinetic and ataxic dysarthria in this chapter).

Pharmacological treatment of hyperkinetic dysarthria

Botulinum toxin injections have produced perhaps the most dramatic effects in improving the functional speech abilities of patients with hyperkinetic dysarthria and associated oromandibular dystonia (Tsui and Calne, 1988; Blitzer *et al.*, 1989; Duffy and Yorkston, 2003), hemifacial spasm (Brin, 1998), spasmodic torticollis (Tsui *et al.*, 1985), spasmodic dysphonia (Duffy, 2005) and palatal myoclonus (Varney *et al.*, 1996). Other drug agents typically used to treat systemic hyperkinetic movement disorders have demonstrated indirect effects on motor speech mechanisms. For example, in treating limb tremor, the use of Inderal, primodone (Mysoline), carbamazepine (Tegretol), baclofen (Lioresal), methazolamide (Neptazane), trihexyphenidyl (Artane) and lithium have been reported to improve vocal and head tremor (Muenter *et al.*, 1991; Rosenfeld, 1991; Koller *et al.*, 2001). Laryngeal and respiratory dystonias are reportedly receptive to Artane (Ludlow *et al.*, 1989). Oromandibular dystonias and spasmodic dysphonias have been reported to improve following administrations of Lioresal, Artane, lithium and alprazolam (Xanax) (Rosenfeld, 1991). Palatal myoclonus is reportedly responsive to clonazepam, carbamazapine or trihexyphenidyl (Frucht, 2003) and choreic dysarthria responsive to Lioresal, resperine and haloperidol (Haldol) (Rosenfeld, 1991).

Behavioural treatment of hyperkinetic dysarthria

The most useful behavioural strategies for this population include the introduction of postural strategies that reduce involuntary movements and subsequently facilitate functional speech production (Duffy, 2005). In addition, rate-reduction therapy has also been reported to improve speech intelligibility in patients with action myoclonus where increased speech rate results in increased myoclonic activity (Duffy, 2005). Augmentative and alternative communication techniques have also been suggested for those patients in whom functional speech intelligibility is difficult to achieve (Beukelman, 1983).

In reference to patients with adductor spasmodic dysphonia, behavourial techniques which encourage the production of a breathy phonation onset or increased vocal pitch have been effective (Duffy, 2005). In contrast, patients with abductor spasmodic dysphonia have benefited from exercises which encourage the production of hard glottal attack at the commencement of phonation, or the voicing of voiceless consonants (Duffy, 2005). There is also some evidence to suggest (i.e. at least in the case of adductor spasmodic dysphonia), that behavioural strategies may be most effective following injections of botulinum toxin (Murray and Woodson, 1995).

Instrumental biofeedback techniques used in the treatment of hyperkinetic dysarthria

The majority of studies which have applied biofeedback techniques to the treatment of hyperkinetic dysarthria have utilized instrumentation which aims to alleviate involuntary muscle movements by providing electromyographic (EMG) information pertaining to muscle activity (Theodoros and Murdoch, 1998a). For example, hemifacial spasms have been able to be reduced in patients with hyperkinetic dysarthria (Rubow et al., 1984), as have excessive oral and facial movements in cases of tardive dyskinesia with EMG feedback techniques (Fudge et al., 1991; Sherman, 1979). Attempts to normalize breathing patterns have also been successful in a case of generalized dystonia, with the aid of visual feedback via inductance plethysmography (La Blance and Rutherford, 1991). Although worthy of further investigation, the limited amount of outcome data pertaining to the effects of biofeedback approaches in the treatment of hyperkinetic dysarthria prohibits the general application of such techniques to the management of this disorder (Duffy, 2005).

Prosthetic devices used in the treatment of hyperkinetic dysarthria

Bite-blocks have been reportedly successful in improving the speech of patients with oromandibular dystonia and other hyperkinetic movements that disrupt jaw stability (Theodoros and Murdoch, 1998a). Preventing excessive jaw movements and enhancing orofacial postural control as a consequence of applying a bite-block has resulted in improved speech proficiency in a small number of patients with hyperkinetic dysarthria (Dworkin, 1996).

Ataxic dysarthria

In comparison to the treatment of other types of dysarthria, the management of ataxic dysarthria has a primary focus on improving overall control of the motor speech apparatus as well as integration of speech movements, in contrast to the remediation of specific deficits in muscle strength and tone (Murdoch and Theodoros, 1998). Surgical and prosthetic treatment approaches have also been labelled as largely irrelevant to the population with ataxic dysarthria (Duffy, 2005). Some benefits of pharmacological therapy have been documented, however, including the reduction of vocal tremor with clonazepam (Cannito and Marquardt, 1997). Consequently, a discussion of behavioural and instrumental techniques commonly applied to the treatment of ataxic dysarthria follows.

Treatment of articulatory dysfunction in ataxic dysarthria

Articulatory deficits typically seen in cases of ataxic dysarthria include imprecise consonant production, vowel distortion and irregular breakdowns in articulation (Darley *et al.*, 1975), resulting from impaired coordination of the range, speed, force and timing of lip, tongue and jaw musculature (McNeil *et al.*, 1990). Recommended articulatory treatment strategies include phoneme drills focusing on improving articulatory coordination (Murray, 1983), integral stimulation, intelligibility drills, exaggeration of articulatory movements, phonetic placement and derivation, as well as minimal contrasts (Duffy, 1995). Biofeedback techniques such as electropalatography (Hardcastle *et al.*, 1991) and articulography (Engelke *et al.*, 1996), which provide information pertaining to the range, force and timing of lip, tongue, palate and/or jaw movements, have also been suggested.

Treatment of phonatory dysfunction in ataxic dysarthria

Phonatory instability and incoordination producing abnormal alterations in pitch and loudness as well as harsh vocal quality, represent the phonatory characteristics of a speaker with ataxic dysarthria (Murdoch and Theodoros, 1998). Treatment approaches which focus on the coordination of breathing and phonation have been recommended on the premise that phonation and respiration are integrally connected (Murdoch and Theodoros, 1998). Vocal drills involving the manipulation of pitch and loudness have also been suggested, including hand-drawn or simulated electronic feedback on instrumentation such as the VisiPitch (Murray, 1983).

The issue of vocal quality is addressed with strategies that aim to reduce vocal fold tension and increase coordination of breathing and voicing to facilitate regular vibration of the vocal folds (Murdoch and Theodoros, 1998). An additional technique used to equilibrate vocal-fold muscle power and expiration is the accent method, which aims to produce rhythmic phonation (Kotby, 1995).

Treatment of respiratory dysfunction in ataxic dysarthria

Respiratory disturbances that manifest as a consequence of ataxic dysarthria are reportedly the result of incoordinated movement of chest-wall components during speech (Murdoch *et al.*, 1991). As a result, treatment strategies which aim to remediate respiratory dysfunction within this population typically focus on the stabilization and coordination of chest-wall movements during expiration (Murdoch and Theodoros, 1998). Chest-wall activity (i.e. rib cage and abdominal wall movements) may be demonstrated with biofeedback techniques such as the Respitrace (i.e. oscillographic display). Other more traditional behavioural approaches include inspiratory checking (Netsell and Hixon, 1992), controlled exhalation tasks, vowel prolongations, timing speech at the onset of expiration, appropriate termination of speech during expiration and optimal breath grouping (Duffy, 1995).

Treatment of prosodic dysfunction in ataxic dysarthria

In contrast to the treatment regimens of other dysarthric subtypes which tackle prosodic disturbances near the termination of therapy, prosodic impairments represent a starting point for patients with ataxic dysarthria (Duffy, 1995). Treatment generally aims to reduce speech rate and to consequently improve speech intelligibility as well as to produce more naturally sounding speech via the development of appropriate stress and intonation patterns (Duffy, 2005).

Given that ataxic dysarthria is characterized by abnormal timing of the components of the motor speech apparatus (Kent *et al.*, 1975), it has been postulated that reducing speech rate permits better coordination of speech subsystems (Murdoch and Theodoros, 1998). Numerous behavioural rate-reduction techniques have been applied successfully to the treatment of ataxic dysarthria, including alphabet (Beukelman and Yorkston, 1977) and pacing boards (Helm, 1979), timed and cued production of single words (Yorkston *et al.*, 1990), hand-tapping, metronomic and word-by-word reading strategies (Rosenbek and La Pointe, 1978), and additive rhythmic and rhythmic cuing of utterances (Yorkston and Beukelman, 1981b; Beukelman *et al.*, 1988; Yorkston *et al.*, 1990).

Biofeedback techniques have also been reportedly successful in reducing speech rate in ataxic dysarthric speakers. For example, oscillographic feedback provides a means of controlling articulatory and pause durations (Yorkston and Beukelman, 1981b; Berry and Goshorn, 1983) as well as vocal intensity (Caligiuri and Murry, 1983), subsequently improving speech intelligibility. In addition, the IBM Speech Viewer has also been demonstrated as effective in improving the modulation of fundamental frequency in patients with ataxic dysarthria (Bougle *et al.*, 1995). Furthermore, clinician-driven rate-reduction techniques (i.e. the clinician instructs the patient to reduce speaking rate during reading of an unfamiliar passage until the optimal rate for maximal intelligibility is determined) (Yorkston and Beukelman, 1981b) and self-monitoring techniques (Yorkston and Beukelman, 1981b) may also represent efficacious rate-reduction methods.

Prosodic impairments may also be improved via the application of contrastive stress and intonation drills (Rosenbek and La Pointe, 1978), and durational contrasts (Yorkston and Beukelman, 1981b; Yorkston, 1999). These drills alter the meaning of utterances on the basis of pitch and loudness levels used, as well as syllable and pause length, respectively.

Treatment of resonatory dysfunction in ataxic dysarthria

Incoordinated movements of the soft palate provide the pathophysiological basis for disorders of nasality (i.e. hypernasality, hyponasality or mixed nasality) which may be seen in patients with ataxic dysarthria, as opposed to weakness of the palatal muscles (Murdoch and Theodoros, 1998). Resonatory treatment techniques may include such approaches as articulation drills, which encourage the contrastive as well as over-emphasized production of nasal and non-nasal consonants as a means of improving the force, timing and range of palatal movement as well as increasing speech intelligibility (Rosenbek and La Pointe, 1978). In addition, exaggerated movements of the lips, tongue and jaw may also be promoted in an effort to enhance oral resonance (Rosenbek and La Pointe, 1978).

Summary

Chapter 12 provided an outline of assessment and treatment strategies commonly employed in the management of subcortical dysarthrias, including hyperkinetic, hypokinetic and ataxic dysarthria. Assessment techniques discussed included history taking, evaluation of motor speech apparatus structure and function, perceptual speech evaluation and speech intelligibility ratings. Treatment strategies were largely discussed in relation to dysarthria-specific subsystem dysfunction, and in the context of applied behavioural, biofeedback, prosthetic and applicable surgical and pharmacological techniques.

References

Adams, S.G. and Lang, A.E. (1992). Can the Lombard effect be used to improve low voice intensity in Parkinson's disease? *European Journal of Disorders of Communication* 27, 121–7.

Barlow, S.M. (1998). The effects of posteroventral pallidotomy on force and speech aerodynamic in Parkinson's disease. In M.P. Cannito, K.M. Yorkston and D.R. Beukelman (eds), *Neuromotor Speech Disorders: Nature, Assessment and Management*. Baltimore, MD: Brookes Publishing.

Berry, W.R. and Goshorn, E.L. (1983). Immediate visual feedback in the treatment of ataxic dysarthria: a case study. In W.R. Berry (ed.), *Clinical Dysarthria* (pp. 253–65). San Diego, CA: College-Hill Press.

Beukelman, D.R. (1983). Treatment of hyperkinetic dysarthria. In W.H. Perkins (ed.), *Current Therapy of Communication Disorders: Dysarthria and Apraxia* (pp. 101–3). New York: Theime-Stratton.

Beukelman, D.R. and Yorkston, K.M. (1977). A communication system for the severely dysarthric speaker with an intact language system. *Journal of Speech and Hearing Disorders* 42, 265–70.

Beukelman, D.R., Yorkston, K.M. and Tice, B. (1988). *Pacer/Tally*. Tucson, AZ: Communication Skill Builders.

Biary, N., Pimental, P.A. and Langenberg, P.W. (1988). A double blind trial of clonazepam in the treatment of Parkinsonian dysarthria. *Neurology* 38, 255.

Blitzer, A., Greene, P.E., Brin, M.F. and Fahn, S. (1989). Botulinum toxin injection for the treatment of oromandibular dystonia. *Annals of Otology, Rhinology, and Laryngology* 98, 93–7.

Bougle, R., Ryalls, J. and Le Dorze, G. (1995). Improving fundamental frequency modulation in head trauma patients: a preliminary comparison of speech-language therapy conducted with and without IBM's Speech Viewer. *Folia Phoniatrica et Logopaedica* 47, 24–32.

Brin, M.F. (1998). Pharmacological treatment of movement disorders. In I. Germano (ed.), *Neurosurgical Treatment of Movement Disorders* (pp. 83–104). Park Ridge, IL: Thieme.

Caligiuri, M.P. and Murry, T. (1983). The use of visual feedback to enhance prosodic control in dysarthria. In W.R. Berry (ed.), *Clinical Dysarthrias* (pp. 267–82). San Diego, CA: College-Hill Press.

Cannito, M.P. and Marquardt, T.P. (1997). Ataxic dysarthria. In M.R. McNeil (ed.), *Clinical Management of Sensorimotor Speech Disorders* (pp. 217–47). New York: Thieme.

Chenery, H.J., Murdoch, B.E. and Ingram, J.C.L. (1988). Studies in Parkinson's disease I: Perceptual speech analysis. *Australian Journal of Human Communication Disorders* 16, 17–29.

Darley, F.E., Aronson, A.E. and Brown, J.R. (1975). *Motor Speech Disorders*. Philadelphia, PA: WB Saunders.

Dromey, C., Ramig, L.O. and Johnson, A.B. (1995). Phonatory and articulatory changes associated with increased vocal intensity in Parkinson's disease: a case study. *Journal of Speech and Hearing Research* 38, 751–64.

Duffy, J.R. (1995). *Motor Speech Disorders: Substrates, Differential Diagnosis and Management*. Baltimore, MD: Mosby-Year Book.

Duffy, J.R. (2005). *Motor Speech Disorders: Substrates, Differential Diagnosis, and Management*, 2nd edn. St. Louis, MO: Elsevier Mosby.

Duffy, J.R. and Yorkston, K.M. (2003). Medical interventions for spasmodic dysphonia and some related conditions: a systematic review. *Journal of Medical Speech Language Pathology* 11, ix.

Dworkin, J.P. (1996). Bite-block therapy for oromandibular dystonia. *Journal of Medical Speech Language Pathology* 4, 47–56.

Enderby, P. (1983). *Frenchay Dysarthria Assessment*. San Diego, CA: College-Hill Press.

Engelke, W., Hoch, G., Bruns, T. and Striebeck, M. (1996). Simultanoeus evaluation of articulatory velo-pharyngeal function under different dynamic conditions with EMA and videoendoscopy. *Folia Phoni-atrica et Logopaedica* 48, 65–77.

Fairbanks, G. (1960). *Voice and Articulation Drillbook*. New York: Harper and Row.

Fox, C., Morrison, C.E., Ramig, L.A. and Sapir, S. (2002). Current perspectives on the Lee Silverman Voice Treatment (LSVT) for individuals with idiopathic Parkinson's disease. *American Journal of Speech Language Pathology* 11, 111–23.

Frucht, S.J. (2003). Myoclonus. In J.H. Noseworthy (ed.), *Neurological Therapeutics: Principles and Practice*, vol. 1, (pp. 2913–20). New York: Martine Dunitz.

Fudge, R.C., Thailer, S.A. and Alpert, M. (1991). The effects of electromyographic feedback training on suppression of the oral-lingual movements associated with tardive dyskinesia. *Biofeedback and Self-regulation* 16, 117–29.

Hand, C.R., Burns, M.O. and Ireland, E. (1979). Treatment of hypertonicity in muscles of lip retraction. *Biofeedback and Self-regulation* 4, 171–81.

Hardcastle, W.J., Gibbon, F.E. and Jones, W. (1991). Visual display of tongue-palate contact: electropala-tography in the assessment and remediation of speech disorders. *British Journal of Communication Disorders* 26, 41–74.

Helm, N.A. (1979). Management of palilalia with a pacing board. *Journal of Speech and Hearing Disorders* 44, 350–3.

Johnson, J.A. and Pring, T.R. (1990). Speech therapy and Parkinson's disease: a review and further data. *British Journal of Disorders of Communication* 25, 183–94.

Kelly, P.J., Ahlskog, J.E., Goerss, S.J., Daube, J.R., Duffy, J.R. et al. (1987). Computer-assisted stereotactic ventralis lateralis thalamotomy with microelectrode recording control in patients with Parkinson's disease. *Mayo Clinic Proceedings* 62, 655–64.

Kent, R. (1989). Toward phonetic intelligibility testing in dysarthria. *Journal of Speech and Hearing Disorders* 54, 482.

Kent, R. and Rosenbek, J.C. (1982). Prosodic disturbance and neurological lesion. *Brain and Language* 15, 259–91.

Kent, R., Netsell, R. and Bauer, L. (1975). Cineradiographic assessment of articulatory mobility in the dysarthrias. *Journal of Speech and Hearing Disorders* 40, 467–80.

Kleinow, J., Smith, A. and Ramig, L.O. (2001). Speech motor stability in IPD: Effects of rate and loudness manipulations. *Journal of Speech Language and Hearing Research* 44, 1041–51.

Koller, W., Graner, D. and Mlcoch, A. (2001). Essential voice tremor: treatment with propranolol. *Neurology* 35, 106–8.

Kotby, M.N. (1995). *The Accent Method of Voice Therapy*. San Diego, CA: Singular Publishing Group.

La Blance, G.R. and Rutherford, D.R. (1991). Respiratory dynamics and speech intelligibility in dysarthric speakers with generalised dystonia. *Journal of Communication Disorders* 24, 141–56.

Limousin, P., Krack, P., Pollak, P., Benazzouz, A., Ardouin, C.M. *et al.* (1998). Electrical stimulation of the subthalamic nucleus in advanced Parkinson's disease. *New England Journal of Medicine* 339(16), 1105–11.

Logemann, J.A. and Fisher, H.B. (1981). Vocal tract control in Parkinson's disease: phonetic feature analysis of misarticulations. *Journal of Speech and Hearing Disorders* 46, 348–52.

Ludlow, C.L., Sedora, S.E. and Fujita, M. (1989). Inspiratory speech with respiratory dystonia. In N. Helm-Estabrooks and J.L. Aten (eds), *Difficult Diagnoses in Communication Disorders*. Boston, MA: College Hill.

Maruska, K.G., Smit, A.B., Koller, W.C. and Garcia, J.M. (2000). Sentence production in Parkinson's disease treated with deep brain stimulation and medication. *Journal of Medical Speech Language Pathology* 8, 265–70.

McFarlane, S.C., Hoh-Romeo, T.L. and Lavorato, A.S. (1991). Unilateral vocal fold paralysis: perceived vocal quality following three methods of treatment. *American Journal of Speech Language Pathology* 1, 45–8.

McNeil, M.R., Weismer, G., Adams, S. and Mulligan, M. (1990). Oral structure nonspeech motor control in normal, dysarthric, aphasic and apraxic speakers: isometric force and static position. *Journal of Speech and Hearing Research* 33, 255–68.

Moncur, J.P. and Brackett, I.P. (1974). *Modifying Vocal Behaviour*. New York: Harper and Row.

Muenter, M.D., Daube, J.R., Caviness, J.N. and Miller, P.M. (1991). Treatment of essential tremor with methazolamide. *Mayo Clinic Proceedings* 66, 991–7.

Murdoch, B.E. and Theodoros, D.G. (1998). Ataxic dysarthria. In B.E. Murdoch (ed.), *Dysarthria: a Physiological Approach to Assessment and Treatment* (pp. 242–65). Cheltenham: Stanley Thornes.

Murdoch, B.E., Chenery, H.J., Stokes, P. and Hardcastle, W.J. (1991). Respiratory kinematics in speakers with cerebellar disease. *Journal of Speech and Hearing Research* 34, 768–80.

Murray, T. (1983). Treatment of ataxic dysarthria. In W.H. Perkins (ed.), *Current Therapy of Communication Disorders: Dysarthria and Apraxia* (pp. 79–89). New York: Thieme-Stratton.

Murray, T. and Woodson, G. (1995). Combined-modality treatment of adductor spasmodic dysphonia with botulinum toxin and voice therapy. *Journal of Voice* 9, 460–5.

Netsell, R. and Cleeland, C.S. (1973). Modification of lip hypertonia in dysarthria using EMG feedback. *Journal of Speech and Hearing Disorders* 38, 131–40.

Netsell, R. and Hixon, T.J. (1992). Inspiratory checking in therapy for individuals with speech breathing dysfunction. *Journal of the American Speech and Hearing Association* 34, 152.

Pinto, S., Ozsancak, C., Tripoliti, E., Thobois, S., Limousin Dowsey, P. *et al.* (2004). Treatments for dysarthria in Parkinson's disease. *Lancet Neurology* 3, 547–56.

Ramig, L.O., Bonitati, C.M., Lemke, J.H. and Horii, Y. (1994). Voice treatment for patients with Parkinson's disease: development of an approach and preliminary efficacy data. *Journal of Medical Speech Language Pathology* 2, 191–209.

Ramig, L.O., Sapir, S. and Countryman, S. (2001a). Intensive voice treatment (LSVT) for patients with Parkinson's disease: a 2 year follow-up. *Journal of Neurology Neurosurgery and Psychiatry* 71, 493–8.

Ramig, L.O., Sapir, S., Fox, C. and Countryman, S. (2001b). Changes in vocal loudness following intensive voice treatment (LSVT) in individuals with Parkinson's disease: a comparison with untreated patients and normal age-matched controls. *Movement Disorders* 16, 79–83.

Robertson, S.J. and Thomson, F. (1984). Speech therapy in Parkinson's disease: a study of the efficacy and long term effects of intensive treatment. *British Journal of Disorders of Communication* 19, 213–24.

Rosenbek, J.C. and La Pointe, L.L. (1978). The dysarthrias: description, diagnosis, and treatment. In D. Johns (ed.), *Clinical Management of Neurogenic Communication Disorders* (pp. 97–152). Boston, MA: Little Brown and Co.

Rosenfeld, D.B. (1991). Pharmacologic approaches to speech motor disorders. In D. Vogel and M.P. Cannito (eds), *Treating Disordered Speech Motor Control: for Clinicians by Clinicians* (pp. 111–52). Austin, TX: Pro-Ed.

Rousseaux, M., Krystkowiak, P., Kozlowski, O., Ozsancak, C., Blond, S. *et al.* (2004). Effects of subthalamic nucleus stimulation on parkinsonian dysarthria and speech intelligibility. *Journal of Neurology* 251, 327–34.

Rubow, R.T. and Swift, E. (1985). A microcomputer-based wearable biofeedback device to improve transfer of treatment in Parkinson's dysarthria. *Journal of Speech and Hearing Disorders* 50, 166–78.

Rubow, R.T., Rosenbek, J.C., Collins, M.J. and Celesia, G.C. (1984). Reduction of hemifacial spasm and dysarthria following EMG biofeedback. *Journal of Speech and Hearing Disorders* 49, 26–33.

Schulz, G., Peterson, C.M., Sapienza, M., Greer, M. and Friedman, W. (1999). Voice and speech characteristics of persons with Parkinson's disease pre- and post-pallidotomy surgery: preliminary findings. *Journal of Speech Language and Hearing Research* 42, 1176–94.

Scott, R.B., Gregory, R., Hines, N., Carroll, C., Hyman, N. *et al.* (1998). Neuropsychological, neurological and functional outcome following pallidotomy for Parkinson's disease: a consecutive series of eight simultaneous bilateral and twelve unilateral procedures. *Brain* 121, 659–75.

Scott, S. and Caird, F.I. (1983). Speech therapy for Parkinson's disease. *Journal of Neurology Neurosurgery and Psychiatry* 46, 140–4.

Shannon, K.M. (2000). Surgical treament of Parkinson's disease. In C.H. Adler and J.E. Ahlskog (eds), *Parkinson's Disease and Movement Disorders: Diagnosis and Treatment Guidelines for the Practicing Physician* (pp. 185–96). Totowa, NJ: Humana Press.

Sherman, R.A. (1979). Successful treatment of one case of tardive dyskinesia with electromyographic feedback from the masseter muscle. *Biofeedback and Self-regulation* 4, 367–70.

Shimizu, M., Watanabe, Y. and Hirose, H. (1982). *Use of the accent method in training for patients with motor speech disorders.* Paper presented at the 22nd World Congress of the International Association of Logopedics and Phoniatrics, Hanover.

Smith, M.E., Ramig, L.O., Dromey, C., Perez, K.S. and Samandari, R. (1995). Intensive voice treatment in Parkinson disease: laryngostroboscopic findings. *Journal of Voice* 9, 453–9.

Theodoros, D.G. and Murdoch, B.E. (1998a). Hyperkinetic dysarthria. In B.E. Murdoch (ed.), *Dysarthria: a Physiological Approach to Assessment and Treatment* (pp. 314–36). Cheltenham: Stanley Thornes.

Theodoros, D.G. and Murdoch, B.E. (1998b). Hypokinetic dysarthria. In B.E. Murdoch (ed.), *Dysarthria: a Physiological Approach to Assessment and Treatment* (pp. 266–313). Cheltenham: Stanley Thornes.

Theodoros, D.G., Ward, E.C., Murdoch, B.E., Silburn, P. and Lethlean, J.B. (2000). The impact of pallidotomy on motor speech function in Parkinson's disease. *Journal of Medical Speech Language Pathology* 8, 315–22.

Tsui, J.K. and Calne, D.B. (1988). Botulinum toxin in cervical dystonia. In J. Jankovic and E. Tolosa (eds), *Advances in Neurology 49: Facial Dyskinesias* (pp. 468–73). New York: Raven Press.

Tsui, J.K., Eisen, E. and Mak, J. (1985). A pilot study in the use of botulimun toxin in spasmodic torticollis. *Canadian Journal of Neurological Sciences* 12, 314–16.

Uitti, R., Wharen, R., Duffy, J.A., Lucas, J.A., Schneider, S.L. *et al.* (2000). Unilateral pallidotomy for Parkinson's disease: speech, motor, and neuropsychological outcome measurements. *Parkinsonism and Related Disorders* 6, 133–43.

Varney, S.M., Demetroulakos, J., Fletcher, M., McQueen, W. and Hamilton, M. (1996). Palatal myoclonus: treatment with *Clostridium botulinum* toxin injection. *Otolarngology Head and Neck Surgery* 114, 317–20.

Yorkston, K.M. (1999). *Management of Motor Speech Disorders in Children and Adults*, 2nd edn. Austin, TX: Pro-Ed.

Yorkston, K.M. and Beukelman, D.R. (1981a). *Assessment of Intelligibility of Dysarthric Speech*. Tigard: CC Publications.

Yorkston, K.M. and Beukelman, D.R. (1981b). Ataxic dysarthria: treatment sequences based on intelligibility and prosodic considerations. *Journal of Speech and Hearing Disorders* 46, 398–404.

Yorkston, K.M. and Beukelman, D.R. (1996). *Sentence Intelligibility Test*. Lincoln: Tice Technology Services.

Yorkston, K.M., Beukelman, D.R. and Bell, K.R. (1988). *Clinical Management of Dysarthric Speakers*. Boston, MA: Little, Brown and Co.

Yorkston, K.M., Hammen, V.L., Beukelman, D.R. and Traynor, C.D. (1990). The effect of rate control on the intelligibility of naturalness of dysarthric speech. *Journal of Speech and Hearing Disorders* 55, 550–60.

Zraick, R.I. and La Pointe, L.L. (2008). Hyperkinetic dysarthria. In M.R. McNeil (ed.), *Clinical Management of Sensorimotor Speech Disorders*, 2nd edn (pp. 152–65). New York: Thieme.

Index

ablative surgical techniques, 112–13
amygdaloid nucleus, 21
anterior spinocerebellar tract, 53
assessment of subcortical language disorders, 200–208
assessment of subcortical speech disorders, 275–7
ataxic dysarthria, *see* subcortical speech disorders
athetosis, *see* subcortical speech disorders, hyperkinetic dysarthria

ballism, *see* subcortical speech disorders, hyperkinetic dysarthria
basal ganglia, 5–7, 10–12, 18–29, 71–2, 77, 83, 97–8, 113–17
  language disorders, historical perspective, 10–12; *see also* striatocapsular aphasia
  neuroanatomy and functional neurology, 18–29, 97–8, 216–19
    blood supply, 25–7, 97–8
    circuitry and neurotransmission mechanisms, 22–3
    pathology, 28–9
    role in movement and cognition, 27
  proposed roles in language, 113–7
  role in Lexical Decision Making model, 77
  role in Response-Release Semantic Feedback model, 71–2
  role in Selective Engagement model, 83
  speech motor control, historical perspective, 5–7
Boston Naming Test, 201, 203–4
brain stem, 35–48
  neuroanatomy and functional neurology, 35–48
    blood supply, 44–5
    pathology, 45–8
    role in movement and cognition, 45

caudate nucleus, 18–20
cerebellum, 7–9, 12–13, 48–58, 162–76
  historical perspectives
    language, 12–13
    speech motor control, 7–9

influence on language, 162–76
  in childhood, 173–4
  clinical studies, 170–173
  functional neuroimaging studies, 166–70
  neuroanatomical evidence, 164–6
  neuroanatomy and functional neurology, 48–58, 219–21
    afferent connections, 53–5
    blood supply, 51
    circuitry, 57
    efferent connections, 55–7
    pathology, 57–8
    role in movement and cognition, 51–7
  speech disorders, *see* subcortical speech disorders, ataxic dysarthria
chorea, *see* subcortical speech disorders, hyperkinetic dysarthria
claustrum, 21
corpus striatum, 18–21
corticopontocerebellar tract, 54
cuneocerebellar tract, 54

deep-brain stimulation, 146–53, 231–7
  effect on speech, 232–7
  impact on language function, 148–53
  treatment for Parkinson's disease, 146–8
degenerative subcortical syndromes, 180–194
  hyperkinetic disorders, 181–2
    essential tremor, 182–3
    dyskinesia, 184
    dystonia, 183–4
    Huntington's disease, 181–2; *see also* Huntington's disease
  hypokinetic disorders, 180–181
    Parkinson's disease, 181, 184–91; *see also* Parkinson's disease
dentothalamic pathway, 56
dyskinesia, *see* degenerative subcortical syndromes
  speech disorders, *see* subcortical speech disorders, hyperkinetic dysarthria
dystonia, *see* degenerative subcortical syndromes
  speech disorders, *see* subcortical speech disorders, hyperkinetic dysarthria

essential tremor, 263
    see also degenerative subcortical syndromes

fastigial reticular pathway, 57
fastigial vestibular pathway, 57
functional neuroimaging, 13–14, 166–70

globose-emboliform-rubral pathway, 56
globus pallidus, 20–21, 114–16
    role in language, 114–16

Huntington's disease, 181–2, 191–4, 256–8
    language disorders, 191–4
    speech disorders, *see* subcortical speech
        disorders, hyperkinetic dysarthria
hyperkinesias, 252–63
    quick, 252–8
    slow, 258–63
hyperkinetic dysarthria, *see* subcortical speech
        disorders
hypokinetic dysarthria, *see* subcortical speech
        disorders

internal capsule, 24–9
    blood supply, 25–7
    pathology, 28–9
    role in movement and cognition, 27

lemnisci, decussation of, 40–42
lentiform nucleus, 20–21
levodopa-induced dyskinesia, 261

medulla oblongata, 39–44, 47–8
    clinical significance, 47–8
midbrain, 35, 45–7
    clinical significance, 45–7
models of subcortical participation in language,
        63–90, 139–46
    future research directions, 87–8
    Lexical Decision Making model, 75–9,
        142–4
    limitations, 85–7
    Response-Release Semantic Feedback model,
        69–75, 141–2
    Selective Engagement model, 79–85, 144–6
    Subcortical White Matter Pathways model,
        67–9
motor speech disorders, 9
myoclonic jerks, *see* subcortical speech
        disorders, hyperkinetic dysarthria

Neurosensory Centre Comprehensive
        Examination for Aphasia, 201–2

pallidotomy, 117–20, 121–9, 230–237
    case study, 127–9
    effect on speech, 232–7

implications for language, 118–20
    neuropsychological findings, 118–20
Parkinson's disease, 87–9, 180–181, 184–91, 245
    language disorders, 184–91
        dopamine, effect of, 189–91
        early investigations, 185–6
        relationship to cognitive status, 186–7
        semantic priming experiments, 187–9
    neurosurgical interventions, 88–9
    ratifying subcortical language theories, 87–8
    subthalamic deep-brain stimulation, *see* deep-
        brain stimulation
phrenology, 3
pons, 35–9
    clinical significance, 47
posterior spinocerebellar tract, 53–4
progressive supranuclear palsy, 245–6
pyramids, decussation of, 40

red nucleus, 22

semantic fluency tasks, 207
spinocerebellar tracts
    anterior, 53
    posterior, 53–4
striatocapsular aphasia, 102–7
    characteristics, 103–4
    cortical dysfunction, 105–7
    levels of language processing, 104–5
    prognosis, 107
subcortical language disorders, 200–210
    assessment of, 200–208
        recommended assessments, 201–208
    treatment of, 208–9
        compensatory and behavioural approaches,
            209
        restorative approaches, 209
    see also striatocapsular aphasia; thalamic
        aphasia
subcortical speech disorders, 221–9, 244–69,
        275–85
    assessment of, 275–7
    ataxic dysarthria, 225–9, 264–8
        cerebellar disease, 265–6
        clinical characteristics, 265–8
        neurological framework, 264–5
        treatment of, 283–5
    hyperkinetic dysarthria, 221–5, 251–63
        athetosis, 258–9
        ballism, 258
        chorea, 255–8
        dyskinesia, 259–61
        dystonia, 261–3
        essential voice tremor, 263
        myoclonic jerks, 252–4
        tics, 254–5
        treatment of, 277–85

hypokinetic dysarthria, 221–5, 245–51
  clinical characteristics, 246–51
  in Parkinson's disease, 245
  in progressive supranuclear palsy, 245–6
  treatment of, 277–81
subcortical structures, 3–14, 18–59, 215–38
  language role, 3–14
    historical perspective, 9–14
    models, see models of subcortical
      participation in language
  neuroanatomy and functional neurology,
    18–59
  role in speech motor control, 5–9, 215–38
    evidence from neurosurgical studies,
      229–37
    models, 223–8
substantia nigra, 21
subthalamic nucleotomy, 153–5
subthalamic nucleus, 21, 137–55
  in deep-brain stimulation, see deep-brain
    stimulation
  role in language, 137–55
Sydenham's chorea, 256

tardive dyskinesia, 259–61
Test of Language Competence-Expanded
  edition, 201, 202–5
Test of Word Knowledge, 201, 206
thalamic aphasia, 98–102
  characteristics, 99–100
  lateralization, 100–101

mechanisms, 101–2
prognosis, 102
thalamotomy, 120–127, 230, 232–7
  case studies, 125–7
  effect on speech, 232–7
  implications for language, 120–121
  neuropsychological findings, 120–121
thalamus, 29–35, 70–71, 76–7, 80–83, 97–102,
    116–17
  language disorders, 98–102; see also thalamic
    aphasia
  neuroanatomy and functional neurology,
    29–35
    blood supply, 31, 97–8
    pathology, 34–5
    role in movement and cognition,
      31–33
  proposed role in language, 116–17
  role in Lexical Decision Making model, 76–7
  role in Response-Release Semantic Feedback
    model, 70–71
  role in Selective Engagement model, 80–83
The Word Test-Revised, 201, 205–6
tics, see subcortical speech disorders,
    hyperkinetic disorders
treatment of subcortical language disorders,
    see subcortical language disorders,
    treatment of

Wiig–Semel Test of Linguistic Concepts, 201,
    207